STEREOTYPES AND STEREOTYPING

STEREOTYPES AND STEREOTYPING

Edited by

C. NEIL MACRAE
CHARLES STANGOR
MILES HEWSTONE

THE GUILFORD PRESS
New York   London

© 1996 The Guilford Press
A Division of Guilford Publications, Inc.
72 Spring Street, New York, NY 10012

Printed in the United States of America

This book is printed on acid-free paper.

Last digit is print number: 9 8 7 6 5 4 3 2 1

Library of Congress Cataloging-in-Publication Data

Macrae, C. Neil.
    Foundations of stereotypes and stereotyping / C. Neil Macrae,
Charles Stangor, Miles Hewstone.
      p. cm.
    Includes bibliographical references and index.
    ISBN 1-57230-053-1
    1. Stereotype (Psychology)   I. Stangor, Charles   II. Hewstone,
Miles.   III. Title.
BF323.S63M33   1996
303.3'85—dc20   95-37283
                                                      CIP

Contributors

Luciano Arcuri, PhD, Instituto Psicologia, Università di Padova, Padova, Italy

Galen V. Bodenhausen, PhD, Department of Psychology, Michigan State University, East Lansing, MI

Marilynn B. Brewer, PhD, Department of Psychology, Ohio State University, Columbus, OH

John C. Brigham, PhD, Department of Psychology, Florida State University, Tallahassee, FL

John F. Dovidio, PhD, Department of Psychology, Colgate University, Hamilton, NY

Jennifer L. Eberhardt, PhD, Department of Psychology, Yale University, New Haven, CT

Susan T. Fiske, PhD, Department of Psychology, University of Massachusetts, Amherst, MA

Christopher Fleming, MA, Department of Psychology, Rutgers University, New Brunswick, NJ

Samuel L. Gaertner, PhD, Department of Psychology, University of Delaware, Newark, DE

David L. Hamilton, PhD, Department of Psychology, University of California, Santa Barbara, Santa Barbara, CA

Miles Hewstone, DPhil, School of Psychology, University of Wales, Cardiff, Cardiff, United Kingdom.

Blair T. Johnson, PhD, Department of Psychology, Syracuse University, Syracuse, NY

Charles M. Judd, PhD, Department of Psychology, University of Colorado, Boulder, CO

Lee Jussim, PhD, Department of Psychology, Rutgers University, Piscataway, NJ

Anne Maass, PhD, Dipartimento di Psicologia, Università di Padova, Padova, Italy

Diane M. Mackie, PhD, Department of Psychology, University of California, Santa Barbara, Santa Barbara, CA

C. Neil Macrae, PhD, School of Psychology, Cardiff University, Cardiff, United Kingdom

Bernadette Park, PhD, Department of Psychology, University of Colorado, Boulder, CO

Francine Rosselli, PhD, Department of Psychology, State University of New York at Buffalo, Amherst, NY

Carey S. Ryan, PhD, Department of Psychology, University of Pittsburgh, Pittsburgh, PA

Mark Schaller, PhD, Department of Psychology, University of Montana, Missoula, MT

David J. Schneider, PhD, Department of Psychology, Rice University, Houston, TX

Charles Stangor, PhD, Department of Psychology, University of Maryland at College Park, College Park, MD

Joshua Susskind, MA, Department of Psychology, University of California, Santa Barbara, Santa Barbara, CA

Leslie A. Zebrowitz, PhD, Department of Psychology, Brandeis University, Waltham, MA

Preface

The idea for this book originated in Bristol, UK, in the spring of 1992 when the three of us attended the Second European Small Group Conference on Social Cognition. During the meeting, we listened to a number of presentations that dealt with basic issues in social stereotyping. We were particularly struck by the diverse approaches and varying perspectives adopted in these presentations, and it occurred to us that a summary of contemporary research on stereotyping could make a potentially useful contribution to the field. To that end, we have collected a series of chapters that, taken together, provide an overview of what social psychologists know about stereotypes and stereotyping in the late 20th century.

One goal of the present book is to bridge the gap created in the literature since the publication of David L. Hamilton's seminal volume (Hamilton, 1981). In the last fourteen years, much ink has flowed on the topic of social stereotyping. During this time, moreover, we have considerably expanded our understanding of how stereotypes impact upon mental life. One important lesson we have learned, for instance, is that stereotypes and stereotyping are more complicated than was assumed at the time of Hamilton's book. As such, conclusions about the structure and function of stereotypes require some modification. In Hamilton's volume, it was generally argued that stereotypes are cognitively driven, inaccurate, harmful, biasing, resistant to change, and that everyone uses them. Recent research, however, has challenged many of these claims. Stereotypes may be positive or negative; moreover, they may be accurate or inaccurate. Some stereotypes seem highly resistant to change; others, however, change quite easily. In some contexts, stereotypes exert a profound influence on people's judgments and behavior; in others, they do not. Finally, some people appear to use stereotypes with regularity, whereas others apparently never at all. One thing that has become increasingly clear in recent years is that stereotypes will never be fully understood in purely cognitive terms. Rather, they are bound into the motivational, emotional, and linguistic behavior of individuals, and theoretical treatments of the topic need to acknowledge this state of affairs. Finally, stereotypes appear to serve an important social, as well as individual, function.

In the present book, we have attempted to cover many of these issues and to capture the diversity and richness of contemporary research on social stereotyping. To achieve this objective, we have secured contributions from many of the leading researchers in the field. They have all done a great job for us, and for this we are grateful. The result, we believe, is a book that documents many of the issues and problems that are currently attracting attention in experimental social psychology laboratories throughout the world.

Finally, for their patience, support, and encouragement, we would like to thank Seymour Weingarten and the folks at The Guilford Press.

C. NEIL MACRAE
CHARLES STANGOR
MILES HEWSTONE

REFERENCES

Hamilton, D. L. (Ed.). (1981). *Cognitive processes in stereotyping and intergroup behavior.* Hillsdale, NJ: Erlbaum.

Contents

I. INTRODUCTION: WHAT ARE STEREOTYPES?

1 Stereotypes as Individual and Collective Representations   3
   Charles Stangor and Mark Schaller

II. STEREOTYPE FORMATION AND DEVELOPMENT

2 Social Psychological Foundations of Stereotype   41
   Formation
   *Diane M. Mackie, David L. Hamilton, Joshua Susskind,
   and Francine Rosselli*

3 Physical Appearance as a Basis of Stereotyping   79
   Leslie A. Zebrowitz

4 Assessing Stereotype Accuracy: Implications for   121
   Understanding the Stereotyping Process
   Carey S. Ryan, Bernadette Park, and Charles M. Judd

III. STEREOTYPE FUNCTION AND USE

5 Self-Fulfilling Prophecies and the Maintenance of Social   161
   Stereotypes: The Role of Dyadic Interactions and Social
   Forces
   Lee Jussim and Christopher Fleming

6 Language and Stereotyping   193
   Anne Maass and Luciano Arcuri

7 The Self-Regulation of Intergroup Perception: 227
   Mechanisms and Consequences of Stereotype
   Suppression
   Galen V. Bodenhausen and C. Neil Macrae

8 When Stereotypes Lead to Stereotyping: The Use of   254
   Stereotypes in Person Perception
   Marilynn B. Brewer

9 Stereotyping, Prejudice, and Discrimination: 276
   Another Look
   *John F. Dovidio, John C. Brigham, Blair T. Johnson,
   and Samuel L. Gaertner*

IV. UNDERMINING STEREOTYPES AND STEREOTYPING

10 Contact and Categorization: Social Psychological   323
    Interventions to Change Intergroup Relations
    Miles Hewstone

11 Motivating Individuals to Change: What Is a Target   369
    to Do?
    Jennifer L. Eberhardt and Susan T. Fiske

V. CONCLUSIONS

12 Modern Stereotype Research: Unfinished Business   419
    David J. Schneider

    Index   455

STEREOTYPES AND STEREOTYPING

I

INTRODUCTION:
WHAT ARE STEREOTYPES?

1

Stereotypes as Individual and Collective Representations

CHARLES STANGOR
MARK SCHALLER

Stop for a moment and think about one of the many social groups that make up a diverse geographic area such as Europe or the United States. You'll easily (perhaps you think too easily!) conjure up a portrait of what the people in the group are like. You may generate an oversimplified impression of the characteristics of the group as a whole—that Greeks are fun-loving, that the Irish drink too much, or that African Americans are boisterous. Or perhaps you will retrieve particular instances of people from the group—maybe an image of Marcello Mastroianni appears, reminding you that Italian men are good looking.

This type of thought process reflects the most traditional conceptualization of stereotypes within social psychology, in which stereotypes are considered to be the "pictures in the head" of individuals looking out into their social worlds (e.g., Lippmann, 1922). But stereotypes also exist from the point of view of the person who is being stereotyped. Consider the African American man who is repeatedly denied employment because the white employers in his neighborhood have decided that blacks are lazy and ignorant. Or the frustration of a Catholic woman in Northern Ireland who is denied admission to a major university because of her religion. In these cases, the effects of stereotyping are much more than the simple "picture in the head" would indicate. Cer-

tainly the discriminating individuals in these scenarios have negative beliefs about the targets of their discrimination, but the real problem for
the individual being stereotyped is that in each case the individuals who
are making the decisions have the *same* pictures in their heads. If stereotyping were only an individual problem, the person could go to another
company and speak to a different employment officer, or enroll in a different university. But when stereotypes are consensually shared within a
society, their consequences become much more pernicious, because they
affect entire groups of people in a common way. As Gardner (1973, p.
134) put it, an ethnic group member "may be somewhat chagrined to
find that a few individuals in the larger community have beliefs about
the characteristics of the group of which he is a member, but it has major implications . . . when such beliefs are relatively widespread in the
community."

The basic theme of this chapter is that stereotypes can be conceptualized from two complementary perspectives, and that a full understanding of the stereotyping process involves looking at both types of
approaches. From one perspective stereotypes are represented within the
mind of the individual person. From the other perspective, stereotypes
are represented as part of the social fabric of a society, shared by the
people within that culture. We will consider the implications of thinking
about stereotypes in these different ways upon the important questions
that researchers ask about stereotypes, including what stereotypes are
and how they should be measured. In doing so, we will consider how
stereotypes are represented (i.e., stored for future use) at both individual
and collective levels.

INDIVIDUAL AND COLLECTIVE APPROACHES: HISTORY AND OVERVIEW

The idea that stereotypes are both individual and cultural phenomena is
not a new one. Indeed, individual and collective approaches to the study
of social psychological issues more generally have long traditions within
psychology, as does the distinction between the two. Wundt (1902)
made a clear distinction between individual and collective psychology,
and this distinction was maintained by McDougall (1920) on the collective side, and Allport (1924) on the individual side.

Historically, these theorists were concerned about whether "social
reality" exists at the level of the individual or at the level of the group
(as a "group mind"). That question is less relevant now; there is no

longer a question that all beliefs, including social beliefs such as stereotypes, exist in the minds of individual persons (cf. Asch, 1952). Rather, the pivotal point of distinction between individual and collective approaches lies in the assumed importance of shared social beliefs, above and beyond that of individual beliefs, as determinants of social behavior. This distinction is particularly important for a complete understanding of stereotypes and stereotyping.

Individual approaches have not been particularly concerned about stereotype consensus, focusing instead on the meaning of the stereotype to the individual. According to this perspective, "neither the definition nor the measurement of stereotypes should be constrained by the necessity of consensual agreement" (Hamilton, Stroessner, & Driscoll, 1994, p. 297). To theorists within the cultural approach, on the other hand, societal consensus is paramount. Because group values and group behavior provide the underlying foundation of stereotyping, stereotypes only have meaning (indeed stereotypes are only stereotypes!) to the extent they are culturally shared (Gardner, Kirby, & Findlay, 1973; Katz & Braly, 1933; Moscovici, 1981; Tajfel, 1981; Tajfel & Forgas, 1981). Moscovici observed that "any reduction to cognitive patterns and constructs, by eliminating the extraordinary richness of collective thought . . . converts an important problem into a mere academic exercise" (p. 208). Let us turn now to a more detailed exploration of the individual and collective approaches to stereotype representation.

STEREOTYPE REPRESENTATION

Stereotypes as Individual Beliefs: A Social Cognitive Perspective

The individual approach to stereotyping has primarily been associated with the dominant social cognitive tradition within North America (cf. Fiske & Taylor, 1991; Markus & Zajonc, 1985). The basic assumption of this approach is that, over time, people develop beliefs about the characteristics of the important social groups in their environment, and this knowledge influences their responses toward subsequently encountered individual members of those groups. Thus stereotypes (as one type of knowledge about the social world), develop as the individual perceives his or her environment. The perceived information about social groups is interpreted, encoded in memory, and subsequently retrieved for use in guiding responses. Furthermore, each of these processes is potentially subject to biases due to the assimilative effects of existing knowledge on information processing.

As mental representations of the world, stereotypes influence what information is sought out (Johnston & Macrae, 1994; Rothbart, 1981; Snyder, 1981), attended to (Belmore & Hubbard, 1987), and remembered (Fyock & Stangor, 1994) about members of social groups, as well as influencing social behavior (cf. Jussim & Fleming, Chapter 5, this volume). Indeed the effectiveness of a given model of stereotype representation at the individual level is judged in terms of its ability to account for these basic processes. Stereotype development (Hamilton & Gifford, 1976; Jussim, 1991; Schaller & O'Brien, 1992; Stangor & Duan, 1991), maintenance (Hamilton & Rose, 1980; Stangor & McMillan, 1992) and change (Hewstone & Brown, 1986; Weber & Crocker, 1983) have all been addressed from this perspective (cf. Hamilton & Sherman, 1994; Stangor & Lange, 1993).

An interest with individual-level beliefs and interpersonal interactions has led researchers within the social cognitive tradition to focus upon the "bottom-up" determinants of stereotypes. It has been assumed within this approach that stereotypes are learned, and potentially changed, primarily through the information that individuals acquire through direct contact with members of other social groups.[1] Hypothesized, data-driven mechanisms through which stereotypes may be acquired involve attention to information (Langer & Imber, 1980; McArthur & Post, 1977), recall of information (Fyock & Stangor, 1994; Hamilton & Gifford, 1976), and integration of information (Schaller & O'Brien, 1992). Given the role of information in stereotype formation, information acquired through intergroup contact is expected to offer the best means of change (Hewstone & Brown, 1986). Although the possibility that stereotypes may also be learned and changed through indirect sources (from leaders, parents, peers, the mass media) is not explicitly denied by the individual approach, little research has focused on this possibility (but see Park & Hastie, 1987).

Three general approaches as to how information about social groups is represented within memory have been proposed. These are *group schemas*, *group prototypes*, and *exemplars*. Because each of these approaches is framed at a different level of specificity and makes different assumptions about how group beliefs are represented, each is thus differentially effective at answering important questions about stereotype development and its subsequent impact on social responses. In addition, each of the different approaches has implications for how stereotypes should be measured.

Group Schemas

The most traditional approach to stereotyping within the individual approach is based on the cognitive schema (Fiske & Linville, 1980; Taylor & Crocker, 1981). Schemas are abstract knowledge structures that specify the defining features and relevant attributes of a given concept. Schemas give meaning to social information and promote parsimonious and effective information processing (Fiske & Taylor, 1991; Markus & Zajonc, 1985). As representations of social groups, *group schemas* are collections of beliefs about the characteristics of a social group.

Once developed within memory, schemas have broad influences upon person perception, including attention, perception, interpretation, and storage of social information, as well as judgments of and behavior toward others. At the attentional stage, schemas allow the individual to ignore what are perceived to be unrelated and unimportant details of a situation and thus reduce informational complexity, rendering more elaborative processing unnecessary (cf. Bartlett, 1932). At the storage stage, schemas result in better memory for stereotype-confirming (in comparison to disconfirming) information, because this information is more easily assimilated into the schema. Schemas also provide a basis for making judgments about others—inferences beyond the information given (Bruner, 1957). These schema-based inferences include social responses, and particularly guessing in the direction of schema consistency when unsure (Locksley, Stangor, Hepburn, Grosovsky, & Hochstrasser, 1984; Markus & Zajonc, 1985; Stangor, 1988) Schemas also guide behavior through activation of relevant behavioral "scripts" (Schank & Abelson, 1977). In addition to knowledge about stereotypic traits of social groups, schemas may also contain affective information (Fiske, 1982; Fiske & Pavelchak, 1986).

The schema concept has had great heuristic value for the study of stereotyping because "schematic processing" provides an underlying mechanism to account for stereotype maintenance and use. Because the schema concept is so broad, however, it is difficult to use it to make specific predictions about stereotyping. In some cases the schema notion overpredicts, and thus becomes nonfalsifiable. For instance, both faster and slower reaction times for schema-relevant decisions have been taken as evidence for schematic processing (Bem, 1981; Markus, Crane, Bernstein, & Sidali, 1982). In other cases, the schema concept underpredicts. Schema models have difficulty accounting for better memory for schema-inconsistent versus schema-consistent information, a common finding in the literature on person perception. One particular limitation of the schema approach is that it does not make clear predictions about how one should measure stereotypes independently of the schematic effects themselves. Although diverse measures, including biased memory (Fyock & Stangor, 1994; Stangor & McMillan, 1992) clustering in recall (Noseworthy & Lott, 1984), reaction times (Bem, 1981; Markus et al., 1982) and release from proactive interference (Mills & Tyrell, 1983) have been used as measures of schematic processing, there is no well established method of validating the existence of the schema independently of its outcomes. As a result the concept often becomes circular, because there is a tendency to attribute any type of information-processing bias to "schematic" processing.

Group Prototypes

Because one of the primary goals of the cognitive approach has been to "get specific" about how information is mentally represented, researchers have recently turned away from the schema and its inherent ambiguity toward a conceptualization of stereotypes in terms of more clearly articulated models of mental representation. One popular concept in this regard is the *group prototype*. Group prototypes are mental representations consisting of a collection of associations between group labels (e.g., Italians) and the features that are assumed to be true of the group (e.g., a feature of Italians might be "romantic").[2] Thus, prototypes are mental representations of social groups, similar to group schemas, but at a lower and more specific level of representation.

One advantage of a feature-based prototype approach is that it makes more explicit predictions about the activation and measurement of social stereotypes than do schema models. Because stereotypes are defined as mental associations between category labels and trait terms, stereotypes can be measured by the extent to which these traits are activated upon exposure to category labels; that is, if the trait "romantic" is stereotypic of Italians, then when thinking about Italians, "romantic" should quickly come to mind through spreading activation (Collins & Loftus, 1975). One approach in this regard is to use reaction time methodology (Diehl & Jonas, 1991; Dovidio, Evans, & Tyler, 1986; Gilbert & Hixon, 1991) to assess stereotypes. When presented with a target label (e.g., "Italians"), subjects should be quicker at identifying stereotypic versus nonstereotypic traits as words. Alternatively, free-response formats may be used in which those attributes generated frequently, or early in a protocol, are considered stereotypic because they are activated in response to the category label.

A second advantage of the prototype approach is that it makes explicit predictions concerning memory for group-relevant information. On the basis of prototype models, one can predict that either stereotype-consistent or stereotype-inconsistent information may be well remembered, depending on any number of factors that determine the development of associative links between category labels and associated stereotypes (cf. Srull & Wyer, 1989; Stangor & McMillan, 1992). Nevertheless, there is a clear memory advantage for expectancy-confirming information about existing social groups (Fyock & Stangor, 1994).

Despite their greater theoretical specificity, prototype models are more limited in scope in comparison to schema approaches, and cannot account for the diverse effects that schemas have been used to understand. For instance, it is not clear how behavior and affect would be linked to the stereotyping process within prototype models.

Exemplars

A final approach to conceptualizing stereotype representation is based on the commonsense notion that, in addition to abstract representations of social groups, people also have memories for specific individuals (exemplars) whom they have previously encountered (Smith & Zárate, 1992). And these memories may influence responses when these memories are activated through encounters with others who are similar to the stored memories (cf. Lewicki, 1985). The exemplar approach has been given impetus by the recent interest in understanding how variability among group members is represented in memory, and (although it is possible for prototype models to account for variability judgments) it appears that such information is stored at least partially through memory for exemplars (Linville, Salovey, & Fischer, 1986; Park & Judd, 1990).

Exemplar models have the ability to account for many of the same phenomena as do schemas and prototype models (cf. Smith & Zárate, 1992). Zebrowitz (Chapter 3, this volume), for instance, presents an exemplar-based approach that can account for many important stereotyping effects, including activation of affect and behavioral responses. However, it is known that stereotyping is a heuristic device, occurring more often when the capacity or motivation to process individuating information is reduced (cf. Bodenhausen, 1993). The notion of activating an abstract prototype or schema from memory, which serves as a simplifying summary judgment, seems well suited to account for these results. People also possess stereotypes about groups of which they have had little or no direct contact (Hartley, 1946), suggesting that stereotyping occurs in the absence of exemplar-based processing. Finally, in contrast to the prototype approach, the exemplar approach has not yet dealt explicitly with the issue of stereotype development, including the important questions of how stereotypic characteristics become associated with individual exemplars in memory, and which of the many possible stereotypes of a person might be so linked.

Stereotypes as Collective Belief Systems: A Cultural Perspective

The individual approach to stereotype representation is framed at a micro-analytic level, delineating the cognitive systems that allow individuals to efficiently store and retrieve stereotypes. Although these models range to some extent in generality from the breadth of group schemas to the narrowness of individual exemplars, they are all intrapersonal in orientation. The cultural approach is broader in scope, transcending the intraindividual perspective. Cultural models consider society itself to be the basis of stored knowledge, and stereotypes as public information about social groups that is shared among the individuals within a culture. In this approach, although stereotypes exist "in the head of the society's perceivers," they exist also in the "fabric of the society" itself.

Consensual stereotypes represent one aspect of the entire collective knowledge of a society. This knowledge includes the society's customs, myths, ideas, religions, and sciences (Boster, 1991; Duveen & Lloyd, 1990; Farr & Moscovici, 1984). Because such concepts are traditionally more sociological or anthropological than psychological in nature, their study has not been the traditional focus of experimental social psychologists. And yet, as Tajfel (1981) argued, because cultural stereotypes represent one part of an individual's social knowledge, and because these beliefs have important effects on social behavior, their consideration is essential for a full understanding of stereotypes and stereotyping.

In addition to considering stereotypes from a different level of analysis, cultural approaches also differ from individual models in terms of the assumed sources of stereotype development and change. Whereas the individual approach has focused on how stereotypes are learned through direct interaction with others, cultural approaches consider the ways that stereotypes are learned, transmitted, and changed through indirect sources—information gained from parents, peers, teachers, political and religious leaders, and the mass media. For this reason, cultural approaches focus explicitly on language as a representation of social groups.

Language

"There is no completely non-verbal social stereotyping," wrote Fishman (1956, p. 48). Indeed, a cultural approach to stereotyping emphasizes that stereotypes are learned, maintained, and potentially changed through the language and communication of a culture. Language transcends the individual and offers a means of storing stereotypic beliefs at a collective, consensual level.

Particularly central to language acquisition are the processes of naming, labeling and categorizing (Anglin, 1977). Thus it is no surprise that language provides a basic mechanism by which individuals are categorized into groups, and by which stereotypes are shared with others (Allport, 1954; Fishman, 1956; Moscovici, 1981). It is well known that stereotypes are learned through communication. Correlations between the stereotypes and prejudices of parents and children are commonly observed (Epstein & Komorita, 1966; Fagot, Leinbach, & O'Boyle, 1992). Furthermore, stereotype change occurs through education (Stephan & Stephan, 1984), which must involve some degree of communication.

Study of the role of language in stereotyping leads to an explicit focus on the content of the category labels and the stereotypes. Within the individual approach, the tendency has been to study generic category labels, such as "women" or "Blacks." But the flexibility of language suggests that these standard labels do not capture the full flavor of stereotypes (cf. Devine & Baker, 1991). The same social groups can be labeled in different ways, ranging from the benign and politically correct ("Black," "homosexual," "woman") to the derogatory ("nigger," "faggot," or "bitch").

Whereas benign labels connote mere category membership, the derogatory slurs connote the flavor of the stereotype itself. This is evident when one recognizes that slurs are typically not applied indiscriminantly to all members of the social category, but primarily to those members who fit a certain stereotypic profile. Users of the word "nigger," for instance, often claim that not all Blacks are "niggers," only some of them. So just as other slang terms often convey a more negative experience or expectation than conveyed by the simple descriptive noun, derogatory group labels convey a particular negative stereotype to a greater degree than less offensive descriptive terms. It is in these labels, then, that the stereotype is most purely and powerfully signified in the transpersonal storage system of language.

In addition to its influence on the representation of category labels, language also affects the nature of the stereotypes themselves. One commonly observed effect concerns the tendency to relabel traits in ways the signify the valence of the preferred belief (cf. Saenger & Flowerman, 1954). Of course, language interacts with stereotyping in other ways as well, for instance when it becomes a category itself, or determines which categories are activated (cf. Giles & Saint-Jacques, 1979).

Despite the clear importance of language as a basis of stereotyping, empirical research has not been as abundant, or as integrated into other approaches to stereotyping, as it might be. The study of derogatory labels, or "ethnophaulisms," has received some research attention. Palmore (1962) observed a relationship between the degree of prejudice directed toward a particular ethnic group and the number of derogatory nicknames that exist for that group in the common language. More recently, Mullen and Johnson (1993) observed a correlation between the size of the ethnic group and the number of nicknames. In both cases, the data were based upon collective repositories of cultural beliefs (e.g., dictionaries of slang).

The content of everyday discourse has also been analyzed as it relates to the transmission and reproduction of stereotypes and prejudice (cf. Giles, 1977; van Dijk, 1987). Although language is transpersonal, language users are individuals. And research has examined the individual use of stereotypic language (see Greenberg & Pyszczynski, 1985; Maass & Arcuri, Chapter 6, this volume).

The Media

In modern society, the form by which most stereotypes are transmitted is through the mass media—literature, television, movies, newspapers, E-mail, leaflets, and bumper stickers. The tangible artifacts of consumable mass media thus comprise an "information highway" for the transmission of social stereotypes. These representations of stereotypes are bought, sold, traded, checked out, and otherwise shared by millions, even billions of people across boundaries of distance and time untraveled by ordinary interpersonal communication.

That the mass media are an important collective repository for group stereotypes is recognized explicitly by individuals who attend to the way that groups and group members are portrayed in the media, and by researchers who codify these representations. Many studies have used qualitative data-analytic techniques to describe the manifestations of stereotypes in such diverse media as television shows (e.g., Hartmann & Husband, 1974; Wilson & Gutierrez, 1985), advertising (e.g., Bell, 1992; Pasadeos, 1987), and children's school texts (e.g., Dixon, 1977; Stinton, 1980; Zimet, 1976). Although these studies typically involve descriptive, qualitative methods of coding content, these measurement schemes are amenable to hypothesis-testing contexts as well. For instance, a number of researchers (e.g., Pasadeos, 1987; Weigel, Loomis, & Soja, 1980) have used such methods to study changes in cultural stereotypes over time. Again, although this type of study is typically out of the realm of the everyday life of the experimental social psychologist, the development of comprehensive models of stereotyping will require the ability to understand and assess stereotype development and transmission at both individual and collective levels.

Social Norms and Roles

The language of a social group is explicitly bound up in the norms and the roles of the individual members of those groups (cf. Crandall, Thompson, Sakalli, & Schiffhauer, 1995). Thus, cultural norms are more than simply contributors to individual beliefs about groups; they are a social system through which stereotypes are represented and perpetuated across individuals, across generations, and across time (cf. Sherif, 1936).

Allport (1954) was well aware of the extent to which stereotypes developed through conformity to prevailing norms. On the basis of stereotypes of American soldiers during the Second World War (Stouffer, Suchman, DeVinney, Star, & Williams, 1949), he calculated that "about half of all prejudiced attitudes are based only on the need to conform to custom" (p. 272). Pettigrew (1958, 1959) found that those people who adhered most strongly to norms were also the most prejudiced against out-groups. Recent theoretical analyses of gender stereotypes also implicate social customs and norms—at least in the form of traditional gender roles—in the formation of gender stereotypes (Eagly, 1987; Hoffman & Hurst, 1990). Indeed, measures of gender-specific norms typically evolved from other measures designed to assess prevailing stereotypic beliefs (e.g., Bem, 1974; Spence, Helmreich, & Stapp, 1975).

The social psychological importance of shared group beliefs is clearly demonstrated by examining the power of consensual stereotypes to influence normative behaviors. Once group stereotypes exist in a culture, expected patterns of behavior for those group members follow, and these expectations determine both responses to group members and the behavior of the group members themselves. Consider the influence of traditional gender roles on the behavior of men and women. The power of these norms is twofold: First, men and women feel pressure to comply with the appropriate gender-based social norms rather than risk the collective derogation attendant on norm violation. When group members willingly (or unwillingly) act in stereotypic ways, their behavior justifies and perpetuates the stereotype. Second, even if particular group members wish to act in ways inconsistent with the norm, their ability to do so may be constrained by the norm-based expectations of others via behavioral confirmation effects (see Jussim & Fleming, Chapter 5, this volume).

One example of the power of cultural stereotypes to influence behavior is demonstrated in recent work by Steele and his colleagues (Spencer & Steele, 1992; Steele, 1992; Steele & Aronson, 1995) concerning the effects of culturally-held stereotypes about women and about African Americans on scholastic achievement. Steele and Spencer argue that there is a consensual stereotype within American culture that women are poor at math in comparison to men, and that African Americans are poor in academic tasks more generally. Because women and Blacks are aware of these shared beliefs, they recognize that failure in relevant academic tasks will perpetrate the damaging stereotype. As a result, they experience extra pressure to defy the stereotype and succeed. But the extra pressure itself may be so great as to sabotage those efforts, ironically diminishing the likelihood of performing well. Steele's analysis is provocative, because it uses the stereotype concept to account for behavioral outcomes in a way that individual-level analyses cannot. The influence of stereotypes on performance exists only because stereotypes are consensual, and members of stereotyped groups are themselves intensely aware of these culturally shared beliefs.

POINTS OF CONTRAST

The approaches to understanding stereotype representation reviewed earlier vary substantially in terms of both level of analysis and basic underlying assumptions. In the next sections we compare the emphases of the individual and collective approaches, noting the strengths and weaknesses of each. Then we turn to a discussion of ways in which the two approaches might be integrated.

Individual Approaches

The individual approach to stereotyping has recently defined how stereotypes are understood within contemporary social psychology (cf. Hamilton & Sherman, 1994; Stangor & Lange, 1993), at least in part because it has provided a unifying theoretical perspective for the study of the stereotyping process. In addition to providing specific answers to the basic questions of how central tendency and variability information about social groups are mentally represented, this approach has unified the study of how stereotypes develop (e.g., Hamilton & Gifford, 1976; Schaller & O'Brien, 1992; Stangor & Ford, 1992; see Mackie, Hamilton, Susskind, & Rosselli, Chapter 2, this volume), influence judgments of others (e.g., Brewer, 1988; Fiske & Neuberg, 1990), and change, particularly when the individual encounters stereotype-disconfirming behaviors (e.g., Rothbart & Lewis, 1988; Weber & Crocker, 1983; see Hewstone, Chapter 10, and Eberhardt & Fiske, Chapter 11, this volume). The individual approach makes it clear that these central questions are all conceptually interrelated. The same basic cognitive processes that are part of stereotype formation also underlie stereotype maintenance and change.

A second advantage of the individual approach is that it provides a conceptual foundation for uniting the study of stereotypes with social knowledge more generally, through the language of mental representation. For instance, conceptualizing stereotypes as the cognitive (belief) component of prejudice provides a way of studying stereotypes within the broader literature on attitudes (Eagly & Chaiken, 1993; Fazio, 1990), and provides a means of linking stereotypes to the study of of discriminatory behavior (see Dovidio, Brigham, Johnson, & Gaertner, Chapter 9, this volume).[3] And the links between stereotyping and the self-concept become clear when self-stereotypes are considered in terms of their positive (Turner, 1975) or negative (Jacobs & Eccles, 1985; Spencer & Steele, 1992) effects on the self.

The individual representational approach also provides a mechanism to account for the often-observed flexibility of stereotyping. Despite possessing stereotype knowledge, people do not always make use of these stereotypes (see Brewer, Chapter 8, this volume). The individual approach explains stereotype flexibility through the concepts of construct accessibility (Higgins & King, 1981; Oakes & Turner, 1990; Stangor, 1988) and spreading activation (Collins & Loftus, 1975). As with any type of mental representation, both stereotype representations (schemas; prototypes) and the contents of those representations (the stereotypical beliefs) may be differentially accessible across individuals and across contexts (Stangor & Lange, 1993). Thus, stereotypes may or may not be used as a basis of judgment, depending upon how the target person is categorized (Stangor, Lynch, Duan, & Glass, 1992), the fit between the target individual and the perceiver's expectations about the group to which he or she belongs (Lord, Lepper, & Mackie, 1984; Turner, 1987, Chapter 6), the strength of association between the stereotype and the category label (Dovidio et al., 1986), the contextual demands of the situation (Bodenhausen & Lichtenstein, 1987), as well as individual differences in stereotype accessibility (Bem, 1981; Markus, Crane, Bernstein, & Sidali, 1982; Stangor, 1988; Stangor et al., 1992).

Despite these important contributions toward understanding stereotyping, the individual approach has overemphasized the role of individual perception and direct contact with target group members as determinants of stereotypes. People do form stereotypes about groups with whom they have had no direct contact (Hartley, 1946)—stereotypes that may be quite rich and well developed. And, despite the basic assumption that stereotypes will change through direct contact with members of other groups, contact has only small effects on stereotypes (Hewstone & Brown, 1986; Rothbart & John, 1992). Furthermore, the individual approach often overlooks the socially important outcomes of stereotyping that do not occur at a purely individual level.

Despite the laudable goal of being specific about how information is mentally represented, there is inherent ambiguity in this process, and it is not clear that more specificity necessarily provides a better understanding of stereotyping. Not only is it virtually impossible to distinguish representational formats at the level of specificity that some researchers have claimed (e.g., Barsalou, 1990, has argued that it may be impossible to distinguish exemplar from prototype representations), but it also may not matter from a practical perspective exactly how social information is stored. The important issues concern what information is activated under what conditions, and how and when stereotypes influence social behavior. More macroanalytic investigations may provide greater insights into these questions.

Collective Approaches

In contrast to the emphasis on cognitive representations within the individual approach, the collective approach emphasizes the transmission and reproduction of stereotypes across individuals and generations, and the social outcomes of stereotyping. One concomitant of this broader social approach is an explicit concern with *content* of stereotypes, in comparison to the emphasis on process that has driven the individual approach (Tajfel, 1981). When a common set of beliefs are internalized within a group, these beliefs begin to influence the group's collective behavior. Indeed, it is the stereotype content, consensually shared across a culture, that makes stereotypes particularly problematic.

It *matters* that the stereotypes of Blacks include "lazy," "athletic," and "musical," rather than some other set of traits, both because these beliefs are involved in determining the social status of Blacks within a society and because these beliefs are determined *by* the social position of Blacks.

Furthermore, the collective approach makes it clear that it is consensual, and not individual, stereotypes that lead to the outcomes that make stereotypes of interest in the first place. These include both the negative consequences of behavioral confirmation, biased interpretation of events, and discrimination, and the positive effects of stereotyping on self esteem (Crocker & Major, 1989; Crocker, Voekl, Testa, & Major, 1991; Turner, 1975). Indeed, arguments that stereotypes do not need to be consensual disregard the fundamental requirement that influences of stereotypes at a group level are based upon interindividual consensus.

Because group consensus is such a central part of the collective approach, it is at first blush problematic that stereotypes often demonstrate a significant degree of cross-individual inconsistency (Katz & Braly, 1933; Stangor & Lange, 1993). For instance, in their classic study of ethnic stereotypes, Katz and Braly found that less than 40% of their subjects considered such putatively central traits as "ignorant" and "musical" to describe "Negroes." And for 5 out of their 10 target groups, there was not a single trait that was considered centrally stereotypic by more than half of their subjects. This lack of consensus is partly what led individual level analyses to ignore it.

Yet, it would naturally be expected that the consensus of group beliefs would vary, both between in-groups and out-groups (Linville et al., 1986), across different cultures, and even in subgroups within a single society (cf. Boster, 1991). Thus, treating consensus as a variable can provide important information about the process of stereotyping. Indeed, consensus in group beliefs is a common dependent measure within cognitive anthropology (cf. Boster & d'Andrade, 1989), and sophisticated approaches to such measurement have been developed (cf. Gardner, et al., 1972, for an example within social psychology).

As one example, interindividual consensus could be used to assess whether the development of a given stereotype is determined by top-down or bottom-up processes. To the extent that stereotypes are culturally transmitted through norms and language, individuals who communicate more often (e.g., within families, jobs, or peer groups) should develop stronger stereotype consensus. On the other hand, if consensus is determined by bottom-up factors, then stereotypes should be based on the number and quality of direct or indirect interactions with out-group members, independently of communication with in-groups.

The collective approach also offers a unique perspective on the question of how to change stereotypes. Because cultural models are based on the assumption that many stereotypes are learned and modified through indirect sources, the role of intergroup contact as a source of attitude change is not emphasized. Rather, the collective approach focuses on stereotype change that occurs through institutional changes (Reicher, 1986), leadership (Bar Tal, 1989) and education (Katz & Zalk, 1978; Stephan & Stephan, 1984).

Indeed, educational intervention represents a mechanism of stereotype change that implicitly integrates individual with collective approaches. Educational interventions may take many forms, including exposure to stereotype-disconfirming information about groups, structured cooperative interactions between members of different groups, and instruction to be more tolerant of others' differences. Such interventions are individualistic in that they are directed toward changing the cognitions of individual minds, rather than changing the cultural institutions that maintain stereotypes. But these interventions are collective in that they are administered to large groups of people at a time. They are also collective in that they often draw on collective values (e.g., cultural values emphasizing cooperation or tolerance). And they are collective in that, if successful in changing the cognitions of individual minds, they may indeed effect changes in the cultural institutions that maintain stereotypes—such as language use and contents of the mass media.

Stereotype change also occurs through the efforts of groups to redefine and relabel themselves. The labels "Negro" and "colored" have fallen out of favor, with the labels "Black," "Afro-American" and finally "African American" replacing them. Similar changes have occurred through the work of those who have struggled to change cultural stereotypes about the roles and stereotypes of women. In this sense, a consensual stereotype may also have positive effects when it motivates a group to band together to overcome it—to create or change its own stereotype. These types of top-down change, which occur without changes in the amount or quality of intergroup contact, have been understudied within social psychology.

Yet, there, are fundamental weaknesses to collective approaches as well. Most important there is not yet a unified theoretical or empirical tradition in the area of culturally determined stereotypes. Although these approaches argue that social values and norms are the important determinants of stereotyping, there is little hard evidence to support these hypotheses. Furthermore, the approaches often rely on individual-level measures of perceptual distortion and bias, without being specific about the underlying cognitive mechanisms that produce them.

POINTS OF CONTACT:
FUNCTIONAL DETERMINANTS OF
STEREOTYPE REPRESENTATION

Despite fundamental differences underlying individual and collective approaches to the study of stereotyping, there is an even greater set of commonalities. In addition to sharing the basic goals of understanding the development, stability, and change of group beliefs, as well as their influence on judgment and behavior, both the individual and collective approaches have adopted an underlying functionalist perspective, based on the fundamental supposition that the format in which stereotypes are represented (as is all knowledge) is determined not only by objective reality, but also by the extent to which that knowledge meets important goals. This assumption dates from earlier formulations of stereotyping (Allport, 1954; Erhlich, 1973; Fishman, 1956; Harding, Proshansky, Kutner, & Chein, 1969) and runs through contemporary theorizing in both individual (Fiske & Neuberg, 1990; Snyder & Miene, 1994; Stangor & Ford, 1992) and collective (Jost & Banaji, 1994; Tajfel, 1981; Turner, 1975, 1987) approaches.

The few theorists who have addressed both individual and collective functions of stereotypes have emphasized the differences between underlying functions at the two levels. For instance, Tajfel (1981; Tajfel & Forgas, 1981) noted that stereotypes serve an individual function by systematizing and simplifying information available to a perceiver, and protecting that perceiver's value structure. At a collective level, Tajfel suggested that stereotypes serve groups by offering culturally accepted explanations for events, by justifying group actions, and by providing a means for groups to differentiate themselves positively from other groups. These two sets of functions are separate enough in perspective that Tajfel (1981) openly doubted whether an all-encompassing theory binding them together would even be possible.

Superficially, the underlying functions implied by the two approaches seem different, and it is true that they are again driven by the respective interests in bottom-up versus top-down processing. In the case of individual beliefs, the focus is on individual perceivers interacting with their environment. This approach has emphasized reliance on stereotypes as cognitive tools to satisfy basic needs for environmental understanding and for self-protection. Within the cultural approach, the focus is more top-down, concerning the influence of motivations to accept and transmit culturally shared values or knowledge upon perception and behavior. In this sense, stereotypes function to meet the needs of the culture, its political or religious structures, and the *zeitgeist* more generally.

But this distinction may be more apparent than real. Despite his pessimism, Tajfel (1981) did hint at theoretical initiatives that may relate individual and collective functions together, essentially suggesting that collective needs inform and guide individual needs. We offer a related, but somewhat different perspective. We argue that, just as both approaches are based upon the same underlying set of cognitive mechanisms (categorization, accentuation and perceptual biases), they are also founded on a similar set of underlying motivational needs. Furthermore, individual and collective needs are inherently intertwined. Just as many individual-level concerns require a collective context (e.g., social acceptance by others requires that the individual be located within a phenomenologically relevant culture), so culturally shared values and beliefs are meaningless if not for the fact that individuals translate those values into specific actions.

Here, then, we encounter a fundamental point of rapprochement between the individual and collective perspectives—a set of overlapping and symbiotic motivations. In this section, we focus on two fundamental human needs (explanation and prediction of the social world, and esteem maintenance) and review evidence highlighting the role of these needs in the development of both individual and culturally shared stereotypes.

Epistemic Functions of Stereotypes

A basic human motive is that of knowing, understanding, and predicting others (cf. Heider, 1958; Kelley, 1967; Kruglanski, 1989), and one of the more basic functions of stereotypes is to provide useful information about others (cf. Oakes & Turner, 1990). At an individual level, stereotypes are useful for making both inductive and deductive judgments (Diehl & Jonas, 1991). People constantly meet new individuals about whom they have little information except their social category memberships, and they use this knowledge in an adaptive manner to draw dispositional inferences about the person. At other times, individuals view the behavior of an individual, using this knowledge in conjunction with his or her stereotypes to predict category memberships ("Is she Jewish?"; "Is he gay?"; cf. Gardener, Kirby, & Finlay, 1973).

The prevailing goal of making informed judgments about individuals suggests that stereotypes will develop in a way that enhances the ability to perform this task. Stereotype representations have informational value to the extent that they maximize "meta-contrast" (Turner, 1987; see also Ashmore & Del Boca, 1981; McCauley, Stitt, & Segal, 1980), such that between-group differences are large and within-group differences are small. For instance, based on the assumptions of Tajfel's accentuation theory, Ford and Stangor (1992) hypothesized and found that stereotypes would develop more strongly to the extent that they maximized group differentiation, regardless of whether that differentiation was the result of high between-group distinctiveness or low within-group variability.

Just as individuals use their beliefs about social groups to help them understand and explain individual behavior, stereotypes also develop at the collective level as a basis for rendering social events more tangible (Hewstone, 1989; Tajfel, 1981; Tajfel & Forgas, 1981). These explanations provide information and structure where formerly there was ignorance and confusion. For instance, in the absence of theories about germs and contagion, European communities in the 16th and 17th centuries reacted to outbreaks of bubonic plague by developing plausible (but deeply misguided) explanations for the fever that ravaged their population. The people in Newcastle believed the Scots had poisoned their wells; Barnstaple residents believed it was the work of a local Independent congregation; and in Oxford they blamed it on the sorcery of the Catholic church (Thomas, 1971, cited in Tajfel & Forgas, 1981). Across communities, explanations differed; but within communities, explanations were consensual, satisfying a collective need to understand the community, misfortune.

Predicting and adequately responding to others requires not only sufficient information, but also some means of simplifying or structuring the over complex and often contradictory data that are manifest in the environment (Kruglanski, 1989; Neuberg & Newsom, 1993). Thus, just as stereotypes sometimes supplement an information-impoverished environment, at other times they may reduce the complexity of an information-rich environment. Research amply demonstrates that the use of social stereotypes increases in cognitively demanding situations (see Bodenhausen & Macrae, Chapter 7, this volume), and also develop more strongly when needs for structure or coherence are enhanced (cf. Kruglanski & Freund, 1983; Stangor & Duan, 1991).

But individual motives for closure or simplification extend beyond use of categories to include needs to bring beliefs about diverse social categories into cognitive consonance. One of the original explanations for stereotypes is that they served to justify the negative attitudes that are held about others (Allport, 1954; Fishman, 1956; Myrdal, 1944; Ryan, 1971). Consistent with this notion is evidence demonstrating the relationship between prejudice and stereotypes (see Dovidio, Brigham, Johnson, & Gaertner, Chapter 9, this volume). Furthermore, just as individuals attempt to justify negative events that befall other individuals

(Lerner & Miller, 1978; Milgram, 1974), people may develop stereotypes about categories of victimized others. Research suggests that just such a justification process operates in the formation of negative stereotypes about the survivors of sexual assault (Mazelan, 1980).

Just as stereotypes function to clarify individual cognitive representations of the world, they also act to simplify communication at the social level, allowing people to enjoy an economy of words when speaking about and to others. A speaker can convey an abundance of information by simply labeling a person as a "Jew," "nigger," or "feminist." The reason that verbal exchange is simplified is, of course, the implicit assurance that the category label will convey information to the recipient of the communication through shared group beliefs. Thus, whereas the surface features of the communication may be simple, the level of interpersonal understanding is rich with implied meaning. Moreover, the stereotype label does not merely imply extensive information, but also extensive information that is evaluatively coherent as well, making the communication both simple and compelling (cf. Graumann & Wintermantel, 1989; van Dijk, 1987).

Needs to simplify and structure understanding may be heightened within societies during times of crisis, such as wars, economic recessions, and natural disasters. During these times, leaders use stereotypes of the enemy to reduce potential ambiguity, stifle dissent, and to provide a clear set of behavioral norms. Thus, dehumanizing stereotypes of Japanese, Koreans, and Vietnamese developed in the United States during prominent wars of the 20th century. Even outside of crisis, stereotypes are promoted by collectives to rationalize or justify existing economic or political conditions. Just as individuals justify the pain suffered by others by derogating them, collectives justify actions toward others groups of people that would otherwise be considered unfair or reprehensible through stereotypes. Demeaning stereotypes of African Americans and Native Americans can be attributed at least partially to the need within the White American community to justify the slavery and genocide that victimized those populations.

Stereotypes not only allow societies to justify collective actions, but also to justify collective inaction as well. Stereotypes serve the status quo. Advantaged groups who feel they are unjustly advantaged by a system that favorably allocates rewards to them may rationalize their advantaged state by blaming the failure of others on their inherent personality weaknesses (Pettigrew, 1979). If disenfranchised, downtrodden, and oppressed populations are viewed in terms of negative stereotypes, these beliefs may justify a collective lack of concern by those responsible for the oppression.

Esteem-Related Functions of Stereotypes

Whereas needs for understanding and simplifying the social environment seem more "coldly" functional, stereotypes also serve "hotter" ego-relevant functions at both the individual and the collective level. In order to function capably, people need to feel good about both themselves (Solomon, Greenberg, & Pyszczynski, 1991; Steele, 1988; Tesser, 1988) and the groups to which they belong (Cialdini et al., 1976; Crocker & Luhtanen, 1990; Greenberg et al., 1990; Turner, 1975). Thus, stereotyping and prejudice have traditionally been considered in terms of their relations with the need to maintain self-esteem or self-valuation.

At the individual level, it has been predicted that those who are chronically low in self-esteem would develop stronger stereotypes as a means of regaining positive regard (e.g., Ehrlich, 1973; Wills, 1981). Nevertheless, research support for this hypothesis is weak (Crocker & Schwartz, 1985), and the validity of the expected theoretical relationship has also been questioned (Abrams & Hogg, 1988; Crocker & Schwartz, 1985). After all, to the extent that derogating out-groups successfully enhances self-esteem, then the expected negative relationship between self-esteem and prejudice would be weakened.

On the other hand, there is evidence that temporary threats to self-esteem cause individuals to make more stereotypic and prejudicial responses (e.g., Brown, Collins, & Schmidt, 1988). These studies lead to the more specific hypothesis that stereotypes will develop more strongly when they satisfy basic motivations for self enhancement. Indeed, in a recent study, Ford (1992) found that subjects who were led to believe that they were a member of a social group that had some negative and some positive characteristics in comparison to a relevant out-group developed stronger stereotypes (as assessed through reaction-time measures) about the dimension upon which they compared favorably with the other group.

The relation between self-valuation and stereotyping cannot be understood from a purely individual perspective; it is necessary to consider group- or collective-level variables (Tajfel, 1981). Several different theoretical perspectives explicitly link self-valuation to stereotyping processes through the mediating link of collective-level variables. One theoretical model suggests that by derogating out-groups or favoring in-groups, one implicitly enhances the relative status of one's in-group, which in turn enhances one's view of oneself (Turner, 1975, 1987). Another model suggests that by derogating out-groups or favoring in-groups, the individual may implicitly uphold the standards of one's own culture, which is alleged to be a fundamental source of self-valuation (Solomon et al., 1991). Both perspectives are consistent with the more general notion that individuals' feelings about themselves are not independent of "group-esteem" (Hinkle, Taylor, & Fox-Cardamone, 1989) or "collective self-esteem" (Luhtanen & Crocker, 1992), or other collective-level values. Collective self-esteem is related to the shared aspects of group identity that group members use to enhance their self perceptions (e.g., "Black is Beautiful"), and appears to have an important effect on in-group bias (Crocker & Luhtanen, 1990).

Because a group's collective self-esteem would be expected to be closely related to its perceived status within a society, it might be expected that the tendency to develop and use stereotypes would be greater for groups with low social status—particularly minority groups. Indeed, there is research showing that, within a minimal group design, members of a minority group expressed greater in-group favoritism than did members of a majority group (Gerard & Hoyt, 1974). However, other work that examines more directly the role of status in intergroup perception indicates that greater prejudice is exhibited by groups of higher status (Sachdev & Bourhis, 1987, 1991). In retrospect, this finding represents an interesting parallel with work on individual self esteem, which has also demonstrated unexpected relationships in this regard.

Parallel to research on individual self-esteem, there is the suggestion that temporary threats to the collective esteem of a high status group might lead to increased incidence of prejudice. For instance, Hovland and Sears (1940; see also Hepworth & West, 1988) found that the rate of race-related lynchings in the American South appeared to be influenced by regional economic threat—which may operate as a temporary threat to the self-valuation of the people in that region. Other analyses also reveal that societal threat is positively related to both attitudes and behavior toward out-group members (Doty, Peterson, & Winter, 1991).

Finally, it is important to recognize that another means of obtaining positive self-regard is through acceptance by significant others. Thus, the need for social acceptance is another powerful motivation underlying both individual and collective behavior (Crowne & Marlowe, 1964; Hill, 1987). By developing and expressing consensual stereotypes of out-groups, individuals may be more readily accepted by other ingroup members. Indeed, "any individual who does *not* know the stereotypes of thought and feeling . . . may be said to be a stranger to [a] culture" (Hayakawa, 1950, p. 209). The expression of stereotypes within language "serves as a peculiarly potent symbol of the social solidarity of those who speak the language" (Sapir, 1933, p. 159). Furthermore, by acting towards out-group members in stereotypical ways, a person symbolically expresses his or her group identifications, and thus may be more likely to reap the rewards of social acceptance from his or her own group (cf. La Violette & Silvert, 1951; Turner, 1987).

CONCLUDING REMARKS

If you were to ask a biologist, "Where does life come from?" you might get one of two different answers. The biologist might tell you how organic life arose in the first place, emerging in the form of some string of nucleotides from a primordial soup. Or the biologist might give you a very different answer, describing how every generation of animal life is reproduced from that before it, through coupling of sperm and egg and recombination of DNA. Although these two answers are very different, they are entirely compatible, representing two complementary perspectives on organic life.

Similarly, the study of group stereotypes can be approached from two different, yet complementary perspectives. The individual approach to stereotyping emphasizes the "beginnings" of stereotypes, focusing on the individual cognitive-motivational processes that account for the fact that stereotypes have to begin somewhere (see Mackie, Hamilton, Susskind, & Rosselli, Chapter 2, this volume). Yet, once a stereotype has emerged within a culture, it takes on a life of its own and influences social behavior in ways beyond that of the actions of any individual. At this point, stereotypes depend not so much on direct perception (and misperception) of the social environment as on the existing manifestations of those stereotypes in the behavior and language of the society (Hartman & Husband, 1974). The collective approach to stereotyping has emphasized the "reproduction" of stereotypes, focusing on the means through which stereotypes are transmitted and maintained, and on the ways in which stereotypes serve culturally shared values.

Throughout the short history of the scientific study of stereotypes, the relative popularity of consensual and individual approaches has changed. This is evident both in the manner in which stereotypes are measured by researchers and in the questions researchers ask about stereotypes and their consequences. Before the cognitive revolution in social psychology, techniques such as those used by Katz and Braly (1933) were prevalent, assessing consensus in cultural beliefs about various ethnic groups (Brigham, 1971). Since then, stereotype measurement techniques have been decidedly individual, assessing the manner in which individual beliefs are cognitively represented (e.g., Devine & Baker, 1991; Dovidio et al., 1986; Ford & Stangor, 1992; Martin, 1987; McCauley & Stitt, 1978; Park & Judd, 1990).

In addition, just as the two perspectives on organic life suggest two rather different sets of questions to be answered, and at different levels, the individual and collective perspectives toward stereotypes also promote different types of inquiry. Because the collective approach attends to the specific *content* of stereotypic beliefs, researchers working within this approach have typically dealt directly with meaningful real-world categories. But this perspective has offered limited insight into the underlying, individual-level stereotyping processes through which stereotypes exert their effects. In contrast, the individualistic perspective on stereotype representation has focused directly on the *processes* of stereotype development and change, offering insights into these processes that could not have emerged in the absence of such a perspective. Of course, researchers working within this perspective have often relied on studies using artificial social groups (e.g., alien beings from other planets, or members of group "A") or real groups of limited social relevance ("Nobel Prize winners").

Complementary lines of inquiry are fine, but an integrated perspective may yield insights that are unlikely to emerge from any single line of inquiry. That the time is ripe for a synthesis is suggested by the recent interest in socially shared cognition (e.g., Levine, Resnick, & Higgins, 1993; Resnick, Levine, & Teasley, 1991; Wegner, 1987), and by concentrated attempts to locate individual cognitions about groups within a broader social context (Oakes, Haslam, & Turner, 1994; Turner, 1991). We do not suppose to identify the form that synthesis will or should take. However, one area of inquiry is suggested by the question of whether cultural consensus is an important part of a stereotype. Rather than debate this question as a matter of definition, it might be more fruitful to treat "consensualness" as an important variable. Some stereotypes are more consensually held than others. What consequences might this variable have on important stereotyping phenomena? This variable might have implications for the development and cognitive representation of stereotypes. Perhaps consensual stereotypes are more likely to be represented as abstractions and schemata, and less likely to be represented as prototypes and exemplars. Because of their relevance to needs for social acceptance, perhaps consensual stereotypes are associated more closely in memory with other socially relevant knowledge structures. Perhaps they are more closely tied to one's self-concept. Consensualness might also have implications for the accessibility of stereotypes, the strength of their effects on judgment, and the conditions under which they might exert those effects. Finally, consensualness of stereotypes may have important consequences for understanding change and revision of stereotypic beliefs. Consensual and nonconsensual stereotypes may be differentially vulnerable to the effects of different interventions.

Whether or not these sketchy speculations are accurate, they do highlight the value of considering multiple levels of inquiry into stereotypes and stereotyping processes. A complete understanding of organic life demands consideration of biological processes that operate at several different levels. A full understanding of stereotypes demands, at the very least, some simultaneous adoption of both individual and collective perspectives.

ACKNOWLEDGMENTS

Preparation of this chapter was partially supported by a Lilly Foundation teaching fellowship to Charles Stangor, and by a MONTS grant from the Montana Science and Technology Alliance to Mark Schaller. We thank Chris Crandall and Penny Oakes for their valuable comments on an earlier draft of this chapter.

NOTES

1. In this sense, the individual approach has implicitly assumed that there is at least a kernel of truth to most stereotypes, although that kernel may be subsequently exaggerated through information processing biases.

2. Prototypes may also be conceptualized as containing the average, most typical, or idealized value of group members (Italians are, on average, more romantic than other groups).

3. In fact, if stereotypes are purely the belief component of attitude, with no other social significance, the concept becomes redundant with that of belief (cf. Gardner, 1973).

REFERENCES

Abrams, D., & Hogg, M. A. (1988). Comments on the motivational status of self-esteem in social identity and intergroup discrimination. *European Journal of Social Psychology, 18,* 317–334.

Allport, F. H. (1924). *Social psychology.* New York: Houghton Mifflin.

Allport, G. W. (1954). *The nature of prejudice.* Reading, MA: Addison-Wesley.

Anglin, J. (1977). *Word, object, and conceptual development.* New York: Norton.

Asch, S. (1952). *Social psychology.* New York: Prentice-Hall.

Ashmore, R. D., & Del Boca, F. K. (1981). Conceptual approaches to stereotypes and stereotyping. In D. L. Hamilton (Ed.), *Cognitive processes in stereotyping and intergroup behavior* (pp. 1–35). Hillsdale, NJ: Erlbaum.

Barsalou, L. W. (1990). On the indistinguishability of exemplar memory and abstraction in category representation. In T. K. Srull & R. S. Wyer, Jr. (Eds.), *Advances in social cognition* (Vol. 3, pp. 61–88). Hillsdale, NJ: Erlbaum.

Bartlett, F. C. (1932). *Remembering.* Cambridge, UK: Cambridge University Press.

Bar-Tal, Y. (1989). Can leaders change followers' stereotypes? In D. Bar-Tal, C. F. Graumann, A. W. Kruglanski, & W. Stroebe (Eds.), *Stereotyping and prejudice: Changing conceptions* (pp. 225–242). New York: Springer-Verlag.

Bell, J. (1992). In search of a discourse on aging: The elderly on television. *Gerontologist, 32,* 305–311.

Belmore, S. M., & Hubbard, M. L. (1987). The role of advance expectancies in person memory. *Journal of Personality and Social Psychology, 53,* 61–70.

Bem, S. L. (1974). The measurement of psychological androgyny. *Journal of Consulting and Clinical Psychology, 42,* 155–162.

Bem, S. L. (1981). Gender schema theory: A cognitive account of sex typing. *Psychological Review, 88,* 354–364.

Bodenhausen, G. V. (1993). Emotions, arousal, and stereotypic judgments: A heuristic model of affect and stereotyping. In D. M. Mackie & D. L. Hamilton (Eds.), *Affect, cognition, and stereotyping: Interactive processes in group perception* (pp. 13–37). San Diego: Academic Press.

Bodenhausen, G. V., & Lichtenstein, M. (1987). Social stereotypes and information processing strategies: The impact of task complexity. *Journal of Personality and Social Psychology, 52,* 871–880.

Boster, J. S. (1991). The information economy model applied to biological similarity judgment. In L. B. Resnick, J. M. Levine, & S. D. Teasley (Eds.), *Perspectives on socially shared cognition* (pp. 203–225). Washington, DC: American Psychological Association.

Boster, J. S., & D'Andrade, R. G. (1989). Natural and human sources of cross-cultural agreement in ornithological classification. *American Anthropologist, 91,* 132–142.

Brewer, M. B. (1988). A dual process model of impression formation. In T. K. Srull & R. S. Wyer (Eds.), *Advances in social cognition* (Vol. 1, pp. 1–36). Hillsdale, NJ: Erlbaum.

Brigham, J. C. (1971). Ethnic stereotypes. *Psychological Bulletin, 76,* 15–33.

Brown, J. D., Collins, R. L., & Schmidt, G. W. (1988). Self-esteem and direct versus indirect forms of self-enhancement. *Journal of Personality and Social Psychology, 55,* 445–453.

Bruner, J. S. (1957). On perceptual readiness. *Psychological Review, 64,* 123–152.

Cialdini, R. B., Borden, R. J., Thorne, A., Walker, M. R., Freeman, S., & Sloane, L. R. (1976). Basking in reflected glory: Three (football) field studies. *Journal of Personality and Social Psychology, 34,* 406–415.

Clark, M. S., & Fiske, S. T. (1982). *Affect and cognition*. Hillsdale, NJ: Erlbaum.

Collins, A. M., & Loftus, E. F. (1975). A spreading-activation theory of semantic processing. *Psychological Review, 82,* 407–428.

Crandall, C. S., Thompson, E. A., Sakalli, N., & Schiffhauer, K. L. (1995). *Creating hostile environments: Name-calling and social norms*. Unpublished manuscript, University of Kansas at Lawrence.

Crocker, J., & Luhtanen, R. (1990). Collective self-esteem and ingroup bias. *Journal of Personality and Social Psychology, 58,* 60–67.

Crocker, J., & Major, B. (1989). Social stigma and self-esteem: The self-protective properties of stigma. *Psychological Review, 96,* 608–630.

Crocker, J., & Schwartz, I. (1985). Prejudice and intergroup favoritism in a minimal intergroup situation: Effects of self-esteem. *Personality and Social Psychology Bulletin, 11,* 379–386.

Crocker, J., Voelkl, K., Testa, M., & Major, B. (1991). Social stigma: The affective consequences of attributional ambiguity. *Journal of Personality and Social Psychology, 60,* 218–228.

Crowne, D. P., & Marlowe, D. (1964). *The approval motive*. New York: Wiley.

Devine, P. G., & Baker, S. M. (1991). Measurement of racial stereotype subtyping. *Personality and Social Psychology Bulletin, 17,* 44–50.

Diehl, M., & Jonas, K. (1991). Measures of national stereotypes as predictors of the latencies of inductive versus deductive stereotypic judgments. *European Journal of Social Psychology, 21,* 317–330.

Dixon, R. (1977). *Catching them young. I. Sex, race, and class in children's fiction*. London: Pluto Press.

Doty, R. M., Peterson, B. E., & Winter, D. G. (1991). Threat and authoritarianism in the United States, 1978–1987. *Journal of Personality and Social Psychology, 61,* 629–640.

Dovidio, J. F., Evans, N. E., & Tyler, R. B. (1986). Racial stereotypes: The contents of their cognitive representations. *Journal of Experimental Social Psychology, 22,* 22–37.

Duveen, G., & Lloyd, B. (1990). *Social representations and the development of knowledge*. Cambridge, UK: Cambridge University Press.

Eagly, A. H. (1987). *Sex differences in social behavior: A social-role interpretation*. Hillsdale, NJ: Erlbaum.

Eagly, A. H., & Chaiken, S. (1993). *The psychology of attitudes*. Fort Worth, TX: Harcourt Brace Jovanovich.

Eagly, A. H., Makhijani, M. G., & Klonsky, B. G. (1992). Gender and evaluation of leaders: A meta-analysis. *Psychological Bulletin, 111,* 3–22.

Ehrlich, H. J. (1973). *The social psychology of prejudice*. New York: Wiley.

Epstein, R., & Komorita, S. S. (1966). Prejudice among Negro children as related to parental ethnocentrism. *Journal of Personality and Social Psychology, 4,* 643–647.

Fagot, B. I., Leinbach, M. D., & O'Boyle, C. (1992). Gender labeling, gender stereotyping, and parenting behaviors. *Developmental Psychology, 28,* 225–230.

Farr, R. M., & Moscovici, S. (1984). *Social representations*. Cambridge, UK: Cambridge University Press.

Fazio, R. H. (1990). The MODE model as an integrative framework. *Advances in Experimental Social Psychology, 23,* 75–109.

Fishman, J. A. (1956). An examination of the process and function of social stereotyping. *Journal of Social Psychology, 43,* 27–64.

Fiske, S. T. (1982). Schema-triggered affect: Applications to social perception. In M. S. Clark & S. T. Fiske (Eds.), *Affect and cognition: The 17th Annual Carnegie Symposium on Cognition* (pp. 55–78). Hillsdale, NJ: Erlbaum.

Fiske, S. T., & Linville, P. W. (1980). What does the schema concept buy us? *Personality and Social Psychology Bulletin, 6,* 543–557.

Fiske, S. T., & Neuberg, S. L. (1990). A continuum of impression formation, from category-based to individuating processes: Influences of information and motivation on attention and interpretation. *Advances in Experimental Social Psychology, 23,* 1–74.

Fiske, S. T., & Pavelchak, M. A. (1986). Category-based versus piecemeal-based affective responses: Developments in schema-triggered affect. In R. M. Sorrentino & E. T. Higgins (Eds.), *Handbook of motivation and cognition: Foundations of social behavior* (Vol. 1, pp. 167–203). New York: Guilford Press.

Fiske, S. T., & Taylor, S. E. (1991). *Social cognition* (2nd ed.). New York: McGraw-Hill.

Ford, T. E. (1992). *The effect of motivation and attribute diagnosticity on stereotype formation*. Unpublished doctoral dissertation, University of Maryland at College Park.

Ford, T. E., & Stangor, C. (1992). The role of diagnosticity in stereotype formation: Perceiving group means and variances. *Journal of Personality and Social Psychology, 63,* 356–367.

Fyock, J., & Stangor, C. (1994). The role of memory biases in stereotype maintenance. *British Journal of Social Psychology, 33,* 331–344.

Gardner, R. C. (1973). Ethnic stereotypes: The traditional approach, a new look. *Canadian Psychologist, 14,* 133–148.

Gardner, R. C., Kirby, D. M., & Findlay, J. C. (1973). Ethnic stereotypes: The significance of consensus. *Canadian Journal of Behavioral Science, 5,* 4–12.

Gardner, R. C., Kirby, D. M., Gorospe, F. H., & Villamin, A. C. (1972). Ethnic stereotypes: An alternative assessment technique, the stereotype differential. *Journal of Social Psychology, 87,* 259–267.

Gerard, H. B., & Hoyt, M. F. (1974). Distinctiveness of social categorization and attitude toward ingroup members. *Journal of Personality and Social Psychology, 29,* 836–842.

Gilbert, D. T., & Hixon, J. G. (1991). The trouble of thinking: Activation and application of stereotypic beliefs. *Journal of Personality and Social Psychology, 60,* 509–517.

Giles, H. (1977). *Language, ethnicity, and intergroup relations*. New York: Academic Press.

Giles, H., & Saint-Jacques, B. (1979). *Language and ethnic relations*. Oxford: Pergamon Press.

Graumann, C. F., & Wintermantel, M. (1989). Discriminatory speech acts: A functional approach. In D. Bar-Tal, C. F. Graumann, A. W. Kruglanski, & W. Stroebe (Eds.), *Stereotyping and prejudice: Changing conceptions* (pp. 183–204). New York: Springer-Verlag.

Greenberg, J., & Pyszczynski, T. (1985). The effects of an overheard ethnic slur on evaluations of the target: How to spread a social disease. *Journal of Experimental Social Psychology, 21*, 61–72.

Greenberg, J., Pyszczynski, T., Solomon, S., Rosenblatt, A., Veeder, M., Kirkland, S., & Lyon, D. (1990). Evidence for terror management theory II: The effects of mortality salience on reactions to those who threaten or bolster the cultural worldview. *Journal of Personality and Social Psychology, 58*, 308–318.

Hamilton, D. L., & Gifford, R. K. (1976). Illusory correlation in interpersonal perception: A cognitive basis of stereotypic judgments. *Journal of Experimental Social Psychology, 12*, 392–407.

Hamilton, D. L., & Rose, T. L. (1980). Illusory correlation and the maintenance of stereotypic beliefs. *Journal of Personality and Social Psychology, 39*, 832–845.

Hamilton, D. L., & Sherman, J. W. (1994). Stereotypes. In R. S. Wyer, Jr., & T. K. Srull (Eds.), *Handbook of social cognition* (2nd ed., Vol. 2, pp. 1–68). Hillsdale, NJ: Erlbaum.

Hamilton, D. L., Stroessner, S. J., & Driscoll, D. M. (1994). Social cognition and the study of stereotyping. In P. G. Devine, D. L. Hamilton, & T. M. Ostrom (Eds.), *Social cognition: Contributions to classic issues in social psychology* (pp. 291–321). New York: Springer-Verlag.

Harding, J., Proshansky, H., Kutner, B., & Chein, I. (1969). Prejudice and ethnic relations. In G. Lindzey & E. Aronson (Eds.), *Handbook of social psychology* (2nd ed., Vol. 5, pp. 1–76). Reading, MA: Addison-Wesley.

Hartley, E. L. (1946). *Problems in prejudice*. New York: King's Crown Press.

Hartmann, P., & Husband, C. (1974). *Racism and the mass media*. London: Davis- Poynter.

Hayakawa, S. I. (1950). Recognizing stereotypes as substitutes for thought. *Etc.: Review of General Semantics, 7*, 208–210.

Heider, F. (1958). *The psychology of interpersonal relations*. Hillsdale, NJ: Erlbaum.

Hepworth, J. T., & West, S. G. (1988). Lynchings and the economy: A time-series reanalysis of Hovland and Sears (1940). *Journal of Personality and Social Psychology, 55*, 239–247.

Hewstone, M. (1989). *Causal attribution: From cognitive processes to cognitive beliefs*. Oxford: Blackwell.

Hewstone, M., & Brown, R. (1986). Contact is not enough: An intergroup perspective on the 'Contact Hypothesis'. In M. Hewstone & R. J. Brown (Eds.), *Contact and conflict in intergroup encounters* (pp. 1–44). London: Blackwell.

Higgins, E. T., & King, G. (1981). Accessibility of social constructs: Information-processing consequences of individual and contextual variability. In N. Cantor & J. F. Kihlstrom (Eds.), *Personality, cognition and social interaction* (pp. 69–121). Hillsdale, NJ: Erlbaum.

Hill, C. A. (1987). Affiliation motivation: People who need people . . . but in different ways. *Journal of Personality and Social Psychology, 52,* 1008–1018.

Hinkle, S., Taylor, L. A., & Fox-Cardamone, D. L. (1989). Intragroup identification and intergroup differentiation: A multicomponent approach. *British Journal of Social Psychology, 28,* 305–317.

Hoffman, C., & Hurst, N. (1990). Gender stereotypes: Perception or rationalization. *Journal of Personality and Social Psychology, 58,* 197–208.

Hovland, C. I., & Sears, R. (1940). Minor studies of aggression: Correlation of lynching with economic indices. *Journal of Psychology, 9,* 301–310.

Jacobs, J., & Eccles, J. S. (1985). Gender differences in math ability: The impact of media reports on parents. *Educational Researcher, 14,* 20–25.

Johnston, L., & Macrae, C. N. (1994). Changing social stereotypes: The case of the information seeker. *European Journal of Social Psychology, 24,* 237–266.

Jost, J. T., & Banaji, M. R. (1994). The role of stereotyping in system-justification and the production of false consciousness. *British Journal of Social Psychology, 33,* 1–27.

Jussim, L. (1991). Social perception and social reality: A reflection-construction model. *Psychological Review, 98,* 54–73.

Katz, D., & Braly, K. (1933). Racial stereotypes in one hundred college students. *Journal of Abnormal and Social Psychology, 28,* 280–290.

Katz, P. A., & Zalk, S. R. (1978). Modification of children's racial attitudes. *Developmental Psychology, 14,* 447–461.

Kelley, H. H. (1967). Attribution theory in social psychology. In D. Levine (Ed.), *Nebraska Symposium on Motivation* (Vol. 15, pp. 192–238). Lincoln: University of Nebraska Press.

Kruglanski, A. W. (1989). *Lay epistemics and human knowledge.* New York: Plenum.

Kruglanski, A. W., & Freund, T. (1983). The freezing and unfreezing of lay inferences: Effects on impressional primacy, ethnic stereotyping, and numerical anchoring. *Journal of Experimental Social Psychology, 19,* 448–468.

La Violette, F., & Silvert, K. H. (1951). A theory of stereotypes. *Social Forces, 29,* 237–257.

Langer, E. J., & Imber, L. (1980). Role of mindlessness in the perception of deviance. *Journal of Personality and Social Psychology, 39,* 360–367.

Lerner, M. J., & Miller, D. T. (1978). Just world research and the attribution process: Looking back and ahead. *Psychological Bulletin, 85,* 1030–1051.

Levine, J. M., Resnick, L. B., & Higgins, E. T. (1993). Social foundations of cognition. *Annual Review of Psychology, 44,* 585–612.

Lewicki, P. (1985). Nonconscious biasing effects of single instances on subsequent judgments. *Journal of Personality and Social Psychology, 48,* 563–574.

Linville, P. W., Salovey, P., & Fischer, G. W. (1986). Stereotyping and perceived distributions of social characteristics: An application to ingroup–out-group perception. In J. F. Dovidio & S. L. Gaertner (Eds.), *Prejudice, discrimination, and racism* (pp. 165–208). Orlando, FL: Academic Press.

Lippman, W. (1922). *Public opinion.* New York: Harcourt Brace.

Locksley, A., Stangor, C., Hepburn, C., Grosovsky, E., & Hochstrasser, M. (1984). The ambiguity of recognition memory tests of schema theories. *Cognitive Psychology, 16,* 421–448.

Lord, C. G., Lepper, M. R., & Mackie, D. (1984). Attitude prototypes as determinants of attitude–behavior consistency. *Journal of Personality and Social Psychology, 46,* 1254–1266.

Luhtanen, R., & Crocker, J. (1992). A collective self-esteem scale: Self-evaluation of one's social identity. *Personality and Social Psychology Bulletin, 18,* 302–318.

Markus, H., Crane, M., Bernstein, S., & Sidali, M. (1982). Self-schemas and gender. *Journal of Personality and Social Psychology, 42,* 38–50.

Markus, H., & Zajonc, R. B. (1985). The cognitive perspective in social psychology. In G. Lindzey & E. Aronson (Eds.), *The handbook of social psychology* (3rd ed., Vol. 1, pp. 137–230). New York: Random House.

Martin, C. L. (1987). A ratio measure of sex stereotyping. *Journal of Personality and Social Psychology, 52,* 489–499.

Mazelan, P. M. (1980). Stereotypes and perceptions of the victims of rape. *Victimology, 5,* 121–132.

McArthur, L. Z., & Post, D. L. (1977). Figural emphasis and person perception. *Journal of Experimental Social Psychology, 13,* 520–535.

McCauley, C., & Tyrrell, D. J. (1983). An individual and quantitative measure of stereotypes. *Journal of Personality and Social Psychology, 36,* 929–940.

McCauley, C., Stitt, C. L., & Segal, M. (1980). Stereotyping: From prejudice to prediction. *Psychological Bulletin, 87,* 195–208.

McDougall, W. (1920). *The group mind.* Cambridge, UK: Cambridge University Press.

Milgram, S. (1974). *Obedience to authority.* New York: Harper & Row.

Mills, C. J., & Tyrrell, D. J. (1983). Sex-stereotypic encoding and release from proactive interference. *Journal of Personality and Social Psychology, 45,* 772–781.

Moscovici, S. (1981). On social representations. In J. Forgas (Ed.), *Social cognition* (pp. 181–209). London: Academic Press.

Mullen, B., & Johnson, C. (1993). Cognitive representation in ethnophaulisms as a function of group size: The phenomenology of being in a group. *Personality and Social Psychology Bulletin, 19,* 296–304.

Myrdal, G. (1944). *An American dilemma: The Negro problem and modern democracy.* New York: Harper.

Neuberg, S. L., & Newsom, J. T. (1993). Personal need for structure: Individual differences in chronic motivation to simplify. *Journal of Personality and Social Psychology, 65,* 113–131.

Noseworthy, C. M., & Lott, A. J. (1984). The cognitive organization of gender-stereotypic categories. *Personality and Social Psychology Bulletin, 10,* 474–481.

Oakes, P. J., Haslam, S. A., & Turner, J. C. (1994). *Stereotyping and social reality.* Oxford: Blackwell

Oakes, P. J., & Turner, J. C. (1990). Is limited information processing capacity the cause of social stereotyping? In W. Stroebe & M. Hewstone (Eds.), *European review of social psychology* (Vol. 1, pp. 111–135). Chichester, UK: Wiley.

Palmore, E. B. (1962). Ethnophaulisms and ethnocentrism. *American Journal of Sociology, 67,* 442–445.

Park, B., & Hastie, R. (1987). Perception of variability in category development: Instance- versus abstraction-based stereotypes. *Journal of Personality and Social Psychology, 53,* 621–635.

Park, B., & Judd, C. M. (1990). Measures and models of perceived group variability. *Journal of Personality and Social Psychology, 59,* 173–191.

Pasadeos, Y. (1987). Changes in television newscast advertising, 1974–1985. *Communication Research Reports, 4,* 43–46.

Pettigrew, T. F. (1958). Personality and sociocultural factors in intergroup attitudes: A cross-national comparison. *Journal of Conflict Resolution, 2,* 29–42.

Pettigrew, T. F. (1959). Regional differences in anti-Negro prejudice. *Journal of Abnormal and Social Psychology, 59,* 28–36.

Pettigrew, T. F. (1979). The ultimate attribution error: Extending Allport's cognitive analysis of prejudice. *Personality and Social Psychology Bulletin, 5,* 461–476.

Reicher, S. (1986). Contact, action and racialization: Some British evidence. In M. Hewstone & R. Brown (Eds.), *Contact and conflict in intergroup encounters* (pp. 152–168). London: Blackwell.

Resnick, L. B., Levine, J. M., & Teasley, S. D. (1991). *Perspectives on socially shared cognition.* Washington, DC: American Psychological Association.

Rothbart, M. (1981). Memory processes and social beliefs. In D. L. Hamilton (Ed.), *Cognitive processes in stereotyping and intergroup behavior* (pp. 145–181). Hillsdale, NJ: Erlbaum.

Rothbart, M., & John, O. (1992). Intergroup relations and stereotype change: A social-cognitive analysis and some longitudinal findings. In P. M. Sniderman & P. E. Tetlock (Eds.), *Prejudice, politics and race in America.* Stanford CA: Stanford University Press.

Rothbart, M., & Lewis, S. (1988). Inferring category attributes from exemplar attributes: Geometric shapes and social categories. *Journal of Personality and Social Psychology, 55,* 861–872.

Ryan, W. (1971). *Blaming the victim.* New York: Random House.

Sachdev, I., & Bourhis, R. Y. (1987). Status differentials and intergroup behavior. *European Journal of Social Psychology, 17,* 277–293.

Sachdev, I., & Bourhis, R. Y. (1991). Power and status differentials in minority and majority group relations. *European Journal of Social Psychology, 21,* 1–24.

Saenger, G., & Flowerman, S. (1954). Stereotypes and prejudicial attitudes. *Human Relations, 7,* 217–238.

Sapir, E. (1933). Language. *Encyclopedia of the Social Sciences, 9,* 55–169.

Schaller, M., & O'Brien, M. (1992). "Intuitive analysis of covariance" and group stereotype formation. *Personality and Social Psychology Bulletin, 18,* 776–785.

Schank, R. C., & Abelson, R. P. (1977). *Scripts, plans, goals, and understanding: An inquiry into human knowledge structures.* Hillsdale, NJ: Erlbaum.

Sherif, M. (1936). *The psychology of social norms.* New York: Harper & Row.

Smith, E. R., & Zárate, M. A. (1992). Exemplar-based model of social judgment. *Psychological Review, 99,* 3–21.

Snyder, M. (1981). On the self-perpetuating nature of social stereotypes. In D. L. Hamilton (Ed.), *Cognitive processes in stereotyping and intergroup behavior* (pp. 183–212). Hillsdale, NJ: Erlbaum.

Snyder, M., & Miene, P. (1994). On the function of stereotypes and prejudice. In M. Zanna & J. M. Olson (Eds.), *The psychology of prejudice: The Ontario Symposium* (Vol. 7, pp. 33–54). Hillsdale, NJ: Erlbaum.

Solomon, S., Greenberg, J., & Pyszczynski, T. (1991). A terror management theory of social behavior: The psychological consequences of self-esteem and cultural worldviews. *Advances in Experimental Social Psychology, 24,* 93–159.

Spence, J. T., Helmreich, R. L., & Stapp, J. (1975). Ratings of self and peers on sex-role attributes and their relations to self-esteem and conceptions of masculinity and femininity. *Journal of Personality and Social Psychology, 32,* 29–39.

Spencer, S. J., & Steele, C. M. (1992, August). *The effect of stereotype vulnerability on women's math performance.* Paper presented at the 100th Annual Convention of the American Psychological Association, Washington, DC.

Srull, T. K., & Wyer, R. S. (1989). Person memory and judgment. *Psychological Review, 96,* 58–83.

Stangor, C. (1988). Stereotype accessibility and information processing. *Personality and Social Psychology Bulletin, 14,* 694–708.

Stangor, C., & Duan, C. (1991). Effects of multiple task demands upon memory for information about social groups. *Journal of Experimental Social Psychology, 27,* 357–378.

Stangor, C., & Ford, T. E. (1992). Accuracy and expectancy-confirming processing orientations and the development of stereotypes and prejudice. *European Review of Social Psychology, 3,* 57–89.

Stangor, C., & Lange, J. (1993). Cognitive representations of social groups: Advances in conceptualizing stereotypes and stereotyping. *Advances in Experimental Social Psychology, 26,* 357–416.

Stangor, C., Lynch, L., Duan, C., & Glass, B. (1992). Categorization of individuals on the basis of multiple social features. *Journal of Personality and Social Psychology, 62,* 207–281.

Stangor, C., & McMillan, D. (1992). Memory for expectancy-congruent and expectancy-incongruent information: A review of the social and social developmental literatures. *Psychological Bulletin, 111*, 42–61.

Steele, C. M. (1988). The psychology of self-affirmation: Sustaining the integrity of the self. *Advances in Experimental Social Psychology, 21*, 261–302.

Steele, C. M. (1992). Race and the schooling of black Americans. *Atlantic Monthly, 269*(4), 68–78.

Steele, C. M., & Aronson, J. (1995). Stereotype threat and the intellectual test performance of African Americans. *Journal of Personality and Social Psychology, 69*, 797–811.

Stephan, W. G., & Stephan, C. W. (1984). The role of ignorance in intergroup relations. In N. Miller & M. B. Brewer (Eds.), *Groups in contact: The psychology of desegregation* (pp. 229–257). Orlando, FL: Academic Press.

Stinton, J. (1980). *Racism and sexism in children's books*. London: Writers & Readers.

Stouffer, S. A., Suchman, E. A., DeVinney, L. C., Star, S. A., & Williams, R. M., Jr. (1949). *The American soldier: Vol. 1. Adjustment during army life*. Princeton, NJ: Princeton University Press.

Tajfel, H. (1981). Social stereotypes and social groups. In J. C. Turner & H. Giles (Eds.), *Intergroup behavior* (pp. 144–167). Chicago: University of Chicago Press.

Tajfel, H., & Forgas, J. P. (1981). Social categorization: Cognitions, values, and groups. In J. P. Forgas (Ed.), *Social cognition: Perspectives on everyday understanding* (pp. 113–140). London & New York: Academic Press.

Taylor, S. E., & Crocker, J. (1981). Schematic bases of social information processing. In E. T. Higgins, C. P. Herman, & M. P. Zanna (Eds.), *Social cognition: The Ontario symposium* (Vol. 1, pp. 89–134). Hillsdale, NJ: Erlbaum.

Tesser, A., (1988). Toward a self-evaluation maintenance model of social behavior. *Advances in Experimental Social Psychology, 21*, 181–227.

Thomas, K. (1971). *Religion and the decline of magic*. London: Weidenfeld & Nicholson.

Turner, J. C. (1975). Social comparison and social identity; Some prospects for intergroup behavior. *European Journal of Social Psychology, 5*, 5–34.

Turner, J. C. (1987). *Rediscovering the social group: A self-categorization theory*. Oxford: Blackwell.

Turner, J. C. (1991). *Social influence*. Milton Keynes, UK: Open University Press.

van Dijk, T. A. (1987). *Communicating racism*. Newbury Park, CA: Sage.

Weber, R., & Crocker, J. (1983). Cognitive processes in the revision of stereotypic beliefs. *Journal of Personality and Social Psychology, 45*, 961–977.

Wegner, D. M. (1987). Transactive memory: A contemporary analysis of the group mind. In B. Mullen & G. R. Goethals (Eds.), *Theories of group behavior* (pp. 185–208). New York: Springer-Verlag.

Weigel, R., Loomis, J., & Soja, M. (1980). Race relations on prime time television. *Journal of Personality and Social Psychology, 39*, 884–893.

Wills, T. A. (1981). Downward social comparison principles in social psychology. *Psychological Bulletin, 90,* 245–271.

Wilson, C. C., & Gutierrez, F. (1985). *Minorities and the media.* Beverly Hills, CA, & London: Sage.

Zimet, S. (1976). *Print and prejudice.* London: Hodder & Stoughton.

II

STEREOTYPE FORMATION
AND DEVELOPMENT

2

Social Psychological Foundations of Stereotype Formation

DIANE M. MACKIE
DAVID L. HAMILTON
JOSHUA SUSSKIND
FRANCINE ROSSELLI

According to professional basketball player Doc Rivers, stereotypes are alive and well in the National Basketball Association. As described in team scouting reports, Black athletes are "athletically gifted," "explosive," and "have great instincts." White athletes, on the other hand, are "determined," "take-charge guys," "floor generals" with a "work ethic" and a "thorough understanding of their games" (Rivers & Brooks, 1993). According to other observers, similar stereotypes were routinely expressed in basketball commentary at the college and professional level in the late 1980s (Jackson, 1993).

Stereotypes are not commonplace in professional sports alone, of course. On the contrary, views about characteristic qualities of ethnic, religious, gender, sexual orientation, age, political, interest, activity, and occupational groups seem to exist in our own culture and many others. This chapter is concerned with the social psychological processes underlying the formation of such social stereotypes. How do stereotypes form, and what mechanisms contribute to their development? How do such views about the nature of groups and their members come to be part of an individual's or a society's everyday beliefs? Our goal in this chapter, then, is to understand the social psychological nature of stereotype formation.

Like most social psychological phenomena, stereotypes are overdetermined. Their content and organization are influenced by the separate and combined influences of cognitive, affective, sociomotivational, and cultural factors operating in social settings. They arise from and are maintained by the way we think and the way we feel, as well as by the ways we interact and relate. A thorough analysis of the formation of stereotypes thus demands that we consider a variety of mechanisms that can instigate or contribute to their development.

We begin our treatment by defining what we mean by the term stereotype, and we briefly discuss several implications of this definition. We then turn to the question of how stereotypes, as mental representations or structures, develop. How does information about or experience with a group or its members become part of a stereotype? We adopt two approaches to answering this question. First, we discuss the social psychological literature relevant to each of several mechanisms by which stereotypes might develop. Second, we examine the results of developmental research regarding when and how the processes we discuss become operational. Finally, in a concluding section, we discuss some of the implications of what we know about how stereotypes develop and some of the problems raised by what we still do not know.

WHAT ARE SOCIAL STEREOTYPES?

We define a stereotype as a cognitive structure containing the perceiver's knowledge, beliefs, and expectancies about some human social group (Hamilton & Trolier, 1986). Our definition of a stereotype, in keeping with those used throughout this volume, is a broad one. A number of its features, however, are worth noting.

First, it defines a stereotype as a cognitive structure, meaning that it resides in the head of the individual perceiver. In contrast to other definitions that emphasize the shared nature of stereotypic belief systems, in our view the degree of consensus of any given belief is an empirical issue, rather than a definitional property. Because each individual's experience and interpretation of experience are unique, each individual's social stereotypes might also be different. At the same time, because so many of the influences on stereotype formation derive from a common social context, the content of many social stereotypes become widely shared among members of various groups, and even within society as a whole.

Second, we intend the "knowledge, beliefs, and expectancies" that comprise the content of the stereotype to be inclusive terms. In contrast to earlier conceptions that confined the content of stereotypes to traits and other abstract attributes, our definition includes not only beliefs about general properties but also knowledge of physical features, attitudes, behaviors, roles, or preferences thought to be typical of the group; specific exemplar-based knowledge gained from personal experiences and interactions; knowledge and beliefs acquired secondhand from others or from media presentations; and expectancies about likely future behaviors, outcomes, and so forth.

Third, we define the phrase "some human social group" to mean two or more people who are perceived as sharing some common characteristic that is socially meaningful to themselves or others (Smith & Mackie, 1995). Stereotypes therefore are not limited to perceptions of racial, national, and gender categories but rather apply to whatever social groupings are salient to the observer, as well as to subgroups within those broader categories. Thus, possible social groups, and hence possible stereotypes, are limited only by the number of attributes human observers may see as socially meaningful.

Finally, although our definition reflects an emphasis on the cognitive nature of stereotypes as mental representations, it is clear that in many cases affect becomes closely linked to these cognitive properties and is of central importance in understanding the formation and functioning of stereotypes.

MECHANISMS OF STEREOTYPE FORMATION

Earlier, we pointed out that stereotypes are overdetermined. Because they develop as the result of the confluence of a number of different mechanisms, they can reflect the combined effect of multiple processes. To investigate the nature of these individual mechanisms and how they function, research has typically focused on one or another process in isolation (although some work has focused specifically on the interface between different systems; see, e.g., Mackie & Hamilton, 1993). In this section, we review the theoretical frameworks and empirical evidence relevant to the role of cognitive, affective, sociomotivational, and cultural processes in stereotype formation.

Cognitive Mechanisms in Stereotype Formation

Categorization

Stereotype formation begins when an aggregate of persons is perceived as comprising a group, an entity. When a set of persons is perceived to be a group, it is likely that the group is also distinguished from other groups. Thus, individuals are categorized into different groups that are somehow perceived in relation to each other (women vs. men; Democrats vs. Republicans; Poles vs. Italians vs. Germans). The importance of this process of categorization for intergroup perceptions was emphasized by Allport (1954) in his seminal analysis of the nature of intergroup prejudice. However, there was relatively little research on this topic until Tajfel's (1969, 1970) work launched an empirical voyage that has continued to explore new domains for over 20 years. This effort has generated entire literatures on such topics as in-group bias (for a review, see Brewer, 1979), in-group/out-group differentiation (reviewed by Diehl, 1990; Messick & Mackie, 1989; Miller & Brewer, 1986), the out-group homogeneity effect (for a review, see Linville, Fischer, & Salovey, 1989; Messick & Mackie, 1989; Ostrom & Sedikides, 1992; Park, Ryan, & Judd, 1992), and cross-categorization (reviewed by Vanbeselaere, 1991). Here, we briefly discuss two important questions germane to the present chapter: Why do people categorize others into groups, and what consequences follow from this process?

Two lines of reasoning have been offered for why perceivers so readily categorize others into groups, rather than cognitively maintaining their individuality. One argument focuses on the cognitive underpinnings of categorization; the other highlights the role of self-beneficial motives for categorization.

The cognitive interpretation emphasizes the adaptive value of cognitive efficiency. People are continuously engaged in a complex, social stimulus world that can make more demands on information processing than the system can handle; we are often confronted with stimulus overload. Consequently, it is efficient to identify the similarities and differences among various stimulus events and to group those stimuli into categories on that basis. For many purposes, members of the same class can be treated as functionally equivalent, and different from stimuli in other categories. Doing so eases the need to cognitively maintain the individuality of each stimulus event. When these stimuli are people, this process leads us to group people into social categories.

Although categorization involves "information loss" through the failure to recognize the individuality of each category member, categorization also provides "information gain" through ascribing group characteristics to individual members. That is, once an individual is categorized as a group member, the observer can assume that that person possesses many features characteristic of group members, even in the absence of empirical evidence about that individual.

In this view, categorization is a cognitive mechanism that is a natural consequence of the perceiver's simultaneous need to both reduce and elaborate available information. It is a strategy that, although sometimes nonoptimal, is highly effective in many contexts in reducing the information processing load while allowing suitable adaptation to one's life tasks without serious errors of judgment, decision, comprehension, and the like. (Cognitive strategies that, although efficient, had proven maladaptive in these regards presumably would have been dropped from one's cognitive repertoire.) Grouping people into social categories, and thereby overlooking their individualities, is viewed as an extension of this more fundamental mechanism.

A second perspective on why people categorize others into groups emphasizes the self-evaluative benefits of differentiating one's own group from other groups. Such in-group/out-group categorization seems inherent in many intergroup situations. According to social identity theory (Tajfel & Turner, 1979), these differentiations are driven by the perceiver's desire for positive self-evaluation. Part of one's self-evaluation derives from one's membership in social groups. To the extent that we have favorable evaluations of our own groups, or can at least derogate other groups, there will be some beneficial consequence for one's own self-regard. In this view, then, intergroup (and particularly in-group/out-group) categorization rests in part on this motive for self-enhancement.

These (and perhaps other) factors account for the fact that perceivers categorize similar entities into groups. Once those cognitive groupings are established, there are a number of consequences that follow from this act of categorization. These outcomes are discussed at length elsewhere (Diehl, 1990; Hamilton & Trolier, 1986; Messick & Mackie, 1989) and can be summarized briefly here.

- Once categorized as a group, individual members are perceived as being more similar to each other than when they simply are seen as an aggregate of individuals, whereas members of different groups are perceived as being more different from each other than when they simply are seen as an aggregate of individuals (Wilder, 1978a, 1978b).
- These effects—within-group assimilation, between-group contrast—also occur when the distinction is between an in-group and an out-group (Allen & Wilder, 1979).

- With in-group/out-group differentiation, the tendency for within-group assimilation is often particularly strong in perceptions of the out-group, producing the out-group homogeneity effect (Ostrom & Sedikides, 1992; Park & Rothbart, 1982; Quattrone & Jones, 1980), although under specific conditions the reverse outcome can also occur (Brewer, 1993; Simon & Hamilton, 1994).

- With in-group/out-group differentiation, the between-group contrast has a strong evaluative tone, producing in-group bias (Brewer, 1979; Tajfel, Billig, Bundy, & Flament, 1971).

- These effects, which derive largely from the mere act of categorizing others into groups, can then have effects on how subsequently acquired information about group members is processed. Such categorization has been shown to influence automatic evaluative reactions (Dovidio & Gaertner, 1993), extremity of perceptions of trait attributes (Linville, 1982; Linville & Jones, 1980), causal attributions (Hewstone, 1990; Pettigrew, 1979), memory for information describing group members (Howard & Rothbart, 1980), the likelihood that a new individual will be perceived as a group member (Park & Hastie, 1987), and behavioral discrimination (Diehl, 1990; Tajfel et al., 1971). Thus, categorizing others into social groups can have a number of important consequences that lay the foundation upon which stereotypes may then be built.

When do children begin to manifest signs that they have categorized others into groups? The answer depends, of course, on the particular social categories, but evidence indicates that children begin categorizing others quite early. This is particularly true for gender categories. Children as young as 7 months old can differentiate between male and female voices (Miller, 1983). By 9 months, children are capable of responding to male and female faces categorically (Leinbach & Fagot, 1991). By the end of the first year, infants are able to integrate these modes and attend more to female faces when listening to female voices (Poulin-Dubois, Serbin, Kenyon, & Derbyshire, 1994). This intermodal knowledge of gender demonstrates that these infants have begun to form clear gender categories. Gender categorization remains salient during the preschool years. Toddlers are capable of labeling others by gender (Fagot & Leinbach, 1993), and even overgeneralize the labels "mommy" and "daddy" to refer to women and men in general (Brooks-Gunn & Lewis, 1979).

For young children, gender seems to be the most salient category for parsing the social environment, for a number of reasons. First, information about gender is constantly provided to the child. Second, in contrast to some other categories (e.g., ethnicity and occupation), gender has only two conditions, male and female. It is probably easier to classify information into dichotomous categories than to make differentiations among several categories. Third, in the case of gender, children have frequent first-hand experience with both in-group and out-group members, whereas such encounters with out-group members are less likely for many other social categories (e.g., ethnic groups).

In fact, research evidence supports the premise that young children classify by gender to a greater extent than by ethnicity. Gender has a greater impact than ethnicity on preschool children's classifications of others (Doke & Risley, 1972), on their doll preference (Katz & Zalk, 1974), and on their memory for stories (Hirschfeld, 1995). One implication of this early use of gender categories is that children may begin to form stereotypic beliefs about gender prior to their forming stereotypes about other social categories.

This is not to say that young children construe the world only in terms of male and female categories. Preschoolers are also capable of classifying by ethnicity (Aboud, 1988), occupation (Blaske, 1984), body type (Lerner, 1973) and age (Edwards, 1984). They base these categorizations on easily identifiable cues, such as hairstyle, skin color, clothing, and language (Aboud, 1988; Katz, 1983). Nevertheless, during the early years, distinctions based on gender seem to predominate.

The saliency of gender categories decreases during middle childhood, when ethnicity is used as a basis for categorizing others to a greater extent than is gender (Davey & Norburn, 1980; Doke & Risley, 1972), at least in the populations studied. Another change that occurs in middle childhood is that children become capable of forming more abstract classifications, such as those based on nationality or religion. Thus, although the tendency to categorize others into social groupings develops quite early in children, the nature of the predominant categories appears to change somewhat in the course of development.

It is important to recognize that categorization does not always eventuate in the formation of a full-blown stereotype. The stereotype itself evolves only when the perceiver acquires knowledge and develops a set of beliefs about that group, beliefs that are held to characterize the group in general terms. An interesting question—and one we know little about—concerns the conditions under which this transition is and is not likely to occur. Of course, the answer to this question may differ according to the perceiver's developmental stage as well as the social group in question.

Correspondence Bias in Forming Group Representations

Perhaps one of the most well documented biases in social perception is the tendency to see behavior as reflecting an actor's inner dispositions, even if the constraints of social roles or situational contingencies are readily apparent. Originally proposed as a bias in the process of making causal attributions (Jones, 1979; Ross, 1977), more recent evidence suggests that perceivers routinely make dispositional inferences from behavioral acts (Bassili, 1989; Gilbert, 1989; Hamilton, 1988; Newman & Uleman, 1989). Although members of independent, individually oriented cultures seem more prone to the bias than members of more interdependent, collectively oriented societies, the matter appears to be more one of degree than qualitative differences, at least in the populations studied (Miller, 1984). Because the correspondence bias involves the spontaneous process of inferring dispositional characteristics, and because stereotyping involves the perception of groups in terms of such attributes, the correspondence bias seems likely to be a particularly powerful mechanism in stereotype acquisition.

Most of the research on correspondence bias and spontaneous trait inferences has focused on perceivers assuming dispositional properties of individual actors. Some studies, however, have extended this line of research to the case in which the actor's behavior is constrained by social roles, yet the inference is made about dispositions of the actor, with consequences for group perceptions (Eagly & Steffen, 1984; Hoffman & Hurst, 1990). For example, women are more likely to be seen in roles calling for nurturing and supportive behaviors, whereas men are more likely to be seen in roles that call for independent and managerial action. Perceptions of men and women in those roles do not, however, recognize the impact and constraining influence of those roles. Instead, perceivers infer that the persons enacting those roles have dispositional characteristics corresponding to the behaviors required for role fulfillment.

This research on the effect of social roles on the nature of perceivers' inferences about others is discussed in more detail in a later section on social factors that contribute to stereotype development. These issues do, however, raise an interesting question that warrants consideration here. Specifically, given that perceivers make dispositional inferences about actors from the behaviors they observe, when will that inference apply to the actor as an individual, and when will the inference extend to a group-level characterization? That is, when do we perceive the individual as an individual, and when do we perceive the individual as a group member? And when we do perceive the individual in terms of some group membership, are spontaneous trait inferences always viewed in terms of the group, or can they simply be dispositional characterizations of the individual actor? These are questions that have received relatively little attention in the social psychological literature, yet seem important for understanding when perceptions of individuals can contribute to the formation of group-level representations.

Do children manifest this tendency to infer dispositions from behaviors? At what age does the correspondence bias appear? The tendency to perceive others' behaviors as reflecting trait dispositions does not emerge until the child is 7 or 8 years of age. Prior to this age, children do not view traits as reflecting stable personality characteristics (Rholes & Ruble, 1984; Rotenberg, 1980). Whereas young children are capable of discerning the trait implications of behavioral information, they do not use this information to describe themselves or others (Livesley & Bromley, 1973), nor do they base predictions of future behavior on trait information (Rholes & Ruble, 1984; Rotenberg, 1980). Thus, although very young children might categorize others, correspondent inference processes apparently do not contribute to stereotyping at this age.

A number of reasons may account for young children's lack of dispositional inferences. In order to form a dispositional inference, the child may have to observe and remember a number of behavioral events reflecting the same trait. These behaviors may be separated in time and/or interspersed with irrelevant behaviors. Young children's cognitive capabilities may not be up to the task of integrating these events, as young children have limited working memory capacity (Austin, Ruble, & Trabasso, 1977) and have difficulty integrating information that is separated over time (Rholes & Ruble, 1986). In addition, it has been proposed that young children do not form trait dispositions because they focus on the target's current behavior and do not relate it to the target's previous actions (Flavell, 1977).

Older children do form dispositional inferences based on behavior, however (Rholes, Newman, & Ruble, 1990). Dispositional inferences are made more frequently and consistently as children realize that trait information has predictive value. In fact, Shantz (1983) described children in middle childhood as being "trait theorists." At this stage of development, children are actually more likely than adults to form dispositional inferences spontaneously and to expect trait-consistent behavior in the future. These children, then, may be more susceptible to the correspondence bias than are adults.

Illusory Correlation and Differential Perceptions of Groups

People are highly responsive to distinctive stimuli in their environment. We notice the strange, the unusual, the out of the ordinary. Although this characterization may imply that this heightened sensitivity is to stimuli that are somehow bizarre, such responsiveness includes a sensitivity to stimuli that are distinctive simply because of their relative infrequency in our experience. We often notice and attend to events that are unusual simply because they do not occur with regularity. In many contexts, this bias to attend to the infrequent is probably highly adaptive. However, as a generalized tendency, it can also generate other effects as well. The implications of this bias for stereotype formation have been demonstrated in research on illusory correlation.

An *illusory correlation* is a judgment by an observer of a relationship between two variables that is not warranted by the information on which that judgment was based. Typically, the observer "perceives" a relationship that did not exist in the information presented—an illusory correlation—and such an association can occur due to the observer's differential attention to distinctive stimuli. Originally demonstrated in an experimental context by Chapman (1967), the role of this bias in stereotype formation was first demonstrated by Hamilton and Gifford (1976) and has been developed in subsequent research (see reviews by Hamilton & Sherman, 1994; Hamilton & Sherman, 1989; Mullen & Johnson, 1990).

In this research, subjects read a series of statements, each of which describes a different person who belongs to one of two groups (identified simply as A and B) as having performed either a desirable or an undesirable behavior. There are approximately twice as many members of Group A as of Group B, and desirable behaviors occur more frequently than undesirable behaviors. However, because the ratio of desirable to undesirable behaviors is identical for both groups, the overall evaluative information presented about the two groups is the same. Therefore subjects' evaluations of the two groups should be comparable. However, the quite reliable finding is that Group A (the larger group) is rated more favorably than is the smaller Group B.

Why is this so? One prominent explanation for this outcome resides in people's inclination, as mentioned earlier, to attend to distinctive (in this case, infrequent) stimulus events. Members of Group B are infrequent (relative to Group A), and undesirable behaviors occur less frequently than desirable behaviors. The co-occurrence of these two categories—Group B persons acting undesirably—is especially infrequent, and hence is particularly salient. These items therefore receive enhanced processing as the information is acquired, making them easily accessible from memory at a later time, such as when judgments about the groups are requested. Because of their greater accessibility, instances of Group B members performing undesirable behaviors come to have disproportionate impact on subjects' evaluative judgments of the two groups.

A substantial amount of research evidence provides support for this account of the illusory correlation bias (cf. Hamilton & Sherman, 1989). The effect can be attributed to processes that transpire as information is encoded and processed, rather than at the time of judgment (Hamilton, Dugan, & Trolier, 1985, Exp. 1; Stroessner, Hamilton, & Mackie, 1992); is due primarily to the differential impact of the infrequent (distinctive) category of stimulus information (Hamilton & Gifford, 1976, Exp. 2; Hamilton et al., 1985, Exp. 2; Johnson & Mullen, 1994; Regan & Crawley, 1984); and reflects judgments that are not formed during on-line processing (Hamilton et al., 1985, Exp. 2), although they probably are not purely memory-based judgments either (cf. McConnell, Sherman, & Hamilton, 1994a, 1994b).

In addition to this distinctiveness-based interpretation of illusory correlation effects, other accounts based on different mechanisms have also been proposed (Fiedler, 1991; Smith, 1991). Although less empirical evidence is available to substantiate these interpretations, they do demonstrate that there may be several mechanisms by which these illusory correlations may be generated. Regardless of the underlying mechanism, the consequence of this process is that, whereas the information describing the two groups is evaluatively equivalent, subjects perceive the groups differently. These differing evaluative perceptions are based not on any actual properties of the information acquired about the groups, but rather are a consequence of a common feature of our information processing mechanisms. And because stereotyping requires, at the very outset, the differential perception of groups, the illusory correlation bias apparently can create, by itself, the initial foundation for the development of a stereotype.

Given the extensive literature on illusory correlations in adults, it is surprising that there is virtually no research evidence on how and when these effects develop in children. This gap needs to be filled in future research.

Affective Mechanisms in Stereotype Formation

Although stereotypes are commonly defined solely in cognitive terms, it is obvious that people often experience strong feelings and emotions when certain groups (including their own) become the focus of attention. Moreover, affective reactions seem central to early conceptions of social groups. Thus, at least in some cases, the affective components of group stereotypes may become established prior to the particulars of their cognitive content. It therefore becomes important to consider the role of affect in stereotype development.

The analysis of this question is complicated by theoretical uncertainties regarding the place of affect in the conceptual definition of stereotypes. The traditional social psychological view of stereotypes is that they are (purely) cognitive structures, that they are belief systems about the properties of groups and their members. If a particular group, as a stimulus entity, has the capacity to arouse emotional reactions in the perceiver, it is because those affective responses have become *associated with* the beliefs about that group. In this view, affect remains a distinct system, but one that can become closely aligned with these cognitive beliefs, knowledge and expectancies. (This interpretation also reflects the historical view of stereotypes, prejudice, and discrimination as the cognitive, affective, and behavioral components of intergroup attitudes, respectively.) An alternative view is that affect is so intrinsically associated with group perceptions that it is *inherent in* the conception of stereotypes and thus that it is difficult to conceive of a stereotype of a group that is totally devoid of affect, and therefore to think of affect as separate from, but merely associated with, the cognitive elements seems implausible. From this perspective, affect is a central component of the stereotype itself. At present, we know of no evidence that clearly favors one view or the other. We suspect that readers of this chapter will have varying opinions, and indeed the present authors are not of one clear mind on this issue. It impresses us as an important question that is likely to generate continuing analysis, both theoretical and empirical.

For purposes of the present chapter, the important question becomes, how does affect become associated with or arise as part of the stereotype? Perhaps because of the traditional emphasis on a trait-based conception of stereotypes, or perhaps because the affective nature of prejudice has been taken for granted, the amount of evidence directly relevant to this question is surprisingly limited. In the following subsections we discuss a variety of mechanisms that are usually thought of as governing the operation of affect and therefore might be implicated in the development of social stereotypes.

Classical Conditioning of Stereotype Emotions

Classical conditioning occurs when a person or object that is repeatedly paired with a particular emotion itself comes to elicit the emotion. Repeated experience of emotion when the group concept is activated can soon transfer to the group itself through this process. For example, even casual interactions with unfamiliar groups are often accompanied by negative affect. When members of one group are asked to report the emotions they experience in everyday dealings with out-groups, the feelings most often reported are anxiety and irritation (Dijker, 1987; Vanman & Miller, 1993). In fact, some evidence suggests that the less frequent the interaction between two groups, the more anxious and irritated their members are likely to feel when they do meet (Stephan & Stephan, 1985). After several uncomfortable interactions, the emotions initially arising from the intergroup encounter can become associated with the group itself, so that negative affect becomes part of the group stereotype.

Positive or negative emotions might also come to be associated with a group because of the reactions of valued others to the group. If mention of immigrant groups reliably produces anger or disgust on the part of a parent, activation of the group concept will be regularly accompanied by the resulting fear or repulsion felt by a child. With repetition, such negative affective reactions become firmly associated with the group until the group itself elicits them, regardless of the reaction, or even the presence, of others.

As a result of classical conditioning, then, seeing group members, hearing the group mentioned, or even thinking about the group will itself generate the distress, fear, or anger initially activated by the emotional experience. At first, experience with or about the group is bad; soon, the group itself seems bad. Because classical conditioning is assumed to be a basic mechanism of learning that requires little sophisticated cognition, its operation could contribute to stereotype formation even in infants and very young children.

Mere Exposure and Stereotype Emotions

An extensive literature attests to the fact that repeated and unreinforced exposure to a stimulus will enhance attitudes toward that stimulus (Zajonc, 1968; for reviews see Bornstein, 1989; Harrison, 1977; Stang, 1974). Such a mechanism seems likely to contribute to positive stereotypes overall and in fact, several studies demonstrate that mere exposure effects can play a role in stereotype formation: Repeated, unreinforced exposure (even minimal amounts of 1 to 2 minutes) to an out-group stimulus does provoke more positive attitudes toward that stimulus (Ball & Cantor, 1974; Bornstein, 1993; Cantor, 1972; Hamm, Baum, & Nikels, 1975).

Nevertheless, in most natural circumstances, the mere exposure mechanism seems more likely to contribute to positive stereotypes about *in-group* members (to whom one is frequently exposed), rather than to positive feelings about out-group members (Gaertner & Dovidio, 1986). This is true for two reasons. First, mere exposure effects appear stronger when stimuli occur in a positive or neutral context (as in-group members might) compared to a negative context (in which out-group members more frequently appear; Perlman & Oskamp, 1971; Zajonc, Markus, & Wilson, 1974). In fact, Perlman and Oskamp found that when out-group stimulus persons were presented in a negative context (e.g., described as a prison inmate) there was a slight *decrease* in evaluative ratings with increasing exposure frequency.

Second, mere exposure effects tend to be strongest when perceivers are unaware of their exposure (Bornstein & D'Agostino, 1992). This again works in favor of the in-group. When in-group members are encountered, they are less likely to be explicitly encoded as group members (Park & Rothbart, 1982; Turner, Hogg, Oakes, Reicher, & Wetherell, 1987), and thus awareness of increased exposure to members of that group is less easily tracked. In contrast, exposure to an out-group member is almost always accompanied by explicit categorization of the individual as a member of the out-group, increasing awareness of exposure and thus undermining the positive consequences of mere exposure.

Is the mere exposure effect a result of "hard-wiring" and thus a mechanism by which early preferences for in-group members could develop? If so, then very young children should show a preference for familar stimuli. The relevant evidence, however, reveals a complex picture. In fact, infants seem more interested in novel than familiar stimuli (Fantz, 1964; see Fantz, Fagan, & Miranda, 1975, for a review). For nonsocial stimuli, this preference for novel items continues into early childhood (Cantor & Cantor, 1966; Cantor & Kubose, 1969; Scholtz & Ellis, 1975), with familiarity leading to positive affect only in middle childhood (Heingartner & Hall, 1974; Kail, 1974). At the same time, however, infants show preferences for familiar over unfamiliar people (e.g., typically exhibiting greater distress in response to strangers at around age 6 months). Both infants and preschool children have more positive interactions with familiar than unfamiliar peers (Doyle, Connolly, & Rivest, 1980; Roopnarine, 1985; Stefani & Camaioni, 1983). The fact that children prefer familiar others does not show that familiarity caused this preference, of course, or that mere exposure caused the familiarity. Children's differential responses to social and nonsocial objects warrant further investigation, as does the issue of when mere exposure triggers changes in either familiarity or liking.

One explanation of mere exposure effects emphasizes the role of perceptual fluency (Bornstein & D'Agostino, 1992; Jacoby & Kelley, 1987). According to this explanation, encoding of the stimulus becomes easier with increasing exposures. Although people may misinterpret this ease of encoding as an indication of their liking for the stimulus, they might also use ease of encoding as an indicator of the extremity of the features associated with the stimulus. Thus, a positive stimulus seems to get more positive as the association between its features and itself becomes increasingly strong and accessible; similarly, a stimulus with negative features becomes more negative.

An alternate explanation of mere exposure effects is the expectancy disconfirmation model proposed by Bornstein (1993). According to this model, a stimulus initially evokes many competing responses, both positive and negative. Mere exposure effects occur as negative expectancies are dispelled by further exposure to the stimulus, and positive responses come to predominate. When stimulus persons are presented in negative contexts, however, this context may prevent the dissipation of the negative expectancies such that negative, rather than positive, responding may increase under these conditions.

With respect to stereotype formation, both the perceptual fluency and expectancy disconfirmation mechanisms suggest that the stereotypes formed about in-group members may be more positive than those associated with out-group members.

Sociomotivational Mechanisms in Stereotype Formation

One of the first systematic theoretical accounts of stereotype formation to appear in the social psychological literature was presented in *The Authoritarian Personality* (Adorno, Frenkel-Brunswik, Levenson, & Sanford, 1950). According to this theory, negative stereotypes of other groups often develop as a result of an individual's need or desire to deal with some inner conflict, discontent, or insecurity. Although empirical shortcomings eventually undermined the theory's explanatory power, the motivational underpinnings of this early theory—that a person's views about out-groups are determined in part by the individual's needs and desires—are reflected in current theorizing about stereotype functions and thus stereotype formation. In contrast to the earlier work, however, the focus of these more recent theories is decidedly group oriented. According to these newer approaches, stereotypes about groups arise from perceptions about and reactions to the relative standing among groups. How one's own group is perceived relative to other groups of importance is seen as a key motivational force in the development of stereotypes.

Social Identity Processes and Stereotype Content

Not since the introduction of realistic conflict theory has a single theory impacted the field of intergroup relations as has social identity theory (Tajfel & Turner, 1979). According to social identity theory, people's memberships in groups contribute to their self esteem, and therefore individuals are motivated to attain and maintain a positive social identity from the groups to which they belong. According to the theory, even membership in a short-term, arbitrarily determined group can provide positive social identity if such an in-group can be perceived to be superior to out-group alternatives. If such an advantage is not immediately obvious, members can strive to create positive distinctiveness by favoring the in-group over the out-group on relevant dimensions. In terms of stereotype formation, then, social identity mechanisms provide motives for attributing positive qualities to the in-group and negative qualities to the out-group (Brewer, 1979).

These effects appear to be both basic and pervasive. Indeed, even when people are assigned to groups on an arbitrary basis, they evaluate their own group more positively and attribute more positive qualities to their in-group than to out-groups (for reviews see Brewer, 1979; Diehl, 1990; Messick & Mackie, 1989). Moreover, the very concept "we" appears to have positive connotations compared to the concept "they" (Dovidio & Gaertner, 1993; Perdue, Dovidio, Gurtman, & Tyler, 1990). And when groups appear not to have any qualities that positively distinguish one from another, group members take the opportunity to create a difference. Thus, subjects asked to allocate units of value (such as money or points) to in-group and out-group members typically respond by favoring the in-group relative to the out-group, even at the cost of overall in-group gain (for a review, see Diehl, 1990). The motivational function of favoring the in-group relative to the out-group is best illustrated by findings that show self-esteem to be enhanced by the opportunity to discriminate against an out-group in this way, at least when group membership is minimal (Lemyre & Smith, 1985).

Motivational desires to view the in-group more positively than the out-group also influence attributions made about groups, and thus the dispositional properties that become associated with the group label. As we noted in an earlier section, people tend to overestimate internal factors and underestimate situational factors as causes of an actor's behavior, a tendency known as the *correspondence bias* (Jones, 1979) or the *fundamental attribution error* (Heider, 1958; Ross, 1977). Pettigrew (1979) proposed an extension of this principle to intergroup perceptions, calling it the ultimate attribution error. According to this analysis, negative acts performed by out-group members are attributed to internal dispositional causes to a greater extent than are negative acts performed by in-group members. In contrast, positive acts performed by out-group members are more likely to be explained away as due to nondispositional factors than if the acts were performed by in-group members. These nondispositional causes might include high motivation or effort, the situational context, luck, or viewing the positive behavior as an exception, a special case. The ultimate attribution error was predicted to have greater intensity when the perceiver was conscious of both the self and the other's group membership.

In a review of the literature on the ultimate attribution error, Hewstone (1990) found support for several components of Pettigrew's argument. First, people are more likely to make internal attributions for positive acts performed by in-group rather than by out-group members, but negative behaviors are more likely to be attributed internally for out-group members. Second, out-group failure is explained as due to a lack of ability to a greater extent than failure by the in-group. When out-group success is observed, it is likely to be explained away as due to luck, effort, or as a reflection of an easy task. And third, people show a bias for in-group-serving over out-group-serving attributions for group differences; differences between groups are typically attributed to a quality or circumstance that marks the in-group, rather than the out-group, as superior (consistent with Brewer's, 1979, conclusion).

The studies reviewed by Hewstone (1990) all used preexisting groups about whom stereotypes had already been formed. Nevertheless, the theory can be applied to explain certain aspects of stereotype formation. Social identity theory posits that people are motivated to hold positive perceptions of their in-group in comparison to other groups. The ultimate attribution error seems to be a mechanism that can facilitate the formation of a differentially positive impression of the in-group. If correspondent inferences are made for positive behaviors performed by in-group members and external attributions are made for negative behaviors performed by in-group members, a positive impression of the in-group will be formed. Similarly, by explaining away the positive behaviors of out-group members and making correspondent inferences based on their negative behaviors, a negative impression is formed of the out-group. Thus even if in-group members and out-group members perform identical behaviors, the ultimate attribution error would lead to a discounting of the in-group's negative behaviors and the out-group's positive behaviors. This cognitive bias would lead to the formation of different stereotypes for the two groups.

Further support for the contribution that this mechanism might make to stereotype formation can be found in the developmental literature. Several studies have provided evidence that biased attributions about in-groups and out-groups are a consistent feature of social perception through early childhood (Albert & Porter, 1983; Fagot, 1985; Huston, 1983; Kuhn, Nash, & Brucken, 1978; Martin & Halverson, 1981). However, the basis for this early tendency to attribute positive characteristics to in-groups rather than out-groups is not clear. It may derive from the motivation to positively distinguish one's in-group from out-groups. Alternatively, it may reflect the motivation to perceive groups with whom one is associated in positive terms.

Stereotypes as Justifications for the Status Quo

In the context of motivational desires to perceive groups in hierarchical relationships, stereotypic beliefs about groups often function to provide a rationale for and justification of status disparities, especially differences favoring the in-group. The roles performed by various groups and the relationships between groups provide a starting point for the naturalistic fallacy that the way things are represents the way things should be. Group members are not only seen as being imbued with characteristics that reflect what they do, but they are seen as naturally suited to perform such roles. Similarly, the relationships between groups are not only seen as reflecting their different abilities and preferences, but also are justified by those differences (Pettigrew, 1980).

As noted earlier, one consequence of the correspondence bias is that group members come to be perceived as being naturally suited for the roles they play. For example, the fact that in most cultures women play nurturing roles leads perceivers to see women as dispositionally nurturing. A dispositional inference, in turn, fosters the perception that women are "naturally" nurturing—their "natural" ability to care for others now provides a justification for their role. By this process, stereotypes provide a rationale for distribution of roles across different groups as right, natural, and inevitable.

Once this process begins, it opens the way for correspondent inferences to reflect not just roles, but role relations—the hierarchical ordering of groups. Correspondent inferences don't just imbue females, say, with traits that reflect their nurturing occupations. In the context of a society that values assertiveness and action, correspondent inference processes also can operate to assign characteristics to females that reflect an inferior position vis-à-vis males. Thus as stereotypes that reflect these differences develop, they become the justification and rationalization for the inequalities in social relations that underlie them (Pettigrew, 1980). Historically, for example, women and African Americans have been seen in ways that justified their treatment—as childlike, unintelligent, weak, and thus in need of direction and guidance (Hacker, 1951).

The effects of these correspondent inference biases converge with a widespread belief that the world is just and that outcomes are usually the just consequences of actions or attributes. Such just world beliefs (Lerner, 1980) lead people to believe that others deserve what they get and get what they deserve. For instance, subjects who watched a woman receive apparently painful electric shocks (Lerner & Simmons, 1966) derogated the victim, concluding that she must have done something to deserve her suffering. Rape victims, victims of spousal abuse, and people with AIDS often suffer the same fate (Carli & Leonard, 1990; Hunter & Ross, 1991), as do those whose social roles confine them to subordinate positions.

Research evidence also indicates that, like adults, children use belief in a just world to blame the victim of a misfortune (Furnham & Proctor, 1989; Stein, 1973; Suls & Gutkin, 1976). Jose (1990), for example, found that even young children (first graders) rated positive outcomes that followed good intentions and negative outcomes that followed bad intentions as fairer than outcomes that did not match intentions. Other studies have cast some doubt on whether just-world beliefs always operate as early as in the first grade (e.g., some studies show that younger children prefer positive outcomes, regardless of the actions of the actors; Fein, 1976; Jose & Brewer, 1984), but most show the effects operating by the third- or fourth-grade level. Just-world effects may be particularly strong among older children, in fact, because they often blame victims, regardless of victim responsibility. In one study (Stein, 1973), fourth and fifth graders read about a person who received a reward, a punishment, or a neutral outcome after a game that the target either chose or was forced to play. The target and the game were devalued in the negative outcome condition, regardless of whether the target had chosen to participate. Suls and Gutkin (1976) also found that children expressed greater liking for an actor who was rewarded rather than punished, regardless of whether the actor deserved the outcome.

Just-world beliefs are maintained both by self-protective motives and by cultural norms. Such beliefs allow perceivers to maintain a view of themselves as good and deserving. It is comforting to believe that bad things happen only to bad people—that AIDS is a punishment for taking drugs or for a gay lifestyle, or that poor people are lazy and shiftless (Furnham & Gunter, 1984; Robinson & Bell, 1978). Without beliefs that justify and rationalize inequalities, we would have to face the unsettling thought that bad things could easily happen to us. At the same time, just world beliefs are nurtured by cultural values, such as individual success derived from individual effort, pulling oneself up by one's bootstraps, and the cultural legend of the "self-made" man or woman. Indeed, two thirds of White Americans believe that African Americans generally have worse jobs, lower income, and poorer quality housing than Whites because they lack the motivation to do better (Kluegel & Smith, 1986). Such norms not only justify the disadvantaged positions of less successful groups, but also let advantaged groups off the hook morally: Believing that inequalities are deserved negates the need to examine one's own privileged position.

The fact that stereotypes develop to justify role relations between groups is also reflected in the acquisition of stereotypes that accompanies the onset of intergroup competition. Suddenly, only the most positive traits are associated with the in-group; the in-group is not only good, but righteous and morally superior (White, 1965, 1984). In contrast, the out-group is seen as embodying the most negative of traits. For example, as the peace of the 1920s and 1930s was replaced by war, the Germans became "Huns" and the Japanese, "Japs." And as war was again replaced by peace, German ruthlessness became German efficiency; Japanese cunning became Japanese ingenuity. In the 1990s, trade tensions between the United States and Japan may once again be turning popular views of the Japanese in negative directions (Mydans, 1992).

Cultural Mechanisms in Stereotype Formation

> Stereotypes about ethnic groups appear as part of the social heritage of society. They are transmitted across generations as a component of the accumulated knowledge of society. They are as true as tradition, as pervasive as folklore. No person can grow up in a society without having learned the stereotypes assigned to the major ethnic groups. (Ehrlich, 1973, p. 35)

Because stereotypes are deeply embedded in the fabric of a group's culture, people learn them as a part of growing up. To participate in a culture means, at least in part, learning and accepting what the culture believes about one's own and other groups. Thus, stereotypic conceptions of groups are often socially transmitted: stereotypes are acquired ready-made and prepackaged.

Social Learning of Stereotype Content

Parents are probably the first and most potent source of a child's information about other social groups, but peers and other members of the contact community are also powerful sources. These valued others need not explicitly transmit stereotypes, although they often do. Stereotypes are also learned by observation and imitation—listening to disparaging group labels or derogatory jokes that elicit approving laughter, abiding by family rules against playing with those "other" children, hearing why targets of discrimination or aggression deserve their fate. Such lessons are apparently well learned. By age 5, most children have begun to develop clear-cut racial attitudes (Goodman, 1952; Rosenfield & Stephan, 1981) and young children's ideas about racial groups are highly similar to those of their parents and friends (Epstein & Komorita, 1966; Patchen, Davidson, Hofmann, & Brown, 1977; Stephan & Rosenfield, 1978).

With the possible exception of family and friends, the media are probably the most powerful transmitters of cultural stereotypes, at least in Western societies. The expression of group norms in art, literature, drama, and film both reflects and transmits the stereotypes deeply ingrained in a culture. When stereotype content is not transmitted directly, media portrayals provide grist for the correspondence bias mill, with characteristics associated with such portrayals being attributed to minority groups.

Content analyses of what appears on the most powerful medium of culture transmission—television—underscore the extent to which programming content provides the raw material for stereotype acquisition. Minority groups are no longer invisible on television; even by the 1980s, for example, African Americans appeared in 20% of prime-time advertisements and 59% of prime-time dramas (Weigel, Loomis, & Soja, 1980), although other groups were less prevalent (Omi, 1989; Rothenberg, 1991). Despite an increase in positive prime-time depictions (Weigel et al., 1980), other media (e.g., news shows, "real-life" crime shows, and magazine advertisements) continue to depict African Americans as poor or violent, as athletes, musicians, or objects of charity (Rothenberg, 1991). Native American men are still mostly portrayed as silent, passive, lazy, drunken, and immoral, while Native American females are shown as beautiful, loyal, and submissive (Trimble, 1988). Asian Americans are likely to be depicted as cunning, whereas Latinos are often portrayed as violent and unstable (Omi, 1989). Whereas prime-time television increasingly depicts females as strong and successful, women in paid commercials are generally cast as subordinate to men, dream-like, emotional, or ill (Courtney & Whipple, 1983).

What impact do such portrayals have on stereotype acquisition? Although we need more quantitative research analyzing media influence on stereotype acquisition, some evidence suggests that media depictions can influence the beliefs associated with groups. For example, Archer, Iritani, Kimes, and Barrios (1983) reported that men's faces were much more likely to be portrayed prominently in magazines (in the United States and 11 other countries) than were women's faces (Nigra, Hill, Gelbein, & Clark, 1988). Moreover, when subjects were asked to evaluate photos of male and female models, those whose heads and faces were visually prominent were judged to be more intelligent and ambitious, regardless of gender (Archer et al., 1983). Thus, media portrayals may produce views of males as more intelligent and ambitious than females.

In another instance, adolescent girls who watch relatively traditional portrayals of female roles on television were found to endorse traditional gender stereotypes (Morgan, 1982). The results of this nonexperimental study are reinforced by experimental research in which college women watched television commercials depicting women in either traditional–subordinate or nontraditional–dominating roles (Geis, Brown, Jennings, & Porter, 1984; Jennings, Geis, & Brown, 1980). Although the dependent measure was one of self-stereotyping, and although these subjects could hardly be said to be acquiring a totally new stereotype, the young women who watched the traditional commercials later expressed lower self-confidence, less independence, and fewer career aspirations than did those watching the nontraditional commercials. Media depictions might have even stronger effects on beliefs about groups other than one's own. The potential power of this medium is perhaps best seen in research showing that heavy viewers are most likely to judge television content as veridical depictions of "the way things are" (Gerbner, Gross, Morgan, & Signorelli, 1986).

Particularly strong evidence that stereotype content is socially transmitted to children comes from developmental research indicating that children acquire and use stereotypes before they can appropriately distinguish groups on the basis of the cues thought to be crucial to such a task. Hirschfeld (1995), for example, argues that preschool children first learn verbal labels of groups and the stereotypes associated with those labels, and only later learn what perceptual cues correspond to those group labels; that is, they know the stereotype before they can identify to whom it applies. Supporting this model, Gelman, Collman, and Maccoby (1986) found that children who were unable to classify individuals based on shared features were nevertheless able to infer stereotypic properties when provided with gender labels.

Conformity Processes and Stereotype Acquisition

Socially transmitted stereotypes usually reflect social norms—the generally accepted ways of thinking, feeling, and behaving that people in a group agree on and endorse as right and proper (Thibaut & Kelley, 1959). Although neglected as a research issue for many years, normative processes seem certain to play an important role in stereotype acquisition. From this perspective, stereotype acquisition is seen as conformity to social norms.

Evidence for the importance of conformity processes in stereotype acquisition focuses on factors that influence conformity in areas other than stereotypic beliefs, and asks if those factors also influence the extent of stereotype acceptance and subsequent prejudice. One aspect of this work focuses on individual differences. If stereotypes come to be endorsed through the same mechanisms as other cultural norms, we would expect individuals who are conformists in other respects also to show greater stereotyping and prejudice. The evidence appears to support this kind of individual variation: Those who show greater tendency to conform to other aspects of a culture's social norms also show the most prejudice (Pettigrew, 1958).

Group differences in conformity also suggest the link between established cultural norms and prejudice. Studies that compare developmental changes in children's conformity to their parents rather than peer groups on prosocial, antisocial, and neutral issues (Berndt, 1984; Bronfenbrenner, 1970) show maximal parental conformity before the third grade. After this time, peer pressure begins to gain the upper hand for antisocial issues (e.g., stealing and cheating), with some studies suggesting a peak in the fifth and sixth grades and a gradual increase in independence from both parental and peer influence in the later high school years (Berndt, 1979, 1984; Gavin & Furman, 1989). These changes—from parental conformity in early childhood to increasing independence—tend to coincide with changes away from high levels of in-group preference around 7–9 years of age toward decreased ethnocentrism, at least in the majority population (Aboud & Mitchell, 1977; Williams, Best, & Boswell, 1975). In the absence of any direct investigation of conformity to parental or peer pressures on stereotyping, these parallels should be considered speculative. They impress us, however, as worthy of further research.

The case is strengthened somewhat, however, by comparisons between cultures as well as within cultures. For example, societies characterized by high levels of interdependence (e.g., some East Asian cultures) also display higher levels of conformity to in-group (but not to outgroup) members (Williams & Sogon, 1984) and higher levels of in-group bias (Leung & Park, 1986) than cultures stressing independence (for a review of both literatures, see Smith & Bond, 1994). Thus, cross-culturally as well, conformity and in-group preferences seem to be related.

A second set of findings supporting conformity's role in stereotyping comes from studies of the impact of social settings on prejudice and stereotypes. When members of a group are accepted as equals in a work setting, for example, but shunned as unsuitable companions outside of work, such inconsistencies in thought and behavior seem due to the impact of situation-specific norms (Minard, 1952). Finally, it appears that the acquisition of negative stereotypes increases under conditions in which conformity pressures are highest. For example, situations of intergroup conflict are marked by demands for loyalty, solidarity, and strict adherence to group norms. Under such circumstances, there is widespread endorsement of particularly negative stereotypes of the outgroup (Sherif, Harvey, White, Hood, & Sherif, 1961; White, 1965).

Social Roles and Stereotypic Content

Earlier we discussed the correspondent inference process whereby perceivers infer the personal characteristics of actors from the behaviors they perform, even when those behaviors may have been determined by social constraints. Accordingly, perceivers may infer that behaviors typically manifested by members of some group reflect dispositional properties inherent in that group, rather than the social constraints that in actuality govern the group's behavior.

To the extent that this happens, the behaviors that groups typically perform in society may become the basis for social stereotypes. Thus, groups whose social status results in their filling the "middleman" economic niche in their societies—Jews in the Middle Ages, the Chinese in Indonesia and Malaysia, Muslim merchants in eastern and southern Africa, Korean merchants in African American neighborhoods, and more recently, Caucasian produce sellers who serve the marketplaces of Russia—soon come to be seen as being inherently "sharp" and "frugal" (Pettigrew, 1968). In the same way, the lowest socioeconomic group in society, regardless of its ethnicity, is often seen as ignorant, lazy, loud, dirty, and carefree (Pettigrew, 1968; Ross & Nisbett, 1991). Personality characteristics correspondent with the role played by these groups are attributed to the group as a whole, and a stereotype is born. What this process ignores, of course, is the crucial role that societal constraints on these groups play in determining the behavior patterns they typically manifest. To the extent that the social occupations of different groups are dictated, either by circumstance or by discrimination, correspondent inference processes will help ensure the acquisition of stereotypes consistent with those occupations. Thus, the fact that stereotypes of particular groups often reflect the social roles occupied by those groups indicates the pervasiveness of the correspondence bias as a mechanism of stereotype acquisition (Campbell, 1967; Eagly, 1987).

Research by Eagly (1987; Eagly & Steffen, 1984) has documented this process in gender stereotyping. Because men and women play somewhat different roles in almost all societies, correspondent inferences based on their differing, but role-determined, behavior patterns contribute to the formation of gender stereotypes (Eagly, 1987). For example, if males are more often employed in positions that demand task orientation, assertiveness, and rationality, correspondent inference processes based on those behaviors would account for why males have traditionally been seen as having these "agentic" characteristics. Similarly, if females are overrepresented in homemaking and nurturing roles, the same processes explain why stereotypes of females might emphasize their sensitive, warm, and gentle "communal" characteristics (Eagly & Steffen, 1984). Correspondence biases make people less likely to realize the impact of role requirements, and more likely to conclude that men are task oriented and women interpersonally oriented *by nature*.

Hoffman and Hurst (1990) provided experimental evidence for the contribution of role-determined behaviors to the acquisition of stereotypes. In their study, subjects read descriptions of fictitious inhabitants of a distant planet—"Orinthians" and "Ackmians." After hearing most Orinthians described as involved in child care, subjects judged them to be typically nurturing, affectionate, and gentle, whereas Ackmians, who were described as mainly employed outside the home, were seen as competitive and ambitious. Each group was seen as having psychological characteristics appropriate for its roles. Additional evidence indicated that true stereotypes of these groups had been acquired. Subjects later applied these stereotypes to individual group members whose occupations clashed with the stereotype: they saw an employed Ackmian as more competitive and ambitious than an employed Orinthian.

Correspondent inference processes of this kind also play a part in the acquisition of negative stereotypes about out-groups that accompany intergroup competition. When antagonistic national or racial groups are engaged in recurring cycles of threat and aggression, neither side is likely to see the role that their own behaviors (or other circumstances) play in the other's actions. Instead, those with whom one is competing are more likely to be seen as stubborn, irrational, and violently aggressive.

CONCLUDING COMMENTS

In describing the various mechanisms that help produce stereotypes, we have tried to categorize them according to the primary nature of the process involved (cognitive, affective, sociomotivational, cultural). But inevitably such a classification is somewhat arbitrary. How we think is influenced by our culture; the ways we interact are changed by how we think and feel. Although some reactions to groups may be innate, most stereotypes are acquired by information processing that occurs in a social context. The information can be gained through face-to-face interaction, or can be transmitted via cultural teaching. We should not make the mistake of thinking, however, that face-to-face (or laboratory simulated) interaction involves only cognitive-affective principles, whereas cultural transmission involves only sociocultural processes. Categorization and correspondent inference processes in all likelihood occur regardless of whether group members are encountered on the street or in a television script. In each case, the interaction is defined socially: on the street, by the roles that each participant plays; via television, by the roles the cultural media sees fit to project. At the same time, sociocultural motivations, like conformity to accepted in-group standards or justification of intergroup differences, are likely to be present regardless of whether information about members of another group is delivered firsthand or through cultural channels. Thus, although cognitive, affective, sociomotivational, and cultural processes may make independent contributions to stereotype formation, most often they work in concert with one another, and their effects are inseparably intertwined.

This intertwining of effects makes the task of differentiating the particular processes that contribute to any specific stereotype particularly difficult. Nevertheless, the practical importance of understanding stereotype formation dictates that research should indeed attempt to identify the various antecedents of particular classes of stereotypes. What difference does it make, for example, if a stereotype is based on personal experience rather than social learning? If it has a largely affective base rather than being the product of cognitive mechanisms or biases? The importance of these questions is highlighted by recent research. Regarding the first question, for example, two studies have reported findings demonstrating that stereotypes transmitted intact have different consequences from those built up by experience. Subjects who received intact stereotypes before learning about individual members of the group were more likely to use stereotypic information in making later judgments (Smith & Zárate, 1990) and perceived less variability in the group overall (Park & Hastie, 1987). Regarding the second question, recent research demonstrates that the most effective strategy for changing an attitude may depend on the cognitive, affective, motivational, or behavioral basis of that attitude (DeBono, 1987; Edwards, 1990; Shavitt, 1989). The same is probably true of stereotypes (Snyder & Miene, 1994). The potentially important consequences of these effects call for systematically investigating them in the stereotype domain. Indeed, the stubbornness that ethnic stereotypes have displayed in the face of informational attempts to change them may in part result from their heavily affective nature.

Our overview of the processes that contribute to stereotype formation highlights a number of other topics about which we have insufficient knowledge. For example, the recent revitalization of interest in affective processes has drawn attention to the many ways in which emotion influences intergroup perception (for a collection of relevant examples, see Mackie & Hamilton, 1993), but this work has barely scratched the surface. Much of the research cited in our discussion of conformity effects seems strangely dated. The application of issues such as heuristic and systematic processing, the impact of group context, informational versus normative appeals, and majority and minority influence processes in stereotype research has yet to occur (for an exception, see Macrae, Shepherd, & Milne, 1992). More research is needed investigating at what age stereotype-relevant processes (of all types) appear, so that a more thorough developmental analysis of stereotype formation can be achieved. New questions about the functions of stereotypes are also potentially important. For example, Deaux (1993) has suggested that group membership may fulfill many needs other than, or in addition to, the self-esteem function emphasized in social identity theory. Exploring the variety of possible functions served by stereotypes could shed new light on the factors involved in both the formation and maintenance of stereotypes. Finally, little is known about the possible role of genetic contributions to attitudes and evaluations (Orr & Lanzetta, 1980; Tesser, 1993) that may have implications for stereotype formation, particularly reactions to in-groups and out-groups.

Even our brief review of the processes that contribute to stereotype formation reveals the complex relationship between stereotypes and prejudice. Some of the processes that we have considered indicate that prejudice, an evaluative orientation toward in-groups and out-groups, can precede the formation of stereotypes. In other cases, these same processes seem to produce stereotypic content that, in turn, can provide a basis for prejudice. This mutual interplay reflects a more complex view than the traditional notion that stereotypes invariably lead to prejudice. Stereotypes contribute to prejudice, but prejudice also contributes to stereotyping.

Despite their complexity, the further elucidation of these relationships is vital. Although much of what we report here comes from the results of basic research, the study of stereotyping is always—if only implicitly—motivated by very practical concerns. An understanding of the bases of stereotype formation can contribute to an understanding of how and when the negative consequences of stereotypes might best be eliminated, as well as when stereotypes might serve positive functions. In no other domain is the inevitable joining together of basic and applied knowledge more important than in the study of stereotypes.

ACKNOWLEDGMENTS

This research was supported by National Science Foundation Grant No. SBR-9209995 to Diane Mackie, by National Institute of Mental Health Grant No. MH-40058 to David Hamilton, by a University of California, Santa Barbara, Humanities Social Sciences Research grant to Joshua Susskind, and by a University of California, Santa Barbara, Graduate Division Dissertation Fellowship Award to Francine Rosselli.

REFERENCES

Aboud, F. E. (1988). *Children and prejudice*. New York: Blackwell.

Aboud, F. E., & Mitchell, F. G. (1977). Ethnic role taking: The effects of preference and self-identification. *International Journal of Psychology, 12*, 1–17.

Adorno, T. W., Frenkel-Brunswik, E., Levenson, D. J., & Sanford, R. N. (1950). *The authoritarian personality*. New York: Harper & Row.

Albert, A. A., & Porter, J. R. (1983). Age patterns in the development of children's gender-role stereotypes. *Sex Roles, 9*, 59–67.

Allen, V. L., & Wilder, D. A. (1979). Group categorization and attribution of belief similarity. *Small Group Behavior, 10*, 73–80.

Allport, G. W. (1954). *The nature of prejudice*. Cambridge, MA: Addison-Wesley.

Archer, D., Iritani, B., Kimes, D. D., & Barrica, M. (1983). Face-ism: Five studies of sex differences in facial prominence. *Journal of Personality and Social Psychology, 45*, 725–735.

Austin, V. D., Ruble, D. N., & Trabasso, T. (1977). Recall and order effects as factors in children's moral judgments. *Child Development, 48*, 470–474.

Ball, P. M., & Cantor, G. N. (1974). White boys' ratings of pictures of Whites and Blacks as related to amount of familiarization. *Perceptual and Motor Skills, 39*, 883–890.

Bassili, J. N. (Ed.). (1989). *On-line cognition in person perception.* Hillsdale, NJ: Erlbaum.

Berndt, T. J. (1979). Developmental changes in conformity to peers and parents. *Developmental Psychology, 15*, 608–616.

Berndt, T. J. (1984). The influence of group discussions on children's moral decisions. In J. C. Masters & K. Yarkin-Levin (Eds.), *Boundary areas in social and developmental psychology* (pp. 195–219). New York: Academic Press.

Blaske, D. (1984). Occupational sex-typing by kindergarten and fourth-grade children. *Psychological Reports, 53*, 795–801.

Bornstein, R. F. (1989). Exposure and affect: Overview and meta-analysis of research, 1968–1987. *Psychological Bulletin, 106*, 265–289.

Bornstein, R. F. (1993). Mere exposure effects with outgroup stimuli. In D. M. Mackie & D. L. Hamilton (Eds.), *Affect, cognition, and stereotyping: Interactive processes in group perception* (pp. 195–211). San Diego: Academic Press.

Bornstein, R. F., & D'Agnostino, P. R. (1992). Stimulus recognition and the mere exposure effect. *Journal of Personality and Social Psychology, 63*, 545–552.

Brewer, M. B. (1979). In-group bias in the minimal intergroup situation: A cognitive-motivational analysis. *Psychological Bulletin, 86*, 307–324.

Brewer, M. B. (1993). Social identity, distinctiveness, and in-group homogeneity. *Social Cognition, 11*, 150–164.

Bronfenbrenner, U. (1970). Reaction to social pressure from adults versus peers among Soviet day school and boarding school pupils in the perspective of an American sample. *Journal of Personality and Social Psychology, 15*, 179–189.

Brooks-Gunn, J., & Lewis, M. (1979). Why mama and papa? The development of social labels. *Child Development, 50*, 1203–1206.

Campbell, D. T. (1967). Stereotypes and the perception of group differences. *American Psychologist, 22*, 817–829.

Cantor, G. N. (1972). Effects of familiarization of children's ratings of pictures of Whites and Blacks. *Child Development, 43*, 1219–1229.

Cantor, G. N., & Kubose, S. K. (1969). Preschool children's ratings of familiarized and nonfamiliarized visual stimuli. *Journal of Developmental Child Psychology, 8*, 74–81.

Cantor, J. H., & Cantor, G. N. (1966). Observing behavior in children as a function of stimulus novelty. *Child Development, 35*, 119–128.

Carli, L. L., & Leonard, J. B. (1990). The effect of hindsight on victim derogation. *Journal of Social and Clinical Psychology, 8*, 331–343.

Chapman, L. J. (1967). Illusory correlation in observational report. *Journal of Verbal Learning and Verbal Behavior, 6*, 151–155.

Courtney, A. E., & Whipple, T. W. (1983). *Sex stereotyping in advertising.* Lexington, MA: Lexington Books.

Davey, A., & Norburn, M. (1980). Ethnic awareness and ethnic differentiation amongst primary school children. *New Community, 8,* 51–60.

Deaux, K. (1993). Reconstructing social identity. *Personality and Social Psychology Bulletin, 19,* 4–12.

DeBono, K. G. (1987). Investigating the social-adjustive and value-expressive functions of attitudes: Implications for persuasion processes. *Journal of Personality and Social Psychology, 52,* 279–287.

Diehl, M. (1990). The minimal group paradigm: Theoretical explanations and empirical findings. In W. Stroebe & M. Hewstone (Eds.), *European review of social psychology* (Vol. 1, pp. 263–292). Chichester, UK: Wiley.

Dijker, A. G. M. (1987). Emotional reactions to ethnic minorities. *European Journal of Social Psychology, 17,* 305–326.

Doke, L. A., & Risley, T. R. (1972). Some discriminative properties of race and sex for children from an all-Negro neighborhood. *Child Development, 43,* 677–681.

Dovidio, J. F., & Gaertner, S. L. (1993). Stereotypes and evaluative intergroup bias. In D. M. Mackie & D. L. Hamilton (Eds.), *Affect, cognition, and stereotyping: Interactive processes in group perception* (pp. 167–193). San Diego: Academic Press.

Doyle, A., Connolly, J., & Rivest, L. (1980). The effect of playmate familiarity on the social interactions of young children. *Child Development, 51,* 217–223.

Eagly, A. H. (1987). *Sex differences in social behavior: A social-role interpretation.* Hillsdale, NJ: Erlbaum.

Eagly, A. H., & Steffen, V. (1984). Gender stereotypes stem from the distribution of women and men into social roles. *Journal of Personality and Social Psychology, 53,* 735–754.

Edwards, C. P. (1984). The age group labels and categories of preschool children. *Child Development, 55,* 440–452.

Edwards, K. (1990). The interplay of affect and cognition in attitude formation and change. *Journal of Personality and Social Psychology, 59,* 202–216.

Ehrlich, H. J. (1973). *The social psychology of prejudice.* New York: Wiley.

Epstein, R., & Komorita, S. S. (1966). Prejudice among Negro children as related to parental ethnocentrism and punitiveness. *Journal of Personality and Social Psychology, 4,* 643–647.

Fagot, B. I. (1985). Changes in thinking about early sex role development. *Developmental Review, 5,* 83–98.

Fagot, B. I., & Leinbach, M. D. (1993). Gender-role development in young children: From discrimination to labeling. Special Issue: Early gender-role development. *Developmental Review, 13,* 205–224.

Fantz, R. L. (1964). Visual experience in infants: Decreased attention to familiar patterns relative to novel ones. *Science, 146,* 668–670.

Fantz, R. L., Fagan, J. F., & Miranda, S. B. (1975). Early perceptual development as shown by visual discrimination, selectivity, and memory with varying stimulus and population parameters. In L. Cohen & P. Salapatek (Eds.), *Infant perception: From sensation to cognition: Basic visual processes* (Vol. 1, pp. 249–345). New York: Academic Press.

Fein, D. (1976). Just world responding in 6- and 9-year-old children. *Developmental Psychology, 12,* 79–80.

Fiedler, K. F. (1991). The tricky nature of skewed frequency tables: An information loss account of distinctiveness-based illusory correlations. *Journal of Personality and Social Psychology, 60,* 24–36.

Flavell, J. H. (1977). *Cognitive development.* Englewood Cliffs, NJ: Prentice-Hall.

Furnham, A., & Gunter, B. (1984). Just world beliefs and attitudes towards the poor. *British Journal of Social Psychology, 23,* 265–269.

Furnham, A., & Proctor, E. (1989). Belief in a just world: Review and critique of the individual difference literature. *British Journal of Social Psychology, 28,* 365–384.

Gaertner, S. L., & Dovidio, J. F. (1986). The aversive form of racism. In J. F. Dovidio & S. L. Gaertner (Eds.), *Prejudice, discrimination, and racism* (pp. 61–90). Orlando, FL: Academic Press.

Gavin, L. A., & Furman, W. (1989). Age differences in adolescents' perceptions of their peer groups. *Developmental Psychology, 25,* 827–834.

Geis, F. L., Brown, V., Jennings, J., & Porter, N. (1984). TV commercials as achievement scripts for women. *Sex Roles, 10,* 513–525.

Gelman, S., Collman, P., & Maccoby, E. E. (1986). Inferring properties from categories versus inferring categories from properties: The case of gender. *Child Development, 57,* 396–404.

Gerbner, G., Gross, L., Morgan, M., & Signorielli, N. (1986). Living with television: The dynamics of the cultivation process. In J. Bryant & D. Zillmann (Eds.), *Perspectives on media effects* (pp. 17–40). Hillsdale, NJ: Erlbaum.

Gilbert, D. T. (1989). Thinking lightly about others: Automatic components of the social inference process. In J. S. Uleman & J. A. Bargh (Eds.), *Unintended thought* (pp. 189–211). New York: Guilford Press.

Goodman, M. (1952). *Race awareness in young children.* Cambridge, MA: Addison-Wesley.

Hacker, H. M. (1951). Women as a minority group. *Social Forces, 30,* 60–69.

Hamilton, D. L. (1988). Causal attribution viewed from an information-processing perspective. In D. Bar-Tal & A. W. Kruglanski (Eds.), *The social psychology of knowledge* (pp. 359–385). Cambridge, UK: Cambridge University Press.

Hamilton, D. L., Dugan, P. M., & Trolier, T. K. (1985). The formation of stereotypic beliefs: Further evidence for distinctiveness-based illusory correlations. *Journal of Personality and Social Psychology, 48,* 5–17.

Hamilton, D. L., & Gifford, R. K. (1976). Illusory correlation in interpersonal perception: A cognitive basis of stereotypic judgments. *Journal of Experimental Social Psychology, 12,* 392–407.

Hamilton, D. L., & Sherman, J. W. (1994). Stereotypes. In R. S. Wyer, Jr., & T.

K. Srull (Eds.), *Handbook of social cognition* (2nd ed., pp. 1–68). Hillsdale, NJ: Erlbaum.

Hamilton, D. L., & Sherman, S. J. (1989). Illusory correlations: Implications for stereotype theory and research. In D. Bar-Tal, C. F. Graumann, A. W. Kruglanski, & W. Stroebe (Eds.), *Stereotypes and prejudice: Changing conceptions* (pp. 59–82). New York: Springer-Verlag.

Hamilton, D. L., & Trolier, T. K. (1986). Stereotypes and stereotyping: An overview of the cognitive approach. In J. F. Dovidio & S. L. Gaertner (Eds.), *Prejudice, discrimination, and racism* (pp. 127–163). Orlando, FL: Academic Press.

Hamm, N. H., Baum, M. R., & Nikels, K. W. (1975). Effects of race and exposure on judgments of interpersonal favorability. *Journal of Experimental Social Psychology, 11,* 14–24.

Harrison, A. A. (1977). Mere exposure. In L. Berkowitz (Ed.), *Advances in experimental social psychology* (Vol. 10, pp. 174–221). New York: Academic Press.

Heider, F. (1958). *The psychology of interpersonal relations.* New York: Wiley.

Heingartner, A., & Hall, J. V. (1974). Affective consequences in adults and children of repeated exposure to auditory stimuli. *Journal of Personality and Social Psychology, 29,* 719–723.

Hewstone, M. (1990). The 'ultimate attribution error'? A review of the literature on intergroup causal attribution. *European Journal of Social Psychology, 20,* 311–335.

Hirschfeld, L. A. (1995). Do children have a theory of race? *Cognition, 54,* 209–252.

Hoffman, C., & Hurst, N. (1990). Gender stereotypes: Perception or rationalization? *Journal of Personality and Social Psychology, 58,* 197–208.

Howard, J. W., & Rothbart, M. (1980). Social categorization and memory for ingroup and outgroup behavior. *Journal of Personality and Social Psychology, 38,* 301–310.

Hunter, C. E., & Ross, M. W. (1991). Determinants of health care workers' attitudes towards people with AIDS. *Journal of Applied Social Psychology, 21,* 947–956.

Huston, A. C. (1983). Sex-typing. In E. M. Hetherington & P. H. Mussen (Eds.), *Handbook of child psychology: Vol. 4. Socialization, personality, and social development* (pp. 387–467). New York: Wiley.

Jackson, D. Z. (1993, March 31). Dunking the stereotypes. *Boston Globe.*

Jacoby, L. L., & Kelley, C. M. (1987). Unconscious influences of memory for a prior event. *Personality and Social Psychology Bulletin, 13,* 314–336.

Jennings, J., Geis, F. L., & Brown, V. (1980). Influence of television commercials on women's self-confidence and independent judgment. *Journal of Personality and Social Psychology, 38,* 203–210.

Johnson, C., & Mullen, B. (1994). Evidence for the accessibility of paired distinctiveness in distinctiveness-based illusory correlation in stereotyping. *Personality and Social Psychology Bulletin, 20,* 65–70.

Jones, E. E. (1979). The rocky road from acts to dispositions. *American Psychologist, 34,* 107–117.

Jose, P. E. (1990). Just-world reasoning in children's imminent justice judgments. *Child Development, 61,* 1024–1033.

Jose, P. E., & Brewer, W. F. (1984). Development of story liking: Character identification, suspense and outcome resolution. *Developmental Psychology, 20,* 911–924.

Kail, R. V., Jr. (1974). Familiarity and attraction to stimuli: Developmental change or methodological artifact? *Journal of Experimental Child Psychology, 18,* 504–511.

Katz, P. A. (1983). Developmental foundations of gender and racial attitudes. In R. Leahy (Ed.), *The child's construction of social inequality* (pp. 41–78). New York: Academic Press.

Katz, P. A., & Zalk, S. R. (1974). Doll preferences: An index of racial attitudes? *Journal of Educational Psychology, 66,* 663–668.

Kluegel, J. R., & Smith, E. R. (1986). *Beliefs about inequality: Americans' views of what is and what ought to be.* New York: deGruyter.

Kuhn, D., Nash, S. C., & Brucken, L. (1978). Sex role concepts of two- and three-year olds. *Child Development, 49,* 445–451.

Leinbach, M. D., & Fagot, B. I. (1993). Categorical habituation to male and female faces: Gender schematic processing in infancy. *Infant Behavior and Development, 16,* 317–332.

Lemyre, L., & Smith, P. M. (1985). Intergroup discrimination and self-esteem in the minimal group paradigm. *Journal of Personality and Social Psychology, 49,* 660–670.

Lerner, M. J. (1980). *The belief in a just world: A fundamental delusion.* New York: Plenum Press.

Lerner, M. J., & Simmons, C. H. (1966). Observers' reaction to the "innocent victim": Compassion or rejection? *Journal of Personality and Social Psychology, 4,* 203–210.

Lerner, R. (1973). The development of personal space schemata towards body build. *Journal of Psychology, 84,* 229–235.

Leung, K., & Park, H. (1986). Effects of interaction goals on choice of allocation rule: A cross-national study. *Organizational Behavior and Human Decision Processes, 37,* 111–120.

Linville, P. W. (1982). The complexity-extremity effect and age based stereotyping. *Journal of Personality and Social Psychology, 42,* 193–211.

Linville, P. W., Fischer, G. W., & Salovey, P. (1989). Perceived distributions of the characteristics of in-group and out-group members: Empirical evidence and a computer simulation. *Journal of Personality and Social Psychology, 57,* 165–188.

Linville, P. W., & Jones, E. E. (1980). Polarized appraisals of out-group members. *Journal of Personality and Social Psychology, 38,* 689–703.

Livesley, W. J., & Bromley, D. B. (1973). *Person perception in childhood and adolescence.* New York: Wiley.

Mackie, D. M., & Hamilton, D. L. (Eds.). (1993). *Affect, cognition, and stereotyping: Interactive processes in group perception.* San Diego: Academic Press.

Macrae, C. N., Shepherd, J. W., & Milne, A. B. (1992). The effects of source credibility on the dilution of stereotype-based judgments. *Personality and Social Psychology Bulletin, 18,* 765–775.

Martin, C. L., & Halverson, C. F. (1981). A schematic processing model of sex typing and stereotyping in children. *Child Development, 52,* 1119–1134.

McConnell, A. R., Sherman, S. J., & Hamilton, D. L. (1994a). Illusory correlation in the perception of groups: An extension of the distinctiveness-based account. *Journal of Personality and Social Psychology, 67,* 414–429.

McConnell, A. R., Sherman, S. J., & Hamilton, D. L. (1994b). The on-line and memory-based aspects of individual and group target judgments. *Journal of Personality and Social Psychology, 67,* 173–185.

Messick, D. M., & Mackie, D. M. (1989). Intergroup relations. In M. R. Rosenzweig & L. W. Porter (Eds.), *Annual review of psychology* (Vol. 40, pp. 45–81). Palo Alto, CA: Annual Reviews.

Miller, C. L. (1983). Developmental changes in male/female voice classifications by infants. *Infant Behavior and Development, 6,* 313–330.

Miller, J. G. (1984). Culture and development of everyday social explanation. *Journal of Personality and Social Psychology, 46,* 961–978.

Miller, N., & Brewer, M. B. (1986). Categorization effects on ingroup and outgroup perception. In J. F. Dovidio & S. L. Gaertner (Eds.), *Prejudice, discrimination, and racism* (pp. 209–230). Orlando, FL: Academic Press.

Minard, R. D. (1952). Race relations in the Pocohontas coal field. *Journal of Social Issues, 8*(1), 29–44.

Morgan, M. (1982). Television and adolescents' sex role stereotypes: A longitudinal study. *Journal of Personality and Social Psychology, 43,* 947–955.

Mullen, B., & Johnson, C. (1990). Distinctiveness-based illusory correlations and stereotyping: A meta-analytic integration. *British Journal of Social Psychology, 29,* 11–28.

Mydans, S. (1992, March 4). New unease for Japanese-Americans. *The New York Times,* p. A11.

Newman, L. S., & Uleman, J. S. (1989). Spontaneous trait inference. In J. S. Uleman & J. A. Bargh (Eds.), *Unintended thought* (pp. 155–188). New York: Guilford Press.

Nigra, G. N., Hill, D. E., Gelbein, M. E., & Clark, C. L. (1988). Changes in the facial prominence of women and men over the last decade. *Psychology of Women Quarterly, 12,* 225–235.

Omi, M. (1989). In living color: Race and American culture. In I. Agnus & S. Jhally (Eds.), *Cultural politics in contemporary America* (pp. 111–122). New York: Routledge.

Orr, S. P., & Lanzetta, J. T. (1980). Facial expressions of emotions as conditioned stimuli for human autonomic responses. *Journal of Personality and Social Psychology, 38,* 278–282.

Ostrom, T. M., & Sedikides, C. (1992). Out-group homogeneity effects in natural and minimal groups. *Psychological Bulletin, 112*, 536–552.

Park, B., & Hastie, R. (1987). Perception of variability in category development: Instance- versus abstraction-based stereotypes. *Journal of Personality and Social Psychology, 53*, 621–635.

Park, B., & Rothbart, M. (1982). Perception of out-group homogeneity and levels of social categorization: Memory for the subordinate attributes of in-group and out-group members. *Journal of Personality and Social Psychology, 42*, 1051–1068.

Park, B., Ryan, C. S., & Judd, C. M. (1992). The role of meaningful subgroups in explaining differences in perceived variability for in-groups and out-groups. *Journal of Personality and Social Psychology, 63*, 553–567.

Patchen, M., Davidson, J. D., Hofmann, G., & Brown, W. R. (1977). Determinants of students' interracial behavior and opinion change. *Sociology of Education, 50*, 55–75.

Perdue, C. W., Dovidio, J. F., Gurtman, M. B., & Tyler, R. B. (1990). Us and them: Social categorization and the process of ingroup bias. *Journal of Personality and Social Psychology, 59*, 475–486.

Perlman, D., & Oskamp, S. (1971). The effect of picture content and exposure frequency on evaluations of Negros and whites. *Journal of Experimental Social Psychology, 7*, 503–514.

Pettigrew, T. W. (1958). Personality and sociocultural factors in intergroup attitudes: A cross-national comparison. *Journal of Conflict Resolution, 2*, 29–42.

Pettigrew, T. W. (1968). Race relations: Social and psychological aspects. In D. L. Sills (Ed.), *The international encyclopedia of the social sciences* (Vol. 13, pp. 277–282). New York: Macmillan.

Pettigrew, T. W. (1979). The ultimate attribution error: Extending Allport's cognitive analysis of prejudice. *Personality and Social Psychology Bulletin, 5*, 461–476.

Pettigrew, T. W. (1980). Prejudice. In S. Thernstrom (Ed.), *Harvard encyclopedia of American ethnic groups*. Cambridge, MA: Harvard University Press.

Poulin-Dubois, D., Serbin, L. A., Kenyon, B., & Derbyshire, A. (1994). Infants' intermodal knowledge about gender. *Developmental Psychology, 3*, 436–442.

Quattrone, G. A., & Jones, E. E. (1980). The perception of variability within in-groups and outgroups: Implications for the law of small numbers. *Journal of Personality and Social Psychology, 38*, 141–152.

Regan, D. T., & Crawley, D. M. (1984, August). *Illusory correlation and stereotype formation: Replication and extension.* Paper presented at American Psychological Association Convention, Toronto, Canada.

Rholes, W. S., Newman, L. S., & Ruble, D. N. (1990). Understanding self and other: Developmental and motivational aspects of perceiving persons in terms of invariant dispositions. In E. T. Higgins & R. M. Sorrentino (Eds.), *Handbook of motivation and cognition: Foundations of social behavior* (Vol. 2, pp. 369–407). New York: Guilford Press.

Rholes, W. S., & Ruble, D. N. (1984). Children's understanding of the dispositional characteristics of others. *Child Development, 55,* 550–560.

Rholes, W. S., & Ruble, D. N. (1986). Children's impressions of other persons: The effects of temporal separation of behavioral information. *Child Development, 57,* 872–878.

Rivers, D., & Brooks, B. (1993). *Those who love the game.* New York: Henry Holt.

Robinson, R. V., & Bell, W. (1978). Equality, success, and social justice in England and the United States. *American Sociological Review, 43,* 125–143.

Roopnarine, J. L. (1985). Changes in peer-directed behaviors following preschool experience. *Journal of Personality and Social Psychology, 48,* 740–745.

Rosenfield, D., & Stephan, W. G. (1981). Intergroup relations among children. In S. Brehm, S. Kassin, & F. Gibbons (Eds.), *Developmental social psychology* (pp. 271–297). New York: Oxford University Press.

Ross, L. (1977). The intuitive psychologist and his shortcomings: Distortions in the attribution process. In L. Berkowitz (Ed.), *Advances in Experimental Social Psychology* (Vol. 10, 174–221). New York: Academic Press.

Ross, L., & Nisbett, R. E. (1991). *The person and the situation: Perspectives of social psychology.* New York: McGraw-Hill.

Rotenberg, K. J. (1980). Children's use of intentionality in judgments of character and disposition. *Child Development, 51,* 282–284.

Rothenberg, R. (1991, July 23). Blacks are found to be still scarce in advertisements in major magazines. *The New York Times,* p. A7.

Scholtz, G. J. L., & Ellis, M. J. (1975). Repeated exposure to objects and peers in a play setting. *Journal of Experimental Child Psychology, 19,* 448–455.

Shantz, C. U. (1983). Social cognition. In J. H. Flavell & M. Markman (Eds.), *Handbook of child psychology* (Vol. 3, pp. 495–455). New York: Wiley.

Shavitt, S. (1989). Operationalizing functional theories of attitude. In A. R. Pratkanis, S. J. Breckler, & A. G. Greenwald (Eds.), *Attitude structure and function* (pp. 311–337). Hillsdale, NJ: Erlbaum.

Sherif, M., Harvey, O. J., White, B. J., Hood, W. E., & Sherif, C. W. (1961). *Intergroup conflict and cooperation: The Robbers Cave experiment.* Norman, OK: University of Oklahoma Press/Book Exchange.

Simon, B., & Hamilton, D. L. (1994). Self-stereotyping and social context: The effects of relative in-group size and in-group status. *Journal of Personality and Social Psychology, 66,* 699–711.

Smith, E. R. (1991). Illusory correlation in a simulated exemplar-based memory. *Journal of Experimental Social Psychology, 27,* 107–123.

Smith, E. R., & Mackie, D. M. (1995). *Social psychology.* New York: Worth.

Smith, E. R., & Zárate, M. A. (1990). Exemplar-based models of social categorization. *Social Cognition, 8,* 243–262.

Smith, P. B., & Bond, M. H. (1994). *Social psychology across cultures: Analysis and perspectives.* Boston: Allyn & Bacon.

Snyder, M., & Miene, P. (1994). On the functions of stereotypes and prejudice.

In M. P. Zanna & J. M. Olson (Eds.), *The psychology of prejudice* (Vol. 7, pp. 33–54). Hillsdale, NJ: Erlbaum.

Stang, D. J. (1974). Methodological factors in mere exposure research. *Psychological Bulletin, 81,* 1014–1025.

Stefani, L. H., & Camaioni, L. (1983). Effects of familiarity on peer interaction in the first year of life. *Early Child Development and Care, 11,* 45–54.

Stein, G. M. (1973). Children's reactions to innocent victims. *Child Development, 44,* 805–810.

Stephan, W. G., & Rosenfield, D. (1978). Effects of desegregation on racial attitudes. *Journal of Personality and Social Psychology, 36,* 795–801.

Stephan, W. G., & Stephan, C. W. (1985). Intergroup anxiety. *Journal of Social Issues, 41*(3), 157–175.

Stroessner, S. J., Hamilton, D. L., & Mackie, D. M. (1992). Affect and stereotyping: The effect of induced mood on distinctiveness-based illusory correlations. *Journal of Personality and Social Psychology, 62,* 564–576.

Suls, J. M., & Gutkin, D. C. (1976). Children's reaction to an actor as a function of expectations and of the consequences received. *Journal of Personality, 44,* 149–162.

Tajfel, H. (1969). Cognitive aspects of prejudice. *Journal of Social Issues, 25*(4), 79–97.

Tajfel, H. (1970). Experiments in intergroup discrimination. *Scientific American, 223,* 96–102.

Tajfel, H., Billig, M., Bundy, R. P., & Flament, C. (1971). Social categorization and intergroup behavior. *European Journal of Social Psychology, 1,* 149–177.

Tajfel, H., & Turner, J. C. (1979). An integrative theory of intergroup conflict. In W. G. Austin & S. Worchel (Eds.), *The social psychology of intergroup relations* (pp. 33–47). Monterey, CA: Brooks/Cole.

Tesser, A. (1993). The importance of heritability in psychological research: The case of attitudes. *Psychological Review, 100,* 129–142.

Thibault, J. W., & Kelley, H. H. (1959). *The social psychology of groups.* New York: Wiley.

Trimble, J. E. (1988). Stereotypic images, American Indians, and prejudice. In P. A. Katz & D. A. Taylor (Eds.), *Eliminating racism: Profiles in controversy* (pp. 181–202). New York: Plenum Press.

Turner, J. C., Hogg, M. A., Oakes, P. J., Reicher, S. D., & Wetherell, M. S. (1987). *Rediscovering the social group: A self-categorization theory.* New York: Blackwell.

Vanbeselaere, N. (1991). The different effects of simple and crossed categorizations: A result of the category differentiation process or of differential category salience? In W. Stroebe & M. Hewstone (Eds.), *European review of social psychology* (Vol. 2, pp. 247–278). Chichester, UK: Wiley.

Vanman, E. J., & Miller, N. (1993). Applications of emotion theory and research to stereotyping and intergroup relations. In D. M. Mackie & D. L. Hamilton (Eds.), *Affect, cognition, and stereotyping: Interactive processes in group perception* (pp. 317–344). San Diego: Academic Press.

Weigel, R. H., Loomis, J. W., & Soja, M. J. (1980). Race relations on prime-time television. *Journal of Personality and Social Psychology, 39*, 884–893.

White, R. K. (1965). Images in the context of international conflict: Soviet perceptions of the U.S. and the U.S.S.R. In H. C. Kelman (Ed.), *International behavior: A social psychological analysis* (pp. 236–276). New York: Holt, Rinehart & Winston.

White, R. K. (1984). *Fearful warriors: A psychological profile in U.S.–Soviet relations.* New York: Free Press.

Wilder, D. A. (1978a). Homogeneity of jurors: The majority's influence depends upon their perceived independence. *Law and Human Behavior, 2,* 363–376.

Wilder, D. A. (1978b). Perceiving persons as a group: Effects on attributions of causality and beliefs. *Social Psychology, 1,* 12–23.

Williams, J. E., Best, D. L., & Boswell, D. A. (1975). The measurement of children's racial attitudes in the early school years. *Child Development, 46,* 494–500.

Williams, T. P., & Sogon, S. (1984). Group composition and conforming behavior in Japanese students. *Japanese Psychological Research, 26,* 231–234.

Zajonc, R. B. (1968). Attitudinal effects of mere exposure. *Journal of Personality and Social Psychology, 9* (Monograph Suppl.), 1–27.

Zajonc, R. B., Markus, H., & Wilson, W. R. (1974). Exposure effects and associative learning. *Journal of Experimental Social Psychology, 10,* 248–263.

3

Physical Appearance as a Basis of Stereotyping

LESLIE A. ZEBROWITZ

> . . . groups that look (or sound) different will seem
> to *be* different.
>
> —ALLPORT (1954, p. 132)

Most stereotyped groups can be differentiated by their appearance. Ethnic and racial groups look different from one another, as do men and women, the elderly and the young. Some groups are stereotyped solely on the basis of their appearance—attractive people, obese people, short people, redheads. Even occupational and social groups may differ in their appearance, often by choice. Thus, the nerds and the jocks found in U.S. high schools are differentiated as much by their grooming and dress as by their traits and activities. Allport's insight notwithstanding, these very obvious group differences in appearance have been largely ignored by researchers attempting to understand the phenomenon of group stereotypes.

Another aspect of stereotyping that, surprisingly, has been neglected by researchers is the specific content of group stereotypes. This was a focus of attention in early research. However, as noted by Hamilton, Stroessner, and Driscoll (1994), research in the field has shown "a shift from the investigation of *content* to the investigation of *process*" (p. 13). Recent investigators have been concerned with identifying the internal cognitive structures that represent organized social knowledge about certain groups of people and have an impact on cognitive processes such as attention, memory, and evaluation. The narrow focus on process in current research is unfortunate. As Zebrowitz (1990, p. 9) argued, "the conceptualization and description of . . . contents is essential to an adequate theory [of social perception]." For example, although we may understand *cognitive processes* better from research that reveals that individuals who are placed into certain social categories are perceived to have the attributes and evaluations associated with that category, we will not understand *group stereotypes* unless we also know who gets placed into what categories and why, and what attributes are associated with the various categories and why.

Some attention has been given to the question of who gets placed into what categories, and it has been noted that an individual's physical appearance plays a central role (e.g., Brewer, 1988; McArthur, 1982). However, the question of which particular physical qualities drive categorization and why has been of less concern. Notable exceptions include work by Brewer and her colleagues (e.g., Brewer & Lui, 1989), who found that physical markers of age and sex are salient bases of categorization. Also, Stangor, Lynch, Duan, and Glass (1992) found that markers of an individual's sex are more salient determinants of categorization than markers of race, and that visible stimulus qualities that provide socially useful information are more likely to serve as a basis of categorization than those that are equal in perceptual salience but less functionally significant. The latter finding is related to the proposal that categorization is most likely to be based on stimulus information that is perceived to mark "natural kinds" who share an underlying biologically determined nature (e.g., Rothbart & Taylor, 1992). What has not been systematically addressed in past research is the question of what stimulus qualities are functionally significant.

The question of what attributes are associated with various social categories has been addressed in research taking the "old" content approach to stereotyping (e.g., Broverman, Vogel, Broverman, Clarkson, & Rosenkrantz, 1972; Karlins, Coffman, & Walters, 1969; Lawson, 1971; Schmidt & Boland, 1986; Sleet, 1969). However, the data describing the contents of various group stereotypes are sparse. Also, little attention has been given to the origins of the documented beliefs regarding various groups' attributes. These beliefs—the content of group stereotypes—are certainly fostered by cultural images, but this explanation begs the question of how those images have arisen in the culture in the first place. Some efforts to understand their origins have provided a functional analysis, focusing on the utility of stereotypes to support cognitive economy, self-esteem, or social identity (e.g., see Allport, 1954, for a review of classic research, and Esses, Haddock, & Zanna, 1994; Snyder & Miene, 1994; and Tajfel & Turner, 1986; for more recent expositions). However, functional explanations cannot account for differences in the content of stereotypes of different groups (e.g., the tendency to view one group as lazy and another as pushy). Other theorists have offered a "kernel of truth" hypothesis to explain such specificity of content. Thus, Eagly and her associates have argued that sex stereotypes may derive from the actual distribution of men and women in different social roles (Eagly & Steffen, 1984; Eagly & Wood, 1982). Similarly, Vinacke (1949, p. 285) postulated that "in part wrong, superficial, and limited, they [national stereotypes] nevertheless generalize some actual cultural traits." Brigham (1971, p. 26) also concluded that "ethnic stereotypes can have 'kernels of truth,' at least in a convergent validity sense."

The present chapter focuses on the two topics that have been neglected in recent stereotyping research—group differences in appearance and stereotype contents—and it considers the possibility that one factor that may contribute to consensual beliefs about various social groups is their physical appearance. More specifically, it is proposed that the specific content of group stereotypes may derive in part from a tendency to overgeneralize the accurate information that physical appearance can provide regarding people's psychological attributes. This proposition will be addressed within the framework of the ecological theory of social perception (McArthur & Baron, 1983).

AN ECOLOGICAL APPROACH TO STEREOTYPING

Drawing on Gibson's (1979) ecological theory of visual perception, the ecological approach to social perception makes the fundamental assumption that perceptible stimulus qualities provided in a person's movements, vocal qualities, and facial appearance provide socially useful information. The stimulus qualities that provide this information are typically configural and dynamic, a much richer source of information than the verbal category labels employed in most "top-down" stereotyping research. What these perceptible qualities reveal is an individual's affordances—the behavioral opportunities that a person provides. Similarly, the affordances perceived in particular social groups—group stereotypes—may arise because group members share common perceptible qualities. Thus, rather than merely serving as a basis for categorization, appearance may itself determine the content of the stereotype. This implies that stereotyping should be fine-grained: Group members will be perceived to share common behavioral attributes insofar as they share common physical attributes.[1]

According to the ecological theory, group differences in the content of stereotypes not only will reflect group differences in perceptible stimulus qualities, but also these stereotype contents should often be accurate. This follows from the ecological assumption that social perceptions serve an adaptive function either for the survival of the species or for the goal attainment of individuals. To explain erroneous perceptions, as stereotypes may be, the ecological theory argues that errors can be traced to the overgeneralization of perceptions that typically are adaptive and accurate. More specifically, it will be argued in the present chapter that the social attributes that are accurately revealed by the functionally significant appearance qualities that mark age, emotion, health, species, and identity may be overgeneralized to those whose appearance resembles a particular age level, emotional state, health status, species, or individual. According to the ecological theory, the Type 1 errors shown in such overgeneralization effects occur because they are more adaptive than the Type 2 errors that might result from failures to respond to age, emotion, health, species, and identity information.[2]

Four points must be demonstrated to support the ecological theory account of physical appearance as a basis of stereotyping. First, it must be shown that people are highly attuned to physical appearance. Second, it must be shown that people's impressions of others are influenced by physical appearance and that this influence is fine-grained rather than merely categorical. Third, it must be shown that appearance-driven impressions are adaptive either because they are themselves accurate or because they reflect the overgeneralization of perceptions that typically are accurate. Fourth, it must be shown that appearance-based impressions, be they accurate or overgeneralized, can explain the content of certain group stereotypes. Although the present chapter will provide evidence to support each of these four points, two caveats are in order. First, much of the supporting evidence will draw on research concerning facial appearance rather than other appearance qualities. Second, the evidence to support the fourth point in the ecological theory account will be more speculative than conclusive, inasmuch as there is little good data documenting the content of group stereotypes. As noted earlier, this state of affairs reflects the top down emphasis in current research that investigates the "how" of stereotyping—perceivers' information processing—more than the "what" of stereotyping—the contents.

ATTUNEMENT TO PHYSICAL APPEARANCE

Consistent with the tenets of ecological theory, there is considerable evidence to indicate that people are highly attuned to the stimulus information provided in others' appearance. Qualities of appearance are typically the first thing mentioned when people are asked to describe a stranger or even their friends and family members. Moreover, the tendency to begin by describing someone in terms of appearance occurs even when people are asked for a description that will help others to know what it is like to be around that person (Fiske & Cox, 1979). This reliance on physical appearance in descriptions of others is present from an early age, and very young children rely almost solely on physical qualities (Livesley & Bromley, 1973).

Not only is physical appearance a salient aspect of social perception, but also people are extraordinarily good at recognizing human faces. In the course of a lifetime, we automatically and effortlessly learn to recognize thousands of faces. Moreover, once we have learned a face, we rarely forget it. Fifty years after graduating from high school, people showed almost perfect accuracy (90% correct) in identifying faces taken from their own high school yearbooks versus those taken from other yearbooks of the same era (Bahrick, Bahrick, & Wittlinger, 1975).

The ability to recognize faces seems to be wired into the primate brain. Electrophysiological recordings made from the brains of monkeys while they are viewing various visual stimuli reveal that certain neurons respond specifically to faces—either monkey faces or human faces. Moreover, some of these neurons respond more to certain faces than to others, thereby providing a basis for the recognition of different individuals (Baylis, Rollis, & Leonard, 1985; Desimone, 1991; Perrett, Rolls, & Caan, 1982). Even sheep brains show specialization of certain cells for face recognition, a finding which is consistent the importance to a sheep of accurate facial recognition (Kendrick & Baldwin, 1987).

Although invasive electrophysiological recordings cannot be performed on humans, developmental and clinical evidence also indicates a neurological basis of face recognition. Newborn infants, 9 minutes old, attend to a moving schematic face, but not to other moving patterns (Johnson & Morton, 1991). Human newborns, only hours old, are capable of recognizing their mother's face, preferring to look at a live or still video image of the mother rather than a stranger (Bushnell, Sai, & Mullin, 1989; Field, Cohen, Garcia, & Greenberg, 1985; Walton, Bower, & Bower, 1992). And, a disorder called prosopagnosia, which means "not knowing people," results from a particular type of brain damage—bilateral lesions that involve the occipitotemporal sector of the central visual system (Damasio & Damasio, 1986). People with such lesions show a perceptual deficit in face recognition. The deficits that prosopagnosics show in face perception are quite specific. These individuals are able to say which two faces are the same and which are different. They are also able to correctly identify facial expressions of emotion. What they cannot do is perceive the identity of a face that should be familiar to them. Generally speaking, people with prosopagnosia have no impairment in intelligence, no language deficits. They may also have no difficulty recognizing colors, pictures, objects, voices, or melodies. However, the loss of face recognition sometimes co-occurs with other recognition deficits, probably because the brain areas in which face recognition cells are found also contain cells responsive to other objects, particularly other parts of the body (Ellis & Young, 1989; Tiberghien & Clerc, 1986). The fact that physical appearance is highly salient to social perceivers, coupled with the evidence of a neural basis of face perception, indicates that perceivers are sufficiently attuned to appearance for it to contribute to person perception and group stereotypes.

JUDGING CHARACTER FROM FACIAL APPEARANCE

In accordance with the ecological theory, not only are people highly attuned to appearance qualities, but also they perceive behavioral propensities in these qualities. Consider, for example, an anecdote from Darwin's autobiography, which reveals that his nose practically cost him passage on the *HMS Beagle,* the ship from which he made many of the observations that spawned his theory: "[the Captain] was convinced that he could judge a man's character by the outline of his features, and he doubted whether anyone with my nose could possess sufficient energy and determination for the voyage" (Darwin, 1958, p. 72). The captain of the *Beagle* is by no means unique in his tendency to "judge a book by its cover." "Face reading," or physiognomy, has persisted from ancient times to the present, with Aristotle and Confucius among its illustrious adherents. The physiognomist Lavater, whose writings almost cost Darwin his voyage on the *Beagle,* was widely read from the time his book *Essays on Physiognomy* was first published in 1772. This book was regularly reprinted for a hundred years, for a total of 151 editions in various languages. It reputedly had such an enormous impact on social interactions that people resorted to wearing masks in public (Liggett, 1974).

Although people no longer walk around in masks, a survey of university students revealed that over 90% do believe that there are important facial guides to character (Liggett, 1974). And, college students show almost as much agreement when judging people's traits from facial photographs as when judging more "objective" physiognomic qualities, such as wideness of eyes or fullness of lips. In fact, people seem to find it much easier to make trait judgments than physiognomic judgments (Secord, Dukes, & Bevan, 1954).

One consequence of the relationship between facial appearance and personality impressions is that people who physically resemble each other are perceived to have similar traits, and those who look different from one another are perceived to have different traits. People's faces influence perceptions of their motives as well as their traits (Goldstein, Chance, & Gilbert, 1984; Hochberg & Galper, 1974). These effects do *not* merely reflect racial, gender, or age stereotypes. The belief that people who look similar on the outside also have inner similarities is manifested when the people being compared do not differ in any obvious category memberships. This suggests that appearance can influence trait impressions in the absence of an effect on categorization. Moreover, there is evidence that even common categorical stereotypes are driven by physical variations. For example, the extent to which men and women are believed to have sex-stereotyped attributes varies directly with the masculinity/femininity of their appearance. Indeed, in some cases, physical appearance was a stronger predictor of stereotyping than gender category (Deaux & Lewis, 1984; Friedman & Zebrowitz, 1992). Similarly, Litman, Powell, and Stewart (1983) found that relatively small differences in body build resulted in notably different personality stereotypes. Thus, for example, individuals categorized as "endomorphs" not only were differentiated from those categorized as "mesomorphs" or "ectomorphs," but also from each other: the greater the endomorphy, the stronger the stereotyping.

In contrast to the foregoing evidence for fine-grained stereotyping driven by subtle variations in appearance, Secord, Bevan, and Katz (1956) reported that Black individuals were not differentiated from each other on the basis of how "White" they appeared: The Black stereotype was equally strong for all members of the category. This study has been widely cited as evidence for the categorical nature of stereotypes. However, it should be noted that no inferential statistics were reported to support the authors' conclusions, and an inspection of the descriptive data suggests that the composite stereotype measure may not even have differentiated individuals in the Black and White categories. If so, then it is not surprising that it would not differentiate individuals within the Black category.

Another intriguing consequence of face–trait correspondences is that people whose facial appearance deviates a lot from average—for example, very wide eyes, very thin lips, and so forth—are also perceived to have more extreme personality traits than those with a more average appearance (McArthur & Solomon, 1978; Secord et al., 1954; Secord & Muthard, 1955). The tendency to attribute more extreme traits to people with salient physical features is similar to the tendency to attribute extreme and negative attributes to people who are members of salient social groups. This is the illusory correlation effect, whereby perceptions of the correlation between group membership and behavior are most influenced by the actor–behavior pairs that are most salient.

One factor that increases salience is the novelty of the person or the behavior. This can create the illusion that minority group members and negative or extreme behaviors, all of which are relatively novel, are more correlated than they really are (e.g., see Hamilton & Sherman, 1989). Because physical appearance frequently identifies minority group members, it thus contributes to the tendency to form negative, extreme stereotypes about them. Another factor that increases salience is associative connections between the person and the behavior (e.g., McArthur & Friedman, 1980). Because particular physical qualities are associatively linked to particular behaviors, this can create the illusion that social groups with those qualities are more likely to perform the associatively linked behaviors than they really are. In this manner, physical appearance contributes to illusory correlations that reinforce the specific contents of stereotypes that is, expectancies regarding appearance–behavior links. It should be noted that such illusory correlations may be strongest when a behavior is associated with salient physical qualities. Such appearance–behavior pairings should draw more attention than those in which the appearance of the group is not salient. Appearance qualities that are likely to be salient are those that reveal social affordances that it is highly adaptive for the perceiver to detect. This includes those qualities that are proposed in this chapter to generate overgeneralizations in judging character from appearance.

Not only does appearance convey character, but also stability in appearance facilitates the perception of a constant character. Thus, people who always look the same may be described as either energetic or relaxed, or dominant or deferential, depending on their particular appearance. However, stable traits such as these are not attributed to people whose appearance varies. Rather, the behavior of these people is perceived to "depend on the situation" (Kassin, 1977). Similarly, perceivers are more apt to change their trait ascriptions to a person whose behavior changes when his or her physical appearance also changes than when it remains constant (Bowman, 1979). The effects of appearance stability on impressions suggest that changing stereotypes may be facilitated by changes in the appearance of the stereotyped group.

In sum, many people do judge character from physical appearance, and appearance can influence impressions in the absence of an effect on categorization. Salient appearance qualities have a particularly strong impact: Impressions of people with such qualities are more extreme, and they are more vulnerable to illusory correlation effects that can contribute to negative and extreme stereotypes of minority groups, as well as to the content of group stereotypes. Finally, changing impressions and group stereotypes may be hampered by constancy in the targets' physical appearance.

ACCURACY IN JUDGING CHARACTER FROM APPEARANCE

People not only judge traits from appearance qualities, but also these appearance-based impressions are often accurate, as the ecological theory would predict. There is high interjudge agreement in trait ratings made on the basis of brief exposure to targets' physical appearance and/or vocal qualities, an effect that has been dubbed "consensus at zero acquaintance." This effect occurs primarily for judgments of exraversion and conscientiousness, although it is also seen in judgments of dominance. Evidence for the accuracy of these consensual judgments is provided by the finding that strangers' ratings are corroborated by ratings of the targets' themselves as well as the targets' acquaintances (Albright, Kenny, & Malloy, 1988; Berry, 1990a, 1991; Funder & Colvin, 1988; Kenny, Albright, Malloy, & Kashy, 1994; Passini & Norman, 1966; Watson, 1989). Accuracy has also been demonstrated by congruence of strangers' and self-ratings with the target's scores on personality tests and the target's behavior (Berry, 1990a; Bond, Berry, & Omar, 1994; Cherulnik, Turns, & Wilderman, 1990; Cherulnik, Way, Ames, & Hutto, 1981; Kalma, 1992; Levesque & Kenny, 1993; Moskowitz, 1990; Terry, 1975). This evidence of accuracy in individual trait impressions suggests that stereotypes of social groups may also be accurate insofar as perceivers are responding to the perceptible stimulus information that can yield veridical impressions.

Appearance–Trait Correlations

Although it is clear that people can accurately judge some traits from physical qualities, less is known about what stimulus information they are responding to. Some traits are communicated by visual cues, others by vocal cues, and still others by both (Berry, 1991; Borkenau & Liebler, 1992). Investigations of the particular visual and vocal qualities that accurately communicate various traits have been carried out by determining what qualities are correlated both with actual traits, as revealed in self-reports and personality tests, and also with trait impressions. Valid facial cues to extraversion include attractiveness; soft facial lineaments; stylish hair; a friendly, self-assured, smiling expression; and, to a lesser extent, thick lips. Facial attractiveness also provides a valid cue to high social competence and high dominance. Nonverbal and vocal cues to extraversion include fast movements, frequent head movements, a relaxed gait with arm swinging, and a loud, powerful voice. Low conscientiousness is communicated by a child-like face, a relaxed posture when seated, and frequent self-touching. Agreeableness is communicated by a voice that is high pitched and easy to understand, as well as by a friendly expression and soft facial lineaments. Such facial and vocal qualities also communicate low aggressiveness, which is associated with a baby face for men and a babyish voice for women (e.g., Berry, 1991; Borkenau & Liebler, 1992; Kenny, Horner, Kashy, & Chu, 1992).

Other research has uncovered additional appearance–trait correspondences, although it is unknown whether the naive observer accurately uses this appearance information. One diagnostic set of appearance cues is minor physical anomalies (e.g., widely spaced eyes, multiple hair whorls, and malformed ears) that predict aggressive and impulsive behavior in males (Bell & Waldrop, 1982; Paulhus & Martin, 1986; Waldrop & Halverson, 1972). There are also physical markers of shyness, including blue eyes and a narrow face (e.g., Arcus & Kagan, 1992; Gary, Davis, & DeVivo, 1977; Markle, Rinn, & Bell, 1984; Rosenberg & Kagan, 1987; Worthy, 1974; but for exceptions, see Lester, 1991; Robinson, 1981). Markers of a Type A personality (hard driving, hostile, and competitive) as opposed to the more easygoing Type B include a greater tendency to have a disgusted facial expression and to glare at an interviewer, lowering the brows, raising the upper eyelid and tensing the lower eyelid (Chesney, Ekman, Friesen, Black, & Hecker, 1990). Following the adage that after age 50 everyone has the face he or she deserves, elderly people whose faces resemble a particular emotional expression, even when they are posing a neutral expression, actually have a related personality disposition (Malatesta, Fiore, & Messina, 1987).

Accuracy of Appearance–Trait Relations as a Basis for Group Stereotypes

The evidence for actual correlations between appearance qualities and behavior indicates that accuracy may be one basis for stereotypes about groups that differ in appearance. Attractiveness is a case in point. People whose faces are judged to be attractive are perceived to have desirable traits, particularly in the domain of social competence (e.g., Eagly,

Ashmore, Makhijani, & Longo, 1991). What is more, there actually are differences between attractive and unattractive individuals in this domain (Feingold, 1992; Longo & Ashmore, 1990; Zebrowitz, Dutta, & Collins, 1995). Thus, some stereotypes about attractive versus unattractive people are accurate. Similarly, any tendency to stereotype blue-eyed ethnic groups as more introverted than dark-eyed groups may have a kernel of truth, as may any tendency to stereotype fast-gesturing, loud talking groups as highly extraverted. (See Ryan, Park, & Judd, Chapter 4, this volume, for a further consideration of stereotype accuracy.)

OVERGENERALIZATIONS IN JUDGING CHARACTER FROM APPEARANCE

Although the content of group stereotypes may sometimes reflect accurate beliefs about the behavioral propensities of the group members, another possibility is that they will reflect the overgeneralization of accurate beliefs about the behavioral propensities of individuals who physically resemble the group members. According to the ecological theory, the physical qualities that would give rise to such overgeneralization effects are those that reveal behavioral propensities that are highly adaptive for the perceiver to detect. These include appearance qualities that are correlated with age, emotion, health, species, and identity. Each of these qualities provides valid information about behavioral propensities, and this information may be overgeneralized to those whose appearance resembles a particular age level, emotional state, health status, species, or individual. Arguments supporting each of these possible overgeneralization effects are provided in this chapter. The ability of overgeneralizations based on age-related appearance qualities to account for the content of various group stereotypes is discussed at length. The applicability to group stereotypes of other overgeneralization effects is also considered, albeit more briefly.

The Babyish Overgeneralization Effect

Perceivers are highly sensitive to actual correlations between age and appearance, and age-related appearance qualities provide information about an individual's behavioral affordances that facilitates adaptive actions, such as nurturing the young and mating with the fertile. Such reactions to the appearance qualities that differentiate people of different ages may be overgeneralized. In particular, reactions to babies may be overgeneralized to adults whose appearance in some way resembles that of an infant.

Age–Appearance Correlations

There are obvious correlations between body size and age from birth through maturity. There are also maturational differences in body proportion. Babies are chubbier as well as shorter than adults, their heads are bigger in proportion to their bodies, and their limbs are proportionately shorter. Movement patterns also covary with age. Young children are distinguished by their toddling gaits and older adults by their slow, shuffling gaits. The face also reveals a person's age. As shown in Figure 3.1, the growth process from birth to maturity is accompanied by changes in facial structure that are reliable cues to age. These maturational changes yield a relatively smaller, more backward sloping forehead, relatively smaller, higher placed eyes, and a relatively bigger, more protrusive chin in the adult face. The head is also smaller relative to the body of an adult than a child, and a child's skin is lighter than that of an adult. Like maturation, the aging process also produces facial changes, most notably in the quality of the skin, which becomes progressively more leathery, crinkled, open-pored, and blemished. Age-related changes in connective tissue, bone loss, and the resorption of fatty tissue also yield a less angular jaw, pouches, sagging skin, and a double chin (Enlow, 1982). Interestingly, some of these changes cause the elderly face to revert to a more infantile appearance. Like facial structure, facial muscle movements also reveal age. This has been demonstrated using a point-light technique in which people's faces are videotaped with small dots of reflective tape affixed to them. The movement of the dots, which is all that can be seen when the tapes are played, add information about the target's age, over and above whatever structural information the dots provide. The precise nature of age differences in facial movement remains to be discovered (Berry, 1990b).

People are highly attuned to age–appearance correlations. Age can be accurately identified from facial information not only during the formative years, when there are pronounced changes in facial appearance, but also in adulthood (Henss, 1989; Mark, Shaw, & Pittenger, 1988; Todd, Mark, Shaw, & Pittenger, 1980). The ability to discern age from facial cues develops very early. By 5 months of age, if not sooner, infants are able to discriminate the faces of children and adults (Brooks & Lewis, 1976; Lasky, Klein, & Martinez, 1974). By the preschool years, children are proficient at using age-category labels to identify people pictured in facial photographs and to rank in terms of age faces that range from infancy to over 70. Moreover, children base their judgments on the same information, such as head shape and facial wrinkling, as adults (Edwards, 1984; Jones & Smith, 1984; Kogan, Stephens, & Shelton, 1961; Montepare & McArthur, 1986).

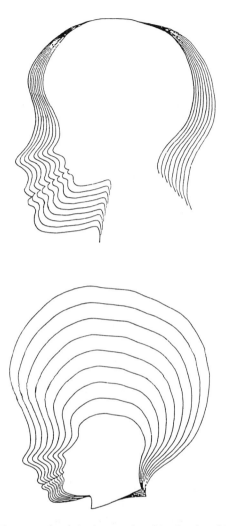

FIGURE 3.1. Top: The growth of the human head is simulated in this compu-
ter-generated sequence of profiles, which were generated using a geometric procedure called a revised cardioidal-strain transformation. Profiles range from infancy (innermost profile) to adulthood (outermost profile). Bottom: The
evolution of the human head is suggested by this sequence, which was generated
by a variation of the revised cardioidal-strain transformation. Profiles range
from a "Neanderthal" man (innermost profile) to a futuristic being (outermost
profile). A computer at the University of Connecticut was used to draw both sequences. From Todd, Mark, Shaw, and Pittenger (1980). Copyright 1980 by Scientific American. Reprinted by permission.

Age-related physical differences not only serve to identify age, but also they play a role in age stereotypes. The gait of elderly people, quite apart from other cues to age, makes them appear weaker and more unhappy than they would if they had a more youthful gait (Montepare & Zebrowitz-McArthur, 1988a). The head shape of infants in and of itself contributes to the impression that they are dependent, lovable, and unthreatening, and their head shape and body proportions elicit protective responses from adults. Smaller body size has the same effect on protective impulses as child-like proportions. When body shape is held constant, people report feeling more compelled to protect the smaller of two figures (Alley, 1983a, 1983b, 1983c). Reactions to such infantile cues are sufficiently strong that they are capitalized on by the entertainment industry in the creation of cartoon characters that have widespread appeal (Gould, 1979; Pittenger, 1990). Similarly, adults whose facial qualities resemble those of infants may be perceived to have child-like traits.

Impressions of Baby-Faced Individuals

People with babyish facial features such as large eyes; small noses; high, thin eyebrows; a small chin; and a round face are indeed seen as more child-like than those with more mature features. More specifically, they are perceived as physically weaker and more submissive, dependent, naive, straightforward, and affectionate than mature-faced people of the same age and attractiveness. Such stereotyped trait impressions are formed of baby-faced individuals of all ages and races in comparison to their more mature-faced peers. They are also manifested by individuals of all races, and they appear in children as young as 3 years of age (Berry & McArthur, 1985, 1986; McArthur & Apatow, 1983–1984; Montepare & Zebrowitz-McArthur, 1989; Zebrowitz & Montepare, 1992; Zebrowitz, Montepare, & Lee, 1993). There is even evidence to indicate that young infants respond positively not only to other babies, but also to baby-faced adults, an effect that suggests the possibility of an innate basis for the babyish overgeneralization effect (Kramer, Zebrowitz, San Giovanni, & Sherak, 1995). The tendency for responses to babies to be overgeneralized to others who resemble them holds true for vocal resemblance as well as for facial resemblance (Berry, 1992; Montepare & Zebrowitz-McArthur, 1988b; Zebrowitz-McArthur & Montepare, 1989). Finally, there is evidence that the perceptions reflected in the babyish overgeneralization effect may sometimes be accurate (Berry, 1990a, 1991; Berry & Brownlow, 1989; Scherer & Scherer, 1981; Zebrowitz & Dutta, 1994).

The strong tendency to overgeneralize our accurate impressions of babies to baby-faced adults suggests that the content of stereotypes about particular social groups may reflect the extent to which they have a babyish appearance. In particular, the babyish overgeneralization effect may contribute to gender stereotypes, height and weight stereotypes, national stereotypes and criminal stereotypes.

Gender Stereotypes

Because the facial characteristics that differentiate babies from adults also tend to differentiate women from men, the babyish overgeneralization effect may contribute to gender stereotypes. Indeed, in discussing sex differences in facial features, Gray's anatomy textbook states that they result from earlier cessation of maturation and growth in females and that "more of the morphological characteristics seen during pre-puberty years are retained in the skull of the adult female than in that of the adult male" (Gray, 1985, p. 178). Thus, men tend to have a larger jaw and thicker, lower eyebrows. Men also have a more prominent browridge and nosebridge, which gives their eyes a more deepset and smaller appearance than women's eyes. Like facial characteristics, the body characteristics which differentiate babies from adults also differentiate women and men. Women, on the average, have more body fat than men do, and they also tend to be shorter.

Although it would be simplistic to propose that stereotypes of women can be completely explained by a babyish overgeneralization effect, it is possible that sex differences in appearance do make some contribution to sex stereotypes. Some support for this possibility is provided by the fact that the character traits attributed to baby-faced adults of either gender parallel stereotypes of women, whereas the traits attributed to mature-faced persons parallel stereotypes of men. Like a baby-faced person, the stereotypic female is perceived as weak, affectionate, dependent, submissive, and naive. Like a mature-faced person, the stereotypic male is perceived as strong, unexpressive, independent, dominant, and shrewd (e.g., Broverman et al., 1972).

Friedman and Zebrowitz (1992) investigated whether typical sex differences in facial maturity may contribute to sex-role stereotypes. We created schematic male and female faces varying in facial maturity, and we asked people to rate these faces on sex-stereotypic traits. Given typical facial maturity, when males were relatively mature-faced and females relatively baby-faced, typical sex stereotypes were obtained. Men were seen as less warm than women and also more powerful, that is, more dominant, strong, and shrewd. However, when the natural association of gender and facial maturity was eliminated or reversed, sex stereotypes were also weakened or reversed. Mature-faced women and baby-faced men were seen as equally warm, and mature-faced women were seen as more powerful than baby-faced men. In short, sex stereotypes can be characterized as a babyish overgeneralization effect. This physical contribution to sex stereotypes is consistent with the finding that they are culturally universal (Williams & Best, 1982). Of course, other explanations, such as different social roles, are also consistent with cultural universality (Eagly, 1987).

There is also evidence that the more child-like height and body type of women may contribute to sex stereotypes. A woman who is described as tall, strong, sturdy, and broad-shouldered is perceived to have stereotypically masculine personality traits, whereas a man who is described as having the more child-like body characteristics of a woman is perceived to have stereotypically feminine traits (Deaux & Lewis, 1984). Such stereotypes persist in social interactions. An investigation of the characteristics of individuals who achieved high-status positions in small-group interactions extending over a five-week period revealed that the tendency for men to attain higher status ranks than women was largely explained by the sex differential in height. When height was equated, the difference in the status of men and women was significantly reduced (Crosbie, 1979).

Height and Weight Stereotypes

Just as the more babyish body type of women contributes to gender stereotypes, so may babyish body types contribute to height and weight stereotypes. Thus, one can look for a babyish overgeneralization effect by examining the character traits attributed to adults who are tall versus short, or chubby versus thin.

The meaning of height is embedded in our language. The terms stature and status suggest that taller people will be viewed as more dominant just as adults are more dominant than children. (See Maass & Arcuri, Chapter 6, this volume, for a discussion of the links between language and stereotyping.) Height is indeed related to status, with shorter people less apt to be in positions of leadership. Shorter people also earn lower incomes, even when age, education, personality, and ethnic identification are controlled. Interestingly, we also tend to perceive lower status people as being shorter, an illusion that reflects the strength of the association between height and status. Just as we "look up" at adults when we are children, we continue to look up to taller adults even after we are grown (Chaiken, 1986; Collins & Zebrowitz, 1994; Roberts & Herman, 1986; Wilson, 1968).

Like impressions of short people, impressions of those who are overweight may reflect an overgeneralization of our reactions to chubby children. Of course, there are other powerful forces contributing to our impressions of chubbiness, namely the premium placed on being thin in Western culture. Nevertheless, it is noteworthy that the stereotypes of overweight "endomorphs," tend to portray them as more child-like than the thin, "ectomorphs" or the average "mesomorphs." There are general evaluative differences in the character traits associated with these three body types, with the mesomorph rated most favorably; however, there are also some specific associations. In particular, the endomorph tends to be rated relatively high on child-like traits such as warm-hearted, agreeable, dependent, and trusting (Kiker & Miller, 1967; Sleet, 1969; Wells & Siegal, 1961) .

National Stereotypes

Nationalities differ in the predominance of two major facial types that have been identified by physical anthropologists (Enlow, 1982). As shown in Figure 3.2, one of these types is structurally similar to a baby face, whereas the other is more mature-faced. The more mature-faced

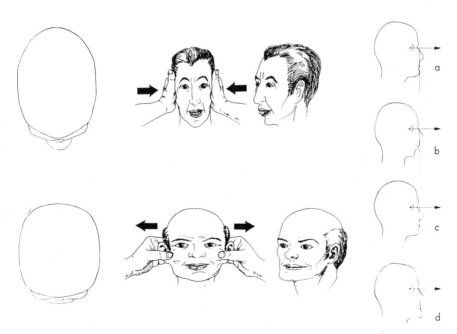

FIGURE 3.2. Views of the dolichocephalic head (top row and *b*) and the brachycephalic head (bottom row and *a* or *d*). From Enlow (1982). Copyright 1982 by W. B. Saunders Co. Reprinted by permission.

type accompanies a long narrow head form, called *dolichocephalic*. This face has a convex profile, like *b* in Figure 3.2. It is narrow, long, and protrusive, with close-set eyes; a relatively thin, longish, and protrusive nose, with a high bridge; and a relatively receding chin. The forehead in this face tends to slope backwards and to jut out over the eyes, which consequently appear deep set. The more baby-faced type accompanies a wide, short, globular head form, called *brachycephalic*. This face has a straight, or even a concave profile, like *a* or *d* in Figure 3.2. It is short, broad, and flat with wide set eyes, and a short, pug-like nose. The forehead in this face tends to be upright, and the eyes are bulging. Although the foregoing features make the brachycephalic face appear more baby-ish, a mature feature of this facial type is its more prominent chin.

Although there is a range of face types within any given group, including mesocephalic faces, which are a mixture of the two basic types, one or the other basic face tends to predominate in different national groups. The dolichocephalic face tends to predominate in Great Britain, Scandinavia, northern Africa, and the Middle Eastern countries of Iran, Afghanistan, Iraq, and Saudi Arabia, as well as in India. The brachycephalic face tends to predominate in middle Europe and the Far East (Enlow, 1982).

Because the facial characteristics that differentiate babies from adults also tend to differentiate one national group from another, the babyish overgeneralization effect may contribute to national stereotypes. Research has shown that national stereotypes actually do differ along the same dimensions as facial maturity stereotypes. One dimension is the degree of dominance or "agency" attributed to the group. National groups that score high on this dimension are perceived as having the same traits that are attributed to mature-faced individuals (and to men)—dominant, assertive, aggressive, ambitious, and independent. Another dimension that differentiates stereotypes of different national groups is empathy and emotionality. National groups that score high on this dimension are perceived as having child-like (and feminine) traits—emotional, sympathetic, and friendly (Eagly & Kite, 1987; Linssen & Hagendoorn, 1994; Peabody, 1985).

There are obviously many factors that contribute to the content of ethnic and national stereotypes (Peabody, 1985; Linssen & Hagendoorn, 1994; Seago, 1947). Interestingly, one predictor is the geographic locale of the nation. People from northern European nations are seen as more dominant, and less emotional and impulsive than those from southern nations (Linssen & Hagendoorn, 1994; Peabody, 1985). A number of explanations for the effects of geographical locale have been suggested, including the effects of climate on social interactions, and a tendency for more enterprising people to migrate to temperate zones

(Linssen & Hagendoorn, 1994). An additional factor that is worthy of exploration is the possibility that the northern national groups, who are stereotyped as dominant and emotionally controlled, show a predominance of the dolichocephalic, mature-faced, facial structure, whereas the southern groups, who are stereotyped as submissive and emotionally expressive, show a predominance of the brachycephalic, baby-faced, structure. Such an effect would be consistent with the finding that national stereotypes are applied more to men than they are to women (Eagly & Kite, 1987). Because adult women retain a more infantile facial configuration than men, the differences between the brachycephalic and dolichocephalic facial types should be more pronounced in men.

Criminal Stereotypes

The babyish overgeneralization effect can also be seen in criminal stereotypes. Lombroso, the founding father of the late 19th-century school of criminal anthropology, argued that criminals could be recognized by their morphological resemblance to apes (Lombroso & Ferrero, 1895). The ape-like facial markers of criminals in this school of thought yield a decidedly nonbabyish appearance. As shown in Figure 3.1, human infants show less resemblance to our evolutionary ancestors than do human adults, who in turn have a more babyish appearance than apes (Gould, 1977; Todd et al., 1980). An analysis of the facial features that Lombroso identified with criminality underscores the fact that they are the antithesis of a baby face. He reported that, compared with normal women, female offenders are more apt to have receding foreheads, overjutting brows, large lower jaws, and prominent cheekbones. Lombroso also reported a relationship between head shape and criminality. Specifically, he claimed that Italian and French provinces marked by a predominance of the mature-looking dolichocephalic faces showed an above average incidence of crimes, whereas those marked by a predominance of the more babyish, brachycephalic faces showed an average crime rate much below that for the country as a whole.

Although Lombroso's tenets may sound outlandish to the modern reader, the assumption that facial appearance and criminality are associated persists. Research has revealed a strong consensus in the general public as to who looks like a criminal (Goldstein et al., 1984; Shoemaker, South, & Lowe, 1973), as well as evidence that more maturefaced individuals are more likely to be convicted of intentional wrongdoing in real as well as in simulated trials (Berry & Zebrowitz-McArthur, 1988; Zebrowitz & McDonald, 1991). Moreover, there is some evidence for accuracy in the associations of appearance and criminal behavior. An early study found that college students did better than chance in guessing which of four crimes had been committed by each of 20 White convicts depicted in photographs (Thornton, 1939). And, there is evidence for a positive association of unattractiveness with criminal behavior (Agnew, 1984; Cavior & Howard, 1973; Cavior, Hayes, & Cavior, 1974; Masters & Greaves, 1967). In the case of women, this association is likely to substantiate Lombroso's assertions, because mature facial features tend to make women unattractive (Friedman & Zebrowitz, 1992; Keating, 1985; McArthur & Apatow, 1983–1984). Also consistent with Lombroso's assertions, preliminary data indicates that juvenile delinquents have a more mature facial appearance than controls matched on age, IQ, ethnicity, and socioeconomic status (Zebrowitz & Blumenthal, 1994).

The Emotion Overgeneralization Effect

Perceivers are highly sensitive to actual correlations between emotion and facial expression, and emotional expressions provide information about an individual's behavioral affordances that facilitates adaptive actions, such as avoiding an angry person and approaching a happy one. Such reactions to the appearance qualities that differentiate people experiencing one or another emotion may be overgeneralized to people whose appearance in some way resembles an emotional expression.

Emotion–Appearance Correlations

Considerable research has demonstrated that at least seven basic emotions can be accurately communicated by facial expressions—happiness, fear, surprise, anger, sadness, disgust, and contempt. In addition to the communication of different emotions by specific facial displays, such as eyebrows raised and drawn together in fear, or pulled down and inward in anger (Ekman, Friesen, & Ellsworth, 1982), the more abstract qualities of curvilinearity versus angularity of the facial configurations are key cues (Aronoff, Barclay, & Stevenson, 1988). There are also dynamic facial cues to emotion, and the point-light technique has demonstrated that movement information itself is sufficient for the accurate identification of emotions, even when no information about the shape and position of facial features is discernible (Bassili, 1979). Perceptual bases of emotion identification are also provided in voice, gait, and gesture (e.g., Mehrabian, 1972; Montepare, Goldstein, & Clausen, 1987; Scherer, 1986).

While there are some cultural differences in emotion recognition, there is also condsiderable evidence for the pancultural generality of emotion reading: people from all corners of the world, including those from an isolated New Guinea tribe, see the same emotion in particular posed facial expressions (see Zebrowitz, 1990, Chap. 4, for a review of relevant research). Insofar as emotion perception from facial expressions is culturally universal, one might expect that this faculty, like facial identification, has an innate, neural basis. Some evidence to support this view is provided by cases of brain damaged individuals as well as normal populations, and the neural basis of emotion recognition seems to be independent of the neural basis of face identification, which was discussed earlier (Benowitz, Bear, Rosenthal, Mesulam, Zaidel, & Sperry, 1983; Ley & Strauss, 1986). Studies of infants also suggest that we are "wired" to perceive particular emotions in particular facial expressions (Ley & Strauss, 1986; Nelson, 1987; Schwartz, Izard, & Ansul, 1985; Sorce, Emde, Campos, & Klennert, 1985).

Impressions of Those Whose Appearance Resembles an Emotional Expression

Given the adaptive value of emotion detection and the strong attunement to appearance correlates of emotion, people may manifest an emotion overgeneralization effect, whereby individuals are perceived to have those traits that are associated with the emotional expressions that their features resemble. Thus, the person whose mouth naturally turns up at the corners may be perceived as happy, and the person with low placed eyebrows may be perceived as angry. Via the processes of temporal extension and nonverbal quasi-communication (Nakdimen, 1984; Secord, 1958), the former individual, who always looks happy, may then be perceived to have the more permanent traits of friendliness and a good sense of humor, whereas the latter individual, who always looks angry, may be perceived as aggressive and dominant. Similarly, because fear drains blood, producing a pallor, the individual or social group with a naturally pale complexion may be perceived as fearful and timid. And, because anger turns the face red, the individual or group with a naturally ruddy complexion may be perceived as angry and aggressive. Some evidence that such "overgeneralizations" may occur is provided by the finding that variations in facial structure yield variations in perceived emotional expression and associated traits. Thus, for example, schematic faces with thick eyebrows are perceived as angrier, as well as less warm and friendly, than the same faces with thin or normal eyebrows. Similarly, more friendliness and a better sense of humor are perceived in people who have more wrinkles at the corner of the eye and more upturned corners on the mouth (Laser & Mathie, 1982; Secord et al., 1954).

Group Stereotypes

Just as the babyish overgeneralization effect may contribute to the content of group stereotypes, so may the emotion overgeneralization effect. Women tend to be "externalizers," showing more facial expressions of emotion than men, whose emotions are expressed more in internal physiological reactions (e.g., Buck, Miller, & Caul, 1974; Hall, 1984). These gender differences in transient facial expressions may, via temporal extension, contribute to the stereotype that women are more emotional and less rational than men (e.g., Broverman et al., 1972). Similarly, the tendency to stereotype some elderly people as despondent and vulnerable (e.g., Schmidt & Boland, 1986) may reflect the resemblance of their lined faces to the emotional expressions of sadness and fear. As noted earlier, such overgeneralizations may sometimes be accurate: Elderly people actually tend to have personality dispositions that match the emotional expressions that their neutral facial expressions resemble (Malatesta et al., 1987).

Sickness Similarities

Fitness-related appearance qualities provide information about an individual's behavioral affordances that facilitates adaptive actions, such as avoiding those with communicable diseases and mating with those who are genetically fit. Such reactions to the appearance qualities that differentiate the fit from the unfit may be overgeneralized to people whose appearance resembles that observed in certain physical or mental disorders. The plausibility of such a basis for stereotyping is bolstered by the fact that many disorders do indeed have visible signs.

Fitness–Appearance Correlations

The traditional medicine of China, Japan, and other Far Eastern cultures emphasizes the face, with physiognomy serving as a principal diagnostic tool (Kushi, 1978). Although the practitioner of traditional Eastern medicine may sound like a witch doctor to many readers, modern diagnosticians continue to utilize physiognomic cues to health, even in the West. Some physiognomic cues may be comprehensible only to the trained physician, such as red discoloration of the cornea and notched teeth in Hutchinson's disease (Goffman, 1963). Others are readily identified by most laymen. For example, bloodshot eyes and a runny nose suggest a cold, allergies, or even drug use.

Facial signs not only may signal a current illness, but they may also aid the diagnosis of an impending one. According to recent press reports, male pattern baldness signals a greater susceptibility to heart disease. People who show low facial expressivity when they are angry reveal symptoms diagnostic of future arthritis, and those who show low facial expressivity when they are sad reveal symptoms indicative of skin problems (Malatesta, Jonas, & Izard, 1987). People with the type of self-healing personality that allows them to achieve health are characterized by unforced, synchronous movements of the eyes, eyebrows, and mouth. They also smile naturally, without holding back the expression of pleasant feelings (Friedman, 1991).

Mental, like physical, fitness may be revealed in the face. Although variations in intelligence within the normal range cannot usually be detected, some forms of mental retardation are accompanied by a distinctive facial appearance (e.g., Down syndrome, cretinism, microcephaly, and hydrocephaly). Mildly retarded children suffering from fetal alcohol syndrome (FAS) also have a distinct pattern of facial malformations, and expert physicians are able to identify FAS children by their looks alone (Clarren, 1981; Clarren et al., 1987). The more minor impairments suffered by the learning disabled may also have visible manifestations, including both dynamic and structural facial qualities (Bryan & Perlmutter, 1979; Bryan & Sherman, 1980; Steg & Rapaport, 1975).

There is a long history to the view that mental illness is manifested in facial appearance. In classical Greek medical theories of the four humors (blood, yellow bile, phlegm, and black bile), melancholics were held to suffer from an excess of black bile, and they were described as bloated and swarthy (Jackson, 1969). The view that insanity has outward manifestations can also be found in art throughout the centuries, and facial images of insanity were as much a part of medical education as of art (Gilman, 1982). Photographs of the insane were scrutinized by Darwin in his seminal study of emotional expressions, and he came to view insanity as characterized by the loss of the ability to control the expression of emotion (Darwin, 1872). Although the emphasis on appearance as a cue to mental illness in past centuries may have been excessive, there seems to be a kernel of truth to this view. Research indicates that mental illness can indeed have visible signs, both in facial structure and facial expression (Campbell, Geller, Small, Petti, & Ferris, 1978; Ekman & Fridlund, 1987; Knight & Valner, 1993; Siegman, 1985).

Group Stereotypes

Social groups whose appearance in some way resembles that of individuals who are physically or mentally unfit may be erroneously perceived as unfit themselves. Thus, similarities between an unattractive and a pained or depressed appearance (e.g., Mueser, Grau, Sussman, &

Rosen, 1984) may contribute to the tendency to stereotype the unattractive as less physically and mentally healthy than the attractive (e.g., Cunningham, 1986; Eagly et al., 1991). This view is reflected not only in the impressions of laypersons, but also in the diagnoses of medical professionals. Unattractive people tend to receive less favorable diagnoses and prognoses from mental health professionals, impressions that may in fact be accurate (Cash, 1985). The physical symptoms of unattractive people are also evaluated more seriously by physicians. Thus, when the same, moderately credible, symptoms were attributed to an attractive and an unattractive woman, doctors perceived the unattractive woman as less healthy and as experiencing more pain and distress (Gilmore & Hill, 1981; Hadjistavropoulos, Ross, & von Baeyer, 1990; Martin, Friedmeyer, & Moore, 1977). Other group stereotypes, such as the view that Blacks are strong (e.g., Zebrowitz et al., 1993), may reflect the obverse of sickness similarities. Insofar as pallor is a sign of illness, dark skin may be taken as a sign of vigor. This may be one of many factors contributing to the less aggressive treatment of illness in Black populations.

Mistaken Identity Effects

As noted earlier, perceivers are highly sensitive to the facial information that reveals an individual's identity, and this ability seems to have a neural basis. The appearance markers of identity provide information about an individual's behavioral affordances that facilitates adaptive actions, such as avoiding potentially dangerous strangers and approaching safe, familiar people. Such reactions to the appearance qualities that identify known individuals may be overgeneralized to adults whose appearance in some way resembles that of the known persons. Such a "mistaken identity" effect is consistent with the exemplar-based model of social judgment, which holds that representations of specific individuals influence judgments about similar persons and groups (Smith & Zárate, 1992).[3] Whereas Smith and Zárate consider many determinants of similarity, arguing that it depends on the perceiver's prior theories and motivation as well as perceptual factors, the mistaken identity effect proposed here focuses on perceptual determinants.

The mistaken identity effect may cause people to be perceived as having the same traits as the significant others or archetypes whom they physically resemble. A Hitler look-alike will have a difficult time convincing people of his warm and nurturant qualities. The woman who resembles Marilyn Monroe will find it hard to convince people of her intellect. And the man who looks like a sleazy politician will have trouble convincing people of his fitness for elective office (Fiske, 1982). A historical illustration of the case of mistaken identity is provided by an account of the initial reactions of the Mexican Indians to the Spanish explorers of the 16th century. They initially viewed the Spaniards as gods, and it has been suggested that they mistook these light-skinned explorers for a white skinned legendary god, Quetzalcoatl, who may have been an early Viking explorer (Prescott, 1966).

The transfer of traits from some significant person to another individual may occur when the person is significant only to the perceiver, a phenomenon akin to the Freudian concept of "transference." Men attribute their own mothers' traits to young women who look like "good mother types," but not to wanton-looking women. Men are also more likely to attribute the traits of a good friend to a woman who physically resembles her than to an equally attractive woman who does not. Young women tend to fall in love with men whose eye color matches their fathers', and they express more positive emotions about a man if he is physically similar to the type of guy they had been attracted to in the past than if he does not physically resemble an old flame, although he may be quite attractive (Andersen & Cole, 1990; Secord & Jourard, 1956; White & Shapiro, 1987; Wilson & Barrett, 1987).

Even a very brief encounter with someone may be sufficient to set in motion the "mistaken identify" effect. When people are asked to choose one of two people for a job requiring a kind and friendly-looking person, their preferences are influenced by whether they had previously interacted with a person resembling one of the job candidates. They are more likely to choose the candidate who resembles someone who had treated them kindly, and they are less likely to choose the candidate who resembles someone who had treated them rudely (Lewicki, 1985). Similarly, Hill, Lewicki, Czyzewska, and Schuller (1990) found that after being exposed to photographs of a few short-faced professors who were known to be fair and a few long-faced professors who were unfair, college students subsequently judged an unknown short-faced professor to be more fair than an unknown long-faced one. They did this even though they were not consciously aware of the correspondence between facial length and fairness among the professors whom they had originally seen.

Because categorization would lose its meaning if it could be evoked by any discriminable difference among people, the findings of Lewicki and his colleagues suggest that exemplars need not influence categorization in order to influence judgments about similar-looking targets. On the other hand, these findings are consistent with the ecological theory assumption that appearance-based stereotyping can be fine grained.

Group Stereotypes

To the extent that there are highly visible individuals from particular social groups, other group members who physically resemble them may be
perceived to have the same traits as those exemplars. In our segregated
society, the Blacks who are most visible to many white Americans are
athletes and musicians, which may contribute to the stereotype of
Blacks as athletic and musical. Similarly, the stereotype that Jews are intelligent and pushy may derive from the fact that the Jews who are most
visible to many Gentile Americans tend to be doctors and lawyers. This
is not so much because a high percentage of Jews occupy these roles, but
rather because these are the only Jews encountered by non-Jews in many
parts of the United States. Thus, a WASP who would describe himself as
liberal and unprejudiced told me at our first meeting that "a Jewish doctor once saved my life," This Jewish exemplar was highly salient to him,
because the doctor was one of the only Jews this small-town Midwest-
erner had known before me. These examples are in some respects akin
to Eagly's (1987) argument that sex stereotypes may derive from the distribution of men and women in different social roles. Thus, women may
be stereotyped as more nurturant than men, because most visible exemplars are in nurturant social roles, whereas men may be stereotyped as
more dominant than women, because they are most visible in leadership
roles.

Animal Analogies

Perceivers are obviously attuned to the appearance of animals. Indeed, a
perusal of children's books reveals that identifying animals is one of the
first things that we are taught, and the investigations of monkeys and
sheep noted earlier as well as animal recognition deficits in brain damaged humans suggest that there may be a neural basis for species recognition (Etcoff, Freeman, & Cave, 1991). Additional evidence for an attunement to animals is provided by the preparedness to develop animal
phobias. There are actually few objects to which people become phobic,
and prime among these are specific animals, particularly snakes and spi-
ders. As Seligman (1971) has noted, the proclivity to develop phobias
toward such objects may be related to the evolutionary survival of the
human species. Differences in appearance among species provides information about behavioral affordances that facilitates adaptive actions,
such as running from dangerous lions, but not from harmless rabbits.
The strength of divergent associations to different animals is under-
scored in humorous depictions such as the Monty Python movie *In
Search of the Holy Grail,* in which a killer monster is a rabbit. Reactions

to the appearance qualities that differentiate one species from another may create an animal overgeneralization effect, whereby people are perceived to have those traits that are associated with the animals that their features resemble.

Although an animal overgeneralization effect may seem a bit farfetched, it is clearly seen in classical writings. A treatise on *Physiognomics* that has been attributed to Aristotle argued that just as animals with coarse hair are brave—the lion, the wildboar, the wolf—so are people with coarse hair. People with smooth, silky hair, on the other hand, Aristotle thought timid as lambs. In the 17th century, Della Porta expressed the logic of animal analogies in the following syllogism: "All parrots are talkers, all men with such noses are like parrots, therefore all such men are talkers" (Della Porta, 1655, quoted in Wechsler, 1982, Chap. 1, p. 179). Lavater, the prominent physiognomist of that era, also endorsed this view, and a 17th century French painter, Charles Le Brun, captured on canvas intriguing similarities between animal and human faces (Lavater, 1879; Le Brun, 1927). The 19th-century novelist, Balzac, drew renowned parallels between the multiplicity of human social types and zoological varieties (Fess, 1924; Marceau, 1976). Further evidence for the propensity to compare humans and animals is provided by Chinese folklore, which categorizes people according to the animal year in which they were born, with individuals born in the year of a particular animal presumed to have traits similar to that animal.

The penchant to draw analogies between the characteristics of animals and humans is not limited to ancient philosophers, physiognomists, and folklorists. It is deeply embedded in our everyday thinking, as evidenced by trait adjectives such as "sheepish," "pigheaded," "bully," "birdbrained," "lionhearted," "catty," "bitchy," "foxy," and metaphors such as "jackass," "dove," "hawk," "bear," "cow," "pig," "wolf." Interestingly, similar terms are used in diverse languages. In Chinese, as in English, a "fox" is cunning, a "sheep" is submissive, and a "wolf" is cruel. And the Chinese, like Americans, call a sharp man "eagle-eyed" and a seductive woman "foxy" (Peng, 1992). Although we usually apply epithets such as "fox" or "leonine" to people whose *behavior* resembles those animals, we may also see "foxy" or "leonine" behavior in people whose faces resemble those animals. Foxes and fox-faced men are judged as shrewd, whereas lions and lion- faced men are seen as dominant and proud (Szymanski & Zebrowitz, 1987).

Group Stereotypes

Stereotyped caricatures of various social groups provide evidence for a tendency to liken them to certain animals. For example, Redfield, a

19th-century physiognomist drew similar profiles of an Irishman and a dog, arguing that the "Irish resemble dogs. Love of contest, love of triumph, and subservience are ruling traits in both characters" (quoted in Appel & Appel, 1974). Of course, a caricaturist can create a physical resemblance where none exists, and it is doubtful that Irish faces truly resemble dogs more than the faces of other ethnic groups (particularly since there are so many different looking dogs). Still, this example underscores a penchant for building stereotypes on physical resemblances to animals, as do caricatures that liken both the Irish and Blacks to apes (Appel & Appel, 1974). Thus, it may be that the resemblance of the stereotypical Jewish nose to the beak of an eagle contributes to the stereotype of Jews as shrewd—possessing the acute perception of the eagle. And, the tendency to stereotype Chinese people as "sly" may reflect in part their foxlike eyes (e.g., Karlins, Coffman, & Walters, 1969; Meenes, 1943).

Functional and Metaphorical Associations

Secord (1958) proposed two additional overgeneralization effects that may contribute to appearance-based stereotyping. One is functional associations. Physical qualities serve certain functions that may be overgeneralized to an associated trait. For example, the finding that people wearing eyeglasses are perceived as more intelligent than those not wearing glasses (e.g., Thornton, 1943, 1944) may derive from associations to the functional properties of glasses: They function to help one read, and such bookish behavior is associated with intelligence. Similarly, the finding that women are perceived as more nurturant than men may derive from associations to the functional properties of breasts: they function to nourish infants, and such activity is overgeneralized to a wide range of nurturant qualities. A second overgeneralization effect proposed by Secord (1958) is metaphorical associations. Physical qualities may be projected to metaphorically associated traits. For example, the stereotype that people with red hair have an excitable temperament may reflect metaphorical associations to the fiery color of their hair, such as "hotheaded." Likewise, semantic associations to the color black may contribute to stereotypes of Black people (Gergen, 1967; Williams, 1964). And the metaphor "crooked" may account for the impression of less honesty in people with more assymetrical faces (Zebrowitz, Voinescu, & Collins, 1995). Like the other determinants of stereotype content proposed in this chapter, it can be argued that functional and metaphorical associations reflect the overgeneralization of accurate information that physical qualities can provide. However, in the case of these two effects, the overgeneralized information does not pertain to the psychological attributes of other people who are physically similar. Rather, it concerns the physical qualities of the stereotyped individuals themselves.

ACCURACY AND OVERGENERALIZATION EFFECTS

It has been argued that the content of group stereotypes may reflect accurate beliefs about the group members, or the overgeneralization of accurate beliefs about individuals who physically resemble the group members, or the overgeneralization of accurate beliefs about physical attributes that the group members possess. One might ask whether most stereotypes are accurate or overgeneralization effects.[4] Although this is an empirical question that is beyond the scope of this chapter, it should be noted that what begins as an overgeneralization effect can end up as an accurate stereotype due to self-fulfilling prophecies. More specifically, different qualities of appearance can cause people to experience different environments, which ultimately cause differences in the character of those who look one way versus another. There are two ways in which this can occur.

First, people's appearance may lead them into situations that reinforce certain behaviors. For example, the physical qualities of women and the obese may cause them to engage in different activities than do men and the slim, and these activities may foster the development of different traits. Second, people's appearance may influence the way they are treated by others (cf. Jussim & Fleming, Chapter 5, this volume). For example, expectancies induced by the babyish overgeneralization effect may cause women and the obese to be treated differently from their male or thin counterparts, which can then elicit the expected behaviors. Self-fulfilling prophecy effects may be fueled by overgeneralized expectations about various stereotyped groups that are expressed in the media and in the popular culture, in addition to those that are expressed in direct interpersonal interactions. The possibility that actual group differences can develop from appearance-based self-fulfilling prophecies indicates that the various overgeneralization effects proposed in this chapter not only can contribute to our understanding of the content of group stereotypes, but also that they may explain actual differences in the behavior of various stereotyped groups.[4]

CONCLUSIONS

The contribution of physical appearance to stereotyping has been considered within McArthur and Baron's (1983) ecological theory of social perception. In support of the ecological position, it has been demonstrated that people are highly attuned to the physical appearance of others, and with good reason. Among other things, appearance provides functionally significant information regarding an individual's age, emotions, health, and identity. Cross-cultural, developmental and physiological research evidence suggests that reading many of these qualities in facial appearance is a fundamental human proclivity that, in some cases, may have a neural basis. Also consistent with the ecological position, appearance exerts a profound impact on trait impressions, and these effects can occur in the absence of appearance-based categorization. Thus, rather than merely serving as a basis for categorization, appearance may itself determine the content of stereotypes about groups who are identified by their appearance. Moreover, as predicted by the ecological theory, such stereotypes may sometimes be accurate, since appearance can provide accurate information about people's traits.

Guided by the ecological question of what socially useful information is provided in perceptible stimulus qualities, the present chapter has identified five overgeneralization effects that may contribute to the content of group stereotypes. Specifically, the functionally significant information that is provided by qualities of appearance associated with age, emotion, health, identity, and species may be overgeneralized to those whose appearance resembles a particular age level (the babyish overgeneralization effect), a particular emotional state (the emotion overgeneralization effect), a particular health status (sickness similarities) a particular individual (mistaken identity effects) or a particular species (animal analogies). Evidence was presented for a possible contribution of each of these overgeneralization effects to the specific content of group stereotypes, including gender stereotypes, height and weight stereotypes, national stereotypes, and criminal stereotypes. Although the accuracy of these group stereotypes is largely unknown, it is possible that some overgeneralization effects may become self-fulfilling prophecies.

The ecological approach to stereotyping developed in the present chapter offers an explanation for the content of beliefs about various social groups, an aspect of stereotyping that has received scant attention from researchers since the ascendance of the social cognition approach. Although stereotype contents are certain to have many determinants, the evidence that has been reviewed indicates that appearance can be a significant contributing factor. This provides a different slant on the "kernel of truth" explanation for the content of group stereotypes: It may reflect the attributes of others whom the group members physically resemble.

ACKNOWLEDGMENT

Preparation of this chapter was supported by National Institute of Mental Health Grant No. MH42684.

NOTES

1. This is not to deny the effects of categorization of stereotyping, but rather to assert that physical qualities can serve as a basis for social impressions in the absence of explicit categorization processes, and that variations in physical qualities should lead to within category variations in social impressions. Research bearing on this assertion will be discussed later
2. An additional tenet of the ecological theory that will not be addressed in the present analysis of stereotyping is that the detection of behavioral affordances and other social properties depends on the perceivers' attunement— the particular stimulus information to which they attend. This, in turn, depends on the perceiver's behavioral capabilities, social goals, and perceptual experience.
3. It is also related to the representativeness heuristic, which can be manifested in a tendency to judge the category membership of people according to their similarity to or "representativeness" of the average person in that category (Kahneman & Tversky, 1973).
4. This question should not be confused with the issue of whether beliefs about a particular social group are generalized to too many members of the group. Rather, the question is whether accurate beliefs about one group of people (babies, angry people, sick people) are overgeneralized to members of another group.
5. It should be noted that a self-fulfilling prophecy effect is only one of several possible relationships between appearance and behavior. Self-defeating prophecy effects may also occur, and behavior may influence appearance (a "Dorian Gray" effect) as well as vice versa. There also may be biologically determined correlations between appearance and behavior.

REFERENCES

Agnew, R. (1984). Appearance and delinquency. *Criminology: An Interdisciplinary Journal, 22,* 421–440.

Albright, L., Kenny, D. A., & Malloy, T. E. (1988). Consensus in personality judgments at zero acquaintance. *Journal of Personality and Social Psychology, 55,* 387–395.

Allport, G. (1954). *The nature of prejudice.* Reading, MA: Addison-Wesley.

Alley, T. R. (1983a). Age-related changes in body proportions, body size and perceived cuteness. *Perceptual and Motor Skills, 56,* 615–622.

Alley, T. R. (1983b). Growth-produced changes in body shape and size as determinants of perceived age and adult caregiving. *Child Development, 54,* 241–248.

Alley, T. R. (1983c). Infantile head shape as an elicitor of adult protection. *Merrill-Palmer Quarterly, 29*, 411- 427.

Andersen, S. M., & Cole, S. W. (1990). "Do I know you?": The role of significant others in general social perception. *Journal of Personality and Social Psychology, 59*, 384–399.

Appel, J. J., & Appel, S. (1974). *The distorted image: Stereotype and caricature in American popular graphics.* New York: Anti-Defamation League of B'nai B'rith.

Arcus, D., & Kagan, J. (1992). *Temperament and craniofacial variation in infants.* Unpublished manuscript, Harvard University.

Aronoff, J., Barclay, A. M., & Stevenson, L. A. (1988). The recognition of threatening facial stimuli. *Journal of Personality and Social Psychology, 54*, 647–655.

Bahrick, H. P., Bahrick, P.O., & Wittlinger, R. P. (1975). Fifty years of memory for names and faces: A cross-sectional approach. *Journal of Experimental Psychology: General, 104*, 54–75.

Bassili, J. N. (1979). Emotion recognition: The role of facial movement. *Journal of Personality and Social Psychology, 37*, 2049–2058.

Baylis, G. C., Rollis, E. T., & Leonard, C. M. (1985). Selectivity between faces in the responses of a population of neurons in the cortex in the superior temporal sulcus of the monkey. *Brain Research, 342*, 91–102.

Bell, R. Q., & Waldrop, M. F. (1982). Temperament and minor physical anomalies. In R. Porter & G. M. Collins (Eds.), *Temperamental differences in infants and young children: CIBA Symposium No. 89* (pp. 206–220). London: Pitman.

Benowitz, L. L., Bear, D. M., Rosenthal, R., Mesulam, M. M., Zaidel, E., & Sperry, R. W. (1983). Hemispheric specialization in nonverbal communication. *Cortex, 19*, 5–11.

Berry, D. S. (1990a). Taking people at face value: Evidence for the kernel of truth hypothesis. *Social Cognition, 8*, 343–361.

Berry, D. S. (1990b). What can a moving face tell us? *Journal of Personality and Social Psychology, 58*, 1004–1014.

Berry, D. S. (1991). Accuracy in social perception: Contributions of facial and vocal information. *Journal of Personality and Social Psychology, 61*, 298–308.

Berry, D. S. (1992). Vocal attractiveness and vocal babyishness: Effects on stranger, self, and friend impressions. *Journal of Nonverbal Behavior, 16*, 41–54.

Berry, D. S., & Brownlow, S. (1989). Were the physiognomists right? Personality correlates of facial babyishness. *Personality and Social Psychology Bulletin, 15*, 266–279.

Berry, D. S., & McArthur, L. Z. (1985). Some components and consequences of a babyface. *Journal of Personality and Social Psychology, 48*, 312–323.

Berry, D. S., & McArthur, L. Z. (1986). Perceiving character in faces: The impact of age-related craniofacial changes on social perception. *Psychological Bulletin, 100*, 3–18.

Berry, D. S., & Zebrowitz-McArthur, L. (1988). What's in a face? Facial maturity and the attribution of legal responsibility. *Personality and Social Psychology Bulletin, 14*, 23–33.

Bond, C. F., Jr., Berry, D. S., & Omar, A. (1994). The kernel of truth in judgments of deceptiveness. *Basic and Applied Social Psychology, 15*, 523–534.

Borkenau, P., & Liebler, A. (1992). Trait inferences: Sources of validity at zero acquaintance. *Journal of Personality and Social Psychology, 62*, 645–657.

Bowman, P. C. (1979). Physical constancy and trait attribution: Attenuation of the primacy effect. *Personality and Social Psychology Bulletin, 5*, 61–64.

Brewer, M. B. (1988). A dual process model of impression formation. In J. K. Srull & R. S. Wyer, Jr. (Eds.), *Advances in social cognition* (Vol. 1, pp. 1–36).

Brewer, M. B., & Lui, L. N. (1989). The primacy of age and sex in the structure of person categories. *Social Cognition, 7*, 262–274.

Brigham, J. C. (1971). Ethnic stereotypes. *Psychology Bulletin, 76*, 15–38.

Brooks, J., & Lewis, M. (1976). Infants' responses to strangers: Midget, adult, and child. *Child Development, 47*, 323–332.

Broverman, I., Vogel, S., Broverman, D., Clarkson, F., & Rosenkrantz, P. (1972). Sex-role stereotypes: A current appraisal. *Journal of Social Issues, 28*, 59–78.

Bryan, J. H., & Perlmutter, B. (1979). Immediate impressions of LD children by female adults. *Learning Disability Quarterly, 2*, 80–88.

Bryan, J. H., & Sherman, R. (1980). Immediate impressions of nonverbal ingratiation attempts by learning disabled boys. *Learning Disability Quarterly, 3*, 19–27.

Buck, R., Miller, R. E., & Caul, W. F. (1974). Sex, personality, and physiological variables in the communication of affect via facial expression. *Journal of Personality and Social Psychology, 30*, 587–596.

Bushnell, I. W. R., Sai, F., & Mullin, J.T. (1989). Neonatal recognition of the mother's face. *British Journal of Developmental Psychology, 7*, 3–15.

Campbell, M., Geller, B., Small, A. M., Petti, T. A., & Ferris, S. H. (1978). Minor physical anomalies in young psychotic children. *American Journal of Psychiatry, 135*, 573–575.

Cash, T. F. (1985). Physical appearance and mental health. In J. A. Graham & A. M. Kligman (Eds.), *The psychology of cosmetic treatments* (pp. 196–216). New York: Praeger.

Cavior, H., Hayes, S., & Cavior, N. (1974). Physical attractiveness of female offenders. *Criminal Justice and Behavior, 1*, 321–331.

Cavior, N., & Howard, L. (1973). Facial attractiveness and juvenile delinquency. *Journal of Abnormal Child Psychology, 1*, 202–213.

Chaiken, S. (1986). Physical appearance and social influence. In C. P. Herman, M. P. Zanna, & E. T. Higgins (Eds.), *Physical appearance, stigma, and social behavior: The Ontario Symposium* (Vol. 3, pp. 143–177). Hillsdale, NJ: Erlbaum.

Cherulnik, P. D., Turns, L. C., & Wilderman, S. K. (1990). Physical appearance and leadership: Exploring the role of appearance-based attribution in leader emergence. *Journal of Applied Social Psychology, 20*, 1530–1539.

Cherulnik, P. D., Way, J. H., Ames, S., & Hutto, D. B. (1981). Impressions of high and low Machiavellian men. *Journal of Personality, 49,* 388–400.

Chesney, M. A., Ekman, P., Friesen, W. V., Black, G. W., & Hecker, M. H. L. (1990). Type A behavior pattern: Facial behavior and speech components. *Psychosomatic Medicine, 52,* 307–319.

Clarren, S. K. (1981). Recognition of fetal alcohol syndrome. *Journal of the American Medical Association, 245,* 2436–2437.

Clarren, S. K., Sampson, P. D., Larsen, J., Donnell, D. J., Barr, H. M., Bookstein, F. L., Martin, D. C., & Streissguth, A. P. (1987). Facial effects of fetal alcohol exposure: Assessment by photographs and morphometric analysis. *American Journal of Medical Genetics, 26,* 651–666.

Collins, M. A., & Zebrowitz, L. A. (1995). The contributions of appearance to occupational outcomes in civilian and military settings. *Journal of Applied Social Psychology, 25,* 129–163.

Crosbie, P. V. (1979). The effects of sex and size on status ranking. *Social Psychology Quarterly, 42,* 340–354.

Cunningham, M. (1986). Measuring the physical in physical attractiveness: Quasi-experiments on the sociobiology of female facial beauty. *Journal of Personality and Social Psychology, 50,* 925–935.

Damasio, A. R., & Damasio, H. (1986). The anatomical substrate of prosopagnosia. In R. Bruyer (Ed.), *The neuropsychology of face perception and facial expression* (pp. 31–38). Hillsdale, NJ: Erlbaum.

Darwin, C. (1872). *The expressions of the emotions in man and animals.* London: John Murray.

Darwin, C. (1958). *The autobiography of Charles Darwin.* New York: Harcourt, Brace, and Co.

Deaux, K., & Lewis, L. L. (1984). Structure of gender stereotypes: Interrelationships among components and gender label. *Journal of Personality and Social Psychology, 46,* 991–1004.

Desimone, R. (1991). Face-selective cells in the temporal cortex of monkeys. *Journal of Cognitive Neuroscience, 3,* 1–18.

Eagly, A. (1987). *Sex differences in social behavior: A social role interpretation.* Hillsdale, NJ: Erlbaum.

Eagly, A. H., Ashmore, R. D., Makhijani, M. G., & Longo, L. C. (1991). What is beautiful is good, but. . ." A meta-analytic review of research on the physical attractiveness stereotype. *Psychological Bulletin, 110,* 109–128.

Eagly, A. H., & Kite, M.E. (1987). Are stereotypes of nationalities applied to both women and men? *Journal of Personality and Social Psychology, 53,* 451–462.

Eagly, A. H., & Steffen, V. J. (1984). Gender stereotypes stem from the distribution of women and men in social roles. *Journal of Personality and Social Psychology, 46,* 735–754.

Eagly, A. H., & Wood, W. (1982). Inferred sex differences in status as a determinant of gender stereotypes about social influence. *Journal of Personality and Social Psychology, 43,* 915–928.

Edwards, C. P. (1984). The age group labels and categories of preschool children. *Child Development, 55,* 440–452.

Ekman, P., & Fridlund, A. J. (1987). Assessment of facial behavior in affective disorders. In J. D. Maser (Ed.), *Depression and expressive behavior* (pp. 37–56). Hillsdale, NJ: Erlbaum.

Ekman, P., Friesen, W. V., & Ellsworth, P. (1982). Does the face provide accurate information? In P. Ekman (Ed.), *Emotion in the human face* (2nd ed., pp. 56–97). Cambridge UK: Cambridge University Press.

Ellis, H., & Young, A. W. (1989). Are faces special? In A. W. Young & H. D. Ellis (Eds.), *Handbook of research on face processing* (pp. 1–26). Amsterdam: North Holland.

Enlow, D. H. (1982). *Handbook of facial growth*. Philadelphia: Saunders.

Esses, V. M., Haddock, G., & Zanna, M. P. (1994). The role of mood in the expression of intergroup stereotypes. In M. P. Zanna & J. M. Olson (Eds.), *The psychology of prejudice: The Ontario symposium* (Vol. 7, pp. 77–102). Hillsdale, NJ: Erlbaum.

Etcoff, N. L., Freeman, R., & Cave, K. R. (1991). Can we lose memories of face? Content specificity and awareness in a prosopagnosic. *Journal of Cognitive Neuroscience, 3,* 25–41.

Feingold, A. (1992). Good looking people are not what we think. *Psychological Bulletin, 111,* 304–341.

Fess, G. M. (1924). *The correspondence of physical and material factors with character in Balzac.* A thesis in romance languages presented to the faculty of the graduate school of the University of Pennsylvania, Philadelphia.

Field, T. M., Cohen, D., Garcia, R., & Greenberg, R. (1985). Mother–stranger face discrimination by the newborn. *Infant Behavior and Development, 7,* 19–25.

Fiske, S. T. (1982). Schema-triggered affect: Applications to social perception. In M. S. Clark & S. T. Fiske (Eds.), *Affect and cognition: The Seventeenth Annual Carnegie Symposium on Cognition.* Hillsdale, N.J.: Erlbaum.

Fiske, S. T., & Cox, M. G. (1979). Person concepts: The effect of target familiarity and descriptive purpose on the process of describing others. *Journal of Personality, 47,* 136–161.

Friedman, H., & Zebrowitz, L. A. (1992). The contribution of typical sex differences in facial maturity to sex-role stereotypes. *Personality and Social Psychology Bulletin, 18,* 430–438.

Friedman, H. S. (1991). *The self-healing personality: Why some people achieve health and others succumb to illness.* New York: Henry Holt.

Funder, D. C., & Colvin, C. R. (1988). Friends and strangers: Acquaintanceship, agreement, and the accuracy of personality judgment. *Journal of Personality and Social Psychology, 55,* 149–158.

Gary, A. L., Davis, L., & DeVivo, P. (1977). Eye color and sex and their effect on counselor self-disclosures. *Journal of Social Psychology, 102,* 247–253.

Gergen, K. J. (1967). The significance of skin color in human relations. *Daedalus, 96,* 391–406.

Gibson, J. J. (1979). *The ecological approach to visual perception.* Boston: Houghton Mifflin.

Gilman, S. L. (1982). *Seeing the insane.* New York: Wiley.

Gilmore, M. R., & Hill, C. T. (1981). Reactions to patients who complain of pain: Effects of ambiguous diagnosis. *Journal of Applied Social Psychology, 11*, 14–22.

Goffman, E. (1963). *Stigma: Notes on the management of spoiled identity.* Englewood Cliffs, NJ: Prentice-Hall.

Goldstein, A. G., Chance, J. E., & Gilbert, B. (1984). Facial stereotypes of good guys and bad guys: A replication and extension. *Bulletin of the Psychonomic Society, 22*, 549–552.

Gould, S.J. (1977). *Ontogeny and phylogeny.* Cambridge, MA: Harvard University Press.

Gould, S.J. (1979). This view of life: Mickey Mouse meets Konrad Lorenz. *Natural History, 88*, 30–36.

Gray, H. (1985). *The anatomy of the human body* (30th American ed.). Philadelphia: Lea & Febiger.

Hadjistavropoulos, H. D., Ross, M. A., & von Baeyer, C. L. (1990). Are physicians' ratings of pain affected by patients' physical attractiveness? *Social Science Medicine, 31*, 69–72.

Hall, J. (1984). *Nonverbal sex differences: Communication accuracy and expressive style.* Baltimore: Johns Hopkins University Press.

Hamilton, D. L., & Sherman, S. J. (1989). Illusory correlations: Implications for stereotype theory and research. In D. Bar-Tal, C. F. Graumann, A. W. Kruglanski, & W. Stroebe (Eds.), *Stereotypes and prejudice: Changing conceptions* (pp. 59–82). New York: Springer-Verlag.

Hamilton, D. L., Stroessner, S. J., & Driscoll, D. M. (1994). Social cognition and the study of stereotyping. In P. G. Devine, D. L. Hamilton, & T. M. Ostrom (Eds.), *Social cognition: Impact on social psychology* (pp. 291–321). San Diego: Academic Press.

Henss, R. (1989). Perceiving age (and attractiveness) in facial photographs. *Arbeiten der Fachrichtung Psychologie,* No. 142, Universitat des Sarrlandes.

Hill, T., Lewicki, P., Czyzewska, M., & Schuller, G. (1990). The role of learned inferential coding rules in the perception of faces. *Journal of Experimental Social Psychology, 26*, 350–371.

Hochberg, J., & Galper, R. E. (1974). Attribution of intention as a function of physiognomy. *Memory and Cognition, 2*, 39–42.

Jackson, S. W. (1969). Galen—On mental disorders. *Journal of the History of the Behavioral Sciences, 5*, 375.

Johnson, M. H., & Morton, J. (1991). *Biology and cognitive development: The case of face recognition.* Oxford: Blackwell.

Jones, G., & Smith, P. K. (1984). The eyes have it: Young children's discrimination of age in masked and unmasked facial photographs. *Journal of Experimental Child Psychology, 38*, 328–337.

Kahneman, D., & Tversky, A. (1973). On the psychology of prediction. *Psychological Review, 80*, 237–251.

Kalma, A. (1992). *Dominance assessment at first glance.* Unpublished manuscript, Institute of Social Psychology, University of Utrecht, The Netherlands.

Karlins, M., Coffman, T. L., & Walters, G. (1969). Fading of stereotypes in three generations of college students. *Journal of Personality and Social Psychology, 13,* 1–16.

Kassin, S.M. (1977). Physical continuity and trait inference: A test of Mischel's hypothesis. *Personality and Social Psychology Bulletin, 3,* 637–640.

Keating, C. F. (1985). Gender and the physiognomy of dominance and attractiveness. *Social Psychology Quarterly, 48,* 61–70.

Kendrick, K. M., & Baldwin, B. A. (1987). Cells in the temporal cortex of sheep can respond preferentially to the sight of faces. *Science, 236,* 448–450.

Kenny, D. A., Horner, C., Kashy, D. A., & Chu, L. (1992). Consensus at zero acquaintance: replication, behavioral cues, and stability. *Journal of Personality and Social Psychology, 62,* 89–97.

Kenny, D. A., Albright, L., Malloy, T. E., & Kashy, D. A. (1994). Consensus in interpersonal perception: Acquaintance and the big five. *Journal of Personality and Social Psychology, 116,* 245–258.

Kiker, V. L., & Miller, A. R. (1967). Perceptual judgment of physiques as a factor in social image. *Perceptual and Motor Skills, 24,* 1013–1014.

Knight, R. A., & Valner, J. B. (1993). Affective deficits in schizophrenia. In C. G. Costello (Ed.), *Symptoms of schizophrenia* (pp. 145–200). New York: Wiley.

Kogan, N., Stephens, J. W., & Shelton, F. C. (1961). Age differences: A developmental study of discriminability and affective response. *Journal of Abnormal and Social Psychology, 62,* 221–230.

Kramer, S. J., Zebrowitz, L. A., San Giovanni, J. P., & Sherak, B. (1995, July 9–14). [Infants' preferences for attractiveness and babyfaceness.] Poster presented at the Eigth International Conference on Perception and Action, Marseilles, France.

Kushi, M. (1978). *Oriental diagnosis.* Boston: Sunwheel.

Laser, P. S., & Mathie, V.A. (1982). Face facts: An unbidden role for features in communication. *Journal of Nonverbal Behavior, 7,* 3–19.

Lasky, R. E., Klein, R. E., & Martinez, S. (1974). Age and sex discrimination in five- and six-month old infants. *Journal of Psychology, 88,* 317–324.

Lavater, J. C. (1879). *Essays on physiognomy.* Translated from German by T. Holcroft. London: William Tegg.

Lawson, E. D. (1971). Hair color, personality, and the observer. *Psychological Reports, 28,* 311–322.

Le Brun, C. (1927). *La physionomie humaine comparée à la physionomie des animaux* (Annotated by L. Metivet). Paris: Henri Laurens.

Lester, D. (1977). Eye color, extraversion, and neuroticism. *Perceptual and Motor Skills, 44,* 1162.

Levesque, M. J., & Kenny, D. A (1993). Accuracy of behavioral predictions at zero acquaintance: A social relations analysis. *Journal of Personality and Social Psychology, 65,* 1178–1187.

Lewicki, P. (1985). Nonconscious biasing effects of single instances on subsequent judgments. *Journal of Personality and Social Psychology, 48,* 563–574.

Ley, R. G., & Strauss, E. (1986). Hemispheric asymmetries in the perception of facial expressions by normals. In R. Bruyer (Ed.), *The neuropsychology of face perception and facial expression* (pp. 269–289). Hillsdale, NJ: Erlbaum.

Liggett, J. (1974). *The human face.* New York: Stein & Day.

Linssen, H., & Hagendoorn, L. (1994). Social and geographical factors in the explanation of the content of European nationality stereotypes. *British Journal of Social Psychology, 33,* 165–182.

Litman, G., Powell, G. E., & Stewart, R. A. (1983). Fine grained stereotyping and the structure of social cognition. *The Journal of Social Psychology, 120,* 45–56.

Livesley, W. J., & Bromley, D. B. (1973). *Person perception in childhood and adolescence.* London: Wiley.

Lombroso, C., & Ferrero, W. (1895). *The female offender.* London: T. Fisher Unwin.

Longo, L. C., & Ashmore, R. D. (1990, August). *The relationship between looks and personality: Strong and general or content specific?* Paper presented at the 98th meeting of the American Psychological Association, Boston.

Malatesta, C. Z., Fiore, M. J., & Messina, J. J. (1987). Affect, personality, and facial expression characteristics of older people. *Psychology and Aging, 2,* 64–69.

Malatesta, C. Z., Jonas, R., & Izard, C. E. (1987). The relation between low facial expressivity during emotional arousal and somatic symptoms. *British Journal of Medical Psychology, 60,* 169–180.

Marceau, F. (1976). *Balzac and his world.* Westport: CT: Greenwood Press. (Original work published 1955 in French under the title *Balzac et son monde.* Paris: Editions Gallimard.)

Mark, L. S., Shaw, R. E., & Pittenger, J. (1988). Natural constraints, scales of analysis, and information for the perception of growing faces. In T. R. Alley (Ed.), *Social and applied aspects of perceiving faces* (pp. 11–50). Hillsdale, NJ: Erlbaum.

Markle, A., Rinn, R. O., & Bell, C. (1984). Eye color as a predictor of outcomes in behavior therapy. *Journal of Clinical Psychology, 40,* 489–495.

Martin, P. J., Friedmeyer, M. H., & Moore, J. E. (1977). Pretty patient—healthy patient? A study of physical attractiveness and psychopathology. *Journal of Clinical Psychology, 33,* 990–994.

Masters, F. W., & Greaves, D. C. (1967). The QuasiModo complex. *British Journal of Plastic Surgery, 20,* 204–210.

McArthur, L. Z. (1982). Judging a book by its cover: A cognitive analysis of the relationship between physical appearance and stereotyping. In A. Hastorf & A. Isen (Eds.), *Cognitive social psychology* (pp. 149–211). New York: Elsevier/North-Holland.

McArthur, L. Z., & Apatow, K. (1983–1984). Impressions of babyfaced adults. *Social Cognition, 2,* 315–334

McArthur, L. Z., & Baron, R. A. (1983). An ecological approach to social perception. *Psychological Review, 90,* 215–238.

McArthur, L. Z., & Friedman, S. (1980). Illusory correlation in impression formation: Variations in the shared-distinctiveness effect as a function of the distinctive person's age, race, and sex. *Journal of Personality and Social Psychology, 39*, 615–624.

McArthur, L.Z., & Solomon, L.K. (1978). Perceptions of an aggressive encounter as a function of the victim's salience and the perceiver's arousal. *Journal of Personality and Social Psychology, 36*, 1278–1290.

Meenes, M. (1943). A comparison of racial stereotypes of 1935 and 1942. *Journal of Social Psychology, 17*, 327–336.

Mehrabian, A. (1972). *Nonverbal communication.* Chicago: Aldine-Atherton.

Montepare, J. M., Goldstein, S. B., & Clausen, A. (1987). The identification of emotions from gait information. *Journal of Nonverbal Behavior, 11*, 33–42.

Montepare, J. M., & McArthur, L. Z. (1986). The influence of facial characteristics on children's age perceptions. *Journal of Experimental Child Psychology, 42*, 303–314.

Montepare, J. M., & Zebrowitz-McArthur, L.(1989). Children's perceptions of babyfaced adults. *Perceptual and Motor Skills, 69*, 467–472.

Montepare, J. M., & Zebrowitz-McArthur, L. (1988a). Impressions of people created by age-related qualities of their gaits. *Journal of Personality and Social Psychology, 55*, 547–556.

Montepare, J.M., & Zebrowitz-McArthur, L. (1988b). Perceptions of adults with childlike voices in two cultures. *Journal of Experimental Social Psychology, 23*, 331–349.

Moskowitz, D. S. (1990). Convergence of self-reports and independent observers: Dominance and friendliness. *Journal of Personality and Social Psychology, 58*, 1096–1106.

Mueser, K. T., Grau, B. W., Sussman, S., & Rosen, A. J. (1984). You're only as pretty as you feel: Facial expression as a determinant of physical attractiveness. *Journal of Personality and Social Psychology, 46*, 469–478.

Nakdimen, K. A. (1984). The physiognomic basis of sexual stereotyping. *American Journal of Psychiatry, 141*, 499–503.

Nelson, C. A. (1987). The recognition of facial expression in the first two years of life: Mechanisms of development. *Child Development, 58*, 889–909.

Passini, F. T., & Norman, W. T. (1966). A universal conception of personality structure? *Journal of Personality and Social Psychology, 4*, 44–49.

Paulhus, D. L., & Martin, C. L. (1986). Predicting adult temperament from minor physical anomalies. *Journal of Personality and Social Psychology, 50*, 1235–1239.

Peabody, D. (1985). *National characteristics.* Cambridge, UK: Cambridge University Press.

Perrett, D. I., Rolls, E. T., & Caan, W. (1982). Visual neurones responsive to faces in the monkey temporal cortex. *Experimental Brain Research, 47*, 329–342.

Pittenger, J. B. (1990). Body proportions as information for age and cuteness: Animals in illustrated children's books. *Perception and Psychophysics, 48*, 124–130.

Prescott, W. H. (1966). *The conquest of Mexico, The conquest of Peru, and other selections.* New York: Twayne.

Roberts, J. V., & Herman, C. P. (1986). The psychology of height: An empirical review. In C. P. Herman, M. P. Zanna, & E. T. Higgins (Eds.), *Physical appearance, stigma, and social behavior: The Ontario Symposium* (Vol. 3, pp. 113–140). Hillsdale, NJ: Erlbaum.

Robinson, T. N. (1981). Eye-color, sex, and personality: A case of negative findings for Worthy's sociability hypothesis. *Perceptual and Motor Skills, 52,* 855–863.

Rosenberg, A., & Kagan, J. (1987). Iris pigmentation and behavioral inhibition. *Developmental Psychobiology, 20,* 377–392.

Rothbart, M., & Taylor, M. (1992). Category labels and social reality: Do we view social categories as natural kinds? In G. R. Semin & K. Fiedler (Eds.), *Language, interaction, and social cognition* (pp. 11–36). London: Sage.

Scherer, K. R. (1986). Vocal affect expression: A review and a model for future research. *Psychological Bulletin, 99,* 143–165.

Scherer, K. R., & Scherer, U. (1981). Speech behavior and personality. In J. K. Darby, Jr. (Ed.), *Speech evaluation in psychiatry* (pp. 115–135). New York: Grune & Stratton.

Schmidt, D. F., & Boland, S. M. (1986). Structure of perceptions of older adults: Evidence for multiple stereotypes. *Psychology and Aging, 1,* 255–260.

Schwartz, G. M., Izard, C.E., & Ansul, S.E. (1985). The 5-month-old's ability to discriminate facial expressions of emotion. *Infant Behavior and Development, 8,* 65–77.

Seago, D. W. (1947). Stereotypes: Before Pearl Harbor and after. *Journal of Psychology, 23,* 55–63.

Secord, P. F. (1958). Facial features and inference processes in interpersonal perception. In R. Taguiri & L. Petrullo (Eds.), *Person perception and interpersonal behavior* (pp. 300–315). Stanford, CA: Stanford University Press.

Secord, P. F., Bevan, W., & Katz, B. (1956). Perceptual accentuation and the Negro stereotype. *Journal of Abnormal and Social Psychology, 53,* 78–83.

Secord, P. F., Dukes, W. F., & Bevan, W. W. (1954). Personalities in faces: I. An experiment in social perceiving. *Genetic Psychology Monographs, 49,* 231–279.

Secord, P. F., & Jourard, S.M. (1956). Mother-concepts and judgments of young women's faces. *Journal of Abnormal and Social Psychology, 52,* 246–250.

Secord, P. F., & Muthard, J. E. (1955). Personalities in faces: IV. A descriptive analysis of the perception of women's faces and the identification of some physiognomic determinants. *Journal of Personality, 39,* 269–278.

Seligman, M. E. P. (1971). Phobias and preparedness. *Behavior Therapy, 2,* 307–320.

Shoemaker, D. J., South, D. R., & Lowe, J. (1973). Facial stereotypes of deviants and judgments of guilt or innocence. *Social Forces, 51,* 427–433.

Siegman, A. W. (1985). Expressive correlates of affective states and traits. In A. W. Siegman & S. Feldstein (Eds.), *Multichannel integrations of nonverbal behavior* (pp. 37–68). Hillsdale, NJ: Erlbaum.

Sleet, D. A. (1969). Physique and social image. *Perceptual and Motor Skills, 28,* 295–299.

Smith, E. R., & Zárate, M. A. (1992). Exemplar-based model of social judgment. *Psychological Review, 99,* 3–21.

Snyder, M., & Miene, P. (1994). On the functions of stereotypes and prejudice. In M.P. Zanna & J. M. Olson (Eds.), *The psychology of prejudice: The Ontario symposium* (Vol. 7, pp. 33–54. Hillsdale, NJ: Erlbaum.

Sorce, J. F., Emde, R. N., Campos, J. J., & Klennert, M. D. (1985). Maternal emotional signaling: Its effects on the visual cliff behavior of 1-year-olds. *Developmental Psychology, 21,* 195–200.

Stangor, C., Lynch, L., Duan, C., & Glass, B. (1992). Categorization of individuals on the basis of multiple social features. *Journal of Personality and Social Psychology, 62,* 207–218.

Steg, J. P., & Rapaport, J. L. (1975). Minor physical anomalies in normal, neurotic, learning-disabled and severely disturbed children. *Journal of Autism and Childhood Schizophrenia, 5,* 299–307.

Szymanski, K., & Zebrowitz, L. A. (1987). *Impressions of male faces as a function of their resemblance to animal faces.* Unpublished research paper, Brandeis University, Waltham, MA.

Tajfel, H., & Turner, J.C. (1986). The social identity theory of intergroup behavior. In S. Worchel & W. G. Austin (Eds.), *Psychology of intergroup relations* (2nd ed., pp. 7–24). Chicago: Nelson-Hall.

Terry, R. (1975). Additional evidence for veridicality of perception based on physiognomic cues. *Perceptual and Motor Skills, 40,* 780–782.

Thornton, G. R. (1939). The ability to judge crimes from photographs of criminals: A contribution to technique. *Journal of Abnormal and Social Psychology, 34,* 378–383.

Thornton, G. R. (1943). The effect upon judgments of personality traits of varying a single factor in a photograph. *Journal of Social Psychology, 18,* 127–148.

Thornton, G. R. (1944). The effect of wearing glasses upon judgment of personality traits. *Journal of Applied Psychology, 28,* 203–207.

Tiberghien, G., & Clerc, I. (1986). The cognitive locus of prosopagnosia. In R. Bruyer (Ed.), *The neuropsychology of face perception and facial expression* (pp. 39–62). Hillsdale, NJ: Erlbaum.

Todd, J. T., Mark, L.S., Shaw, R.E., & Pittenger, J. B. (1980). The perception of human growth. *Scientific American, 242,* 106–114.

Vinacke, W. E. (1949). Stereotyping among national–racial groups in Hawaii: A study in ethnocentrism. *Journal of Social Psychology, 30,* 265–291.

Waldrop, M. F., & Halverson, C. F. (1972). Minor physical anomalies: Their incidence and relation to behavior in a normal and a deviant sample. In R. C. Smart & M. S. Smart (Eds.), *Readings in child development and relationships* (pp. 146–155). New York: Macmillan.

Walton, G. E., Bower, N. J. A., & Bower, T. G. R. (1992). Recognition of familiar faces by newborns. *Infant Behavior and Development, 15,* 265–269.

Watson, D. (1989). Strangers' ratings of the five robust personality factors: Evidence of a surprising convergence with self-report. *Journal of Personality and Social Psychology, 57,* 120–128.

Wechsler, J. (1982). *A human comedy: Physiognomy and caricature in 19th century Paris.* Chicago: University of Chicago Press.

Wells, W. D., & Siegal, B. (1961). Stereotyped somatotypes. *Psychological Reports, 8,* 77–78.

White, G. L., & Shapiro, D. (1987). Don't I know you? Antecedents and social consequences of perceived familiarity. *Journal of Experimental Social Psychology, 23,* 75–92.

Williams, J. E. (1964). Connotations of color names among negroes and caucasions. *Perceptual and Motor Skills, 18,* 121–131.

Williams, J. E., & Best, D. L. (1982). *Measuring sex stereotypes: A thirty-nation study.* Beverly Hills, CA: Sage.

Wilson, G. D., & Barrett, P. T. (1987). Parental characteristics and partner choice: Some evidence for Oedipal imprinting. *Journal of Biosocial Science, 19,* 157–161.

Wilson, P. R. (1968). The perceptual distortion of height as a function of ascribed academic status. *Journal of Social Psychology, 74,* 97–102.

Worthy, M. (1974). *Eye color, sex, and race.* Anderson, SC: Droke House/Hallux.

Zebrowitz, L. A. (1990). *Social perception.* Pacific Grove, CA: Brooks/Cole.

Zebrowitz, L. A., & Blumenthal, J. (1995). *The facial appearance of delinquent and non-delinquent adolescent boys.* Unpublished research paper, Brandeis University, Waltham, MA

Zebrowitz, L. A., Dutta, R., & Collins, M. A. (1995)). *The relationship between facial appearance and personality across the life span.* Unpublished manuscript, Brandeis University, Waltham, MA.

Zebrowitz-McArthur, L., & Montepare, J. M. (1989). Contributions of a babyface and a childlike voice to impressions of moving and talking faces. *Journal of Nonverbal Behavior, 13,* 189–203.

Zebrowitz, L. A., & McDonald, S. M. (1991). The impact of litigants' babyfacedness and attractiveness on adjudications in small claims courts. *Law and Human Behavior, 15,* 603–623.

Zebrowitz, L. A., & Montepare, J. M. (1992). Impressions of babyfaced males and females across the lifespan. *Developmental Psychology, 28,* 1143–1152.

Zebrowitz, L. A., Montepare, J. M., & Lee, H. K. (1993). They don't all look alike: Individuated impressions of other racial groups. *Journal of Personality and Social Psychology, 65,* 85–101.

Zebrowitz, L. A., Voinescu, L., & Collins, M. A. (1995). *Wide-eyed and crooked-faced: Determinants of perceived and real honesty across the lifespan.* Unpublished manuscript, Brandeis University, Waltham, MA.

4

Assessing Stereotype Accuracy: Implications for Understanding the Stereotyping Process

CAREY S. RYAN
BERNADETTE PARK
CHARLES M. JUDD

The accuracy with which we perceive our social world has been a central focus of social perception research. From a practical standpoint, the importance of the accuracy question seems obvious. Employers make judgments about the character and competence of job applicants, clinicians make judgments about the nature of their clients' impairment, social policy makers make judgments about the needs of "special populations," and new acquaintances evaluate each other as potential friends or mates. From a more theoretical standpoint, examining accuracy and errors in social perception can reveal much about the cognitive processes that underlie judgments of social stimuli (e.g., Nisbett & Ross, 1980).

Most of the empirical work on the accuracy of social perceptions has come from the field of person perception. Accuracy research virtually ceased following Cronbach's (1955) classic critique of the methodological problems associated with the assessment of accuracy. Since that time, however, researchers have devoted considerable attention to the development of more sophisticated methods for defining and assessing accuracy. For example, person perception researchers have debated the merits of defining accuracy in terms of consensus between judges (Funder, 1987; Kenny, 1991), correspondence between lay judgments and a normative criterion (Funder, 1987; Kruglanski, 1989; Swann, 1984), correspondence between subjects' judgments and their own internally defined criteria (Kruglanski, 1989), the instrumental value or pragmatic utility of judgments in circumscribed interpersonal contexts (Swann, 1984), and the ability of judgments to predict behavior in realistic social situations (Funder, 1987).

Although it has certainly received far less attention, the issue of accuracy is also important to the study of our perceptions of groups, that is, to the study of stereotypes. Social psychologists have approached the study of stereotyping and prejudice from a variety of theoretical perspectives over the years, and each of these approaches has been accompanied by an implicit assumption about the accuracy of stereotypes. In the early 1900s, for example, scientists believed that the subjugation of Blacks and other minorities was the natural result of their inferiority to Whites. The primary scientific goal was to demonstrate and explain the inferiority of Blacks and other minorities (Duckitt, 1992). The assumption at that time, then, was that the belief in White superiority was accurate, and problems of intergroup relations therefore lay in the inferior qualities of other races. A dramatic reversal soon took place, however; prejudice emerged as an important area of study and the scientific focus shifted to explaining Whites' negatively biased attitudes towards Blacks.

Four major perspectives have dominated the study of prejudice since that time. And, although these perspectives argue that stereotypes serve different purposes, all of them assume that stereotypes are inaccurate. The psychodynamic perspective, for example, argued that prejudice was a result of universal intrapsychic processes such as scapegoating (Dollard, Doob, Miller, Mowrer, & Sears, 1939). Stereotypes were conceptualized as unjustly negative beliefs that served to rationalize an individual's displaced hostility toward some group. According to individual differences perspectives, perhaps best exemplified by the authoritarian personality (Adorno, Frenkel-Brunswik, Levinson, & Sanford, 1950), stereotypes were believed to be the result of a propensity for rigid thinking, which was manifested in the tendency to grossly overgeneralize and exaggerate the attributes of group members (Ashmore & Del Boca, 1981). Sociocultural perspectives, such as realistic group conflict theory (Sherif & Sherif, 1953), conceptualized stereotypes as negative beliefs about a group that serve to legitimize the existing social structure. Most recently, the cognitive perspective has viewed prejudice as a result of social categorization and the limitations of cognitive structures (Allport, 1954; Hamilton, 1981; Hamilton & Trolier, 1986; Tajfel, 1969, 1970). According to the cognitive approach, human beings have a limited capacity for processing information. Stereotypes serve to organize and simplify a complex social world and thus are often likely to take the form of overgeneralizations.

The purpose of this chapter is to explore the long-standing assumption of stereotype inaccuracy. We start with a brief review of previous research on stereotype accuracy, arguing that additional work is necessary to capitalize on the recent advances in the measurement of stereotypes and the assessment of accuracy. We then outline a method to guide the study of stereotype accuracy and review recent empirical research concerning in-group and out-group stereotypes and their accuracy. Finally, we discuss the implications of this work for understanding the stereotyping process and identify directions for future research.

PREVIOUS RESEARCH ON STEREOTYPE ACCURACY

Although inaccuracy has typically been a defining feature of stereotypes, there have been surprisingly few attempts to study the issue empirically. Furthermore, the focus of previous research has been primarily limited to determining whether a particular stereotype under- or overestimated a group's location on stereotypic attribute dimensions. For example, La Piere (1936) wanted to determine whether the stereotype of Armenian laborers as dishonest and overreliant on charity was accurate. He compared perceptions of Armenian laborers with public records indicating the Armenian laborers' actual credit rating and use of public hospitals. La Piere found that people underestimated the group's actual credit rating and overestimated the group's use of public hospitals; he therefore concluded that people's stereotypes of Armenian laborers were exaggerations.

Similarly, McCauley and Stitt (1978) asked White subjects to estimate the percentage of Black Americans and Americans in general who possessed demographic attributes that are generally associated with the stereotype of Blacks (e.g., illegitimate, unemployed, and living in a female headed household). McCauley and Stitt computed "diagnostic ratios" that essentially compared subjects' judgments of the groups with census data indicating the "actual" values of these attributes for each group. They concluded that White subjects underestimated the actual differences between Black Americans and Americans in general. Other researchers have similarly examined accuracy in the stereotypes of regional groups in East Pakistan (Schuman, 1966), hawks and doves on the Vietnam War (Dawes, Singer, & Lemons, 1972), supporters of the women's rights movement (Goldberg, Gottesdeiner, & Abramson,

1975), and gender groups (Martin, 1987). Interestingly, although it is often assumed that the stereotypes of out-groups are particularly likely to be inaccurate, only a few studies have attempted to examine in-group/out-group differences in stereotype accuracy (e.g., Dawes et al., 1972). (See Judd & Park, 1993, for a more detailed review of previous research on stereotype accuracy.)[1]

These studies of stereotype accuracy have essentially focused on the accuracy of subjects' perceptions of the central tendency of a group. This focus is consistent with early approaches in which stereotypes were conceptualized simply as sets of attributes perceived to be characteristic of group members. For example, in the classic study of Katz and Braly (1933), ethnic stereotypes were identified by asking college students to select those traits they considered to be most characteristic of particular ethnic groups. However, more recent conceptualizations of stereotypes include not only perceptions of the modal attributes, or central tendency, of a group but also the variability, or diversity, of group members with respect to those attributes. For example, a fairly extensive literature has demonstrated that in-groups are generally perceived to be more variable than out-groups (e.g., Jones, Wood, & Quattrone, 1981; Judd & Park, 1988; Judd, Ryan, & Park, 1991; Linville, Fischer, & Salovey, 1989; Linville, Salovey, & Fischer, 1986; Park & Judd, 1990; Park & Rothbart, 1982; Park, Ryan, & Judd, 1992). Other research indicates that perceived group variability moderates the extent to which a stereotype is used in making various group-relevant judgments (Krueger & Rothbart, 1988; Park & Hastie, 1987; Ryan, Judd, & Park, in press). In addition, researchers have demonstrated that individuals are generally quite sensitive to the variability of social groups (Nisbett & Kunda, 1985; Park & Hastie, 1987). In short, social scientists have amassed a rather large literature indicating that perceived variability is an important component of social stereotypes. Assessing the accuracy of individuals' perceptions of group variability is therefore important to the study of stereotype accuracy.

In addition to a limited conceptualization of stereotypes, previous research on stereotype accuracy suffers from serious methodological flaws, including response-language confounds and inadequate accuracy criteria, that make it difficult to reach meaningful conclusions. We now turn to a discussion of these methodological problems.

Response-Language Confounds

Extending Cronbach's (1955) classic critique of the assessment of accuracy in person perception, Judd and Park (1993) have identified three types of confounds that make it difficult to interpret the discrepancy between a judgment and a criterion as a measure of stereotype inaccuracy. These confounds result from (1) a judgment-elevation bias, that is, a tendency to provide systematically higher or lower ratings on the response scale; (2) a judgment-positivity bias, that is, a tendency to provide systematically higher central tendency ratings on positive versus negative attributes; and (3) a judgment-extremity bias, that is, a tendency to provide extremity or variability judgments that are either high or low. These biases may be induced by the nature of the judgment task, or they may occur as a result of systematic differences among subjects in their use of the response scales. For example, the standard deviation that is used to assess perceived group dispersion results in systematically higher judgments than does the range measure (Judd et al., 1991). However, this type of judgment-elevation bias may also occur when there are differences among subjects in their use of the response scales, such that some subjects provide higher estimates than others.

Previous research on stereotype accuracy has relied heavily on discrepancy scores to assess accuracy. However, because these three types of confounds in response language preclude meaningful interpretations of the absolute magnitude of discrepancy scores, conclusions from past accuracy research are problematic. Recall, for example, that La Piere (1936) compared perceptions of Armenian laborers with public records indicating the Armenian laborers' "actual" credit rating and use of public hospitals. La Piere found that people underestimated the group's actual credit rating and overestimated the group's use of public hospitals, and concluded that people's stereotypes of Armenian laborers were exaggerations. This sort of stereotype exaggeration may have been due to a general tendency to perceive all groups as dishonest and overreliant on charity, that is, a judgment-extremity bias (Judd & Park, 1993). In short, most of the previous research on stereotype accuracy suffers from these sorts of methodological flaws, that is, the three types of response language confounds. These confounds make it difficult to assess absolute levels of stereotype accuracy. The use of a "full-accuracy" design (Judd & Park, 1993), however, allows the researcher to address a number of important questions concerning stereotype accuracy. In a subsequent section, we describe the full-accuracy design in some detail and identify the sorts of questions that we believe researchers should be asking about the nature of stereotype accuracy.

The Accuracy Criterion

A second methodological problem that has plagued the assessment of stereotype accuracy is the use of invalid accuracy criteria. Using target group members' self-report measures to compute the accuracy criterion has been particularly problematic, because self-report judgments have often not been obtained from a probability sample of group members (e.g., Abate & Berrien, 1967; Dawes et al., 1972; Goldberg et al., 1975; Martin, 1987; Nisbett & Kunda, 1985). This is a serious problem, because there is simply no reason to presume that characteristics derived from the self-reports of a haphazard sample of group members accurately represent the characteristics of the group as a whole.

So how does one determine the group's "actual" central tendency or the "actual" amount of dispersion among group members on a given dimension? In order to empirically assess stereotype accuracy, there must be some way of determining these values. Unfortunately, there is not a simple answer. A number of criteria could be used, each of which has certain biases associated with it. One could eliminate the problem identified earlier by using self-report judgments provided by a probability sample of group members (e.g., Judd & Park, 1993; Judd et al., 1991; McCauley & Stitt, 1978; Schuman, 1966). However, such judgments may still be biased by differences in question wording, context, and response formats. They may also be biased because subjects lack reliable information on which to base their judgments. For example, it may be difficult for subjects to assess their location on attributes such as "analytical" or "nurturant." This may be less problematic, however, when subjects are asked to provide certain attitude judgments, for example, to indicate whether they favor government-subsidized abortions. Biases due to the desire to appear socially acceptable may also be problematic. Although such biases may be minimal for questions that assess preferences or attitudes for which there is not a "right" response (e.g., the extent to which group members enjoy listening to rock music), it seems likely that self-presentational biases will be serious when heavily valenced or socially desirable attributes are assessed (e.g., whether group members engage in illegal activities).

More "objective" accuracy criteria could be used, for example, standardized tests, expert judgments, or public records. These criteria, however, are also subject to biases, including self-presentational issues. For example, records indicating use of mental health centers are likely to be affected by the prevalence and severity of mental health problems as well as the willingness and ability to seek treatment. It may also be difficult to obtain measures using standardized tests or expert judgments for a probability sample of group members. Furthermore, such measures may not exist for many attributes (e.g., personality traits) that define a group's stereotype. Consider, for example, the difficulty of obtaining an "objective" measure of the degree to which group members are "nurturant." In short, although selecting an appropriate accuracy criterion is obviously critical to assessing stereotype accuracy, a correct criterion does not exist. It is therefore important that researchers carefully consider the limitations of the particular criterion they have chosen and, to the extent possible, minimize the biases that are likely to occur. Moreover, when interpreting their results, researchers need to keep the limitations of the criterion in mind.

In our recent work, we have assessed stereotype accuracy for business and engineering majors (Judd et al., 1991) and Democrats and Republicans (Judd & Park, 1993), using self-ratings provided by probability samples of group members as the accuracy criterion. We attempted to minimize biases due to differences in question wording, context, and response formats by asking the same subjects to provide judgments of the target groups and self-ratings on identical attributes, using similar response formats. Note, however, that as we begin to examine the accuracy of stereotypes about such groups as African Americans and White Americans (Ryan, 1994), self-presentational biases associated with self-ratings are likely to be more problematic. Such groups have a long history of conflict, and stronger group loyalties are likely to exist. The attributes contained in these groups' stereotypes tend to be evaluatively loaded; indeed, researchers must inevitably select attributes that vary in their valence in order to examine whether stereotype accuracy depends on the valence of the attributes. However, as we have pointed out, every accuracy criterion has certain biases associated with it.

Consider, for example, the difficulty of assessing the accuracy of perceived intelligence. One could compute an accuracy criterion from group members' self-reports of their own intelligence. Or, one could use a more objective criterion, such as scores on an IQ test. In either case, the criterion must come from a probability sample of group members in order to provide an unbiased estimate of the group's actual self-reported intelligence or, in the latter case, an unbiased estimate of the group's actual score on the intelligence test. Whereas it may not be easy to obtain self-reports from a probability sample of group members, it will often be impossible to administer an IQ test to a probability sample. In addition, although we certainly expect self-presentational biases to be stronger in the case of self-reports, such biases are not eliminated by the use of IQ tests. Performance on an IQ test may be affected by concern about the outcome of the test, as well as by the expertise, interpersonal skills, and even stereotypic beliefs of the individual administering the test. Finally, although the validity of self-reports of intelligence is certainly questionable, the validity of IQ scores may also be questioned, particularly for certain ethnic groups. To reiterate, there is no perfect accuracy criterion; each one is subject to certain biases. Furthermore, the degree to which judgments of a group correspond to group members' self-perceptions seems important, given that it has largely been assumed that stereotypes, by their very nature, are unfair representations of a group. Certainly, the results of such research must be interpreted cautiously, emphasizing that this type of accuracy refers to the extent to which subjects' judgments of the group mirror the aggregated self-perceptions of the members of that group. It is possible that different results would be obtained using a different accuracy criterion.

To summarize, although inaccuracy has long been assumed and has strongly influenced the motivation to study stereotyping, the issue has seldom been examined. Furthermore, there have been recent developments in the conceptualization and assessment of stereotypes that make it possible to examine additional questions about stereotype accuracy. Finally, previous accuracy research has been plagued by serious methodological problems. In the following section, we outline a method for assessing the accuracy of social stereotypes that addresses these methodological problems, and discuss the types of accuracy questions that researchers might be asking. The development of this method has been largely guided by our own and others' work on perceived group variability. We therefore begin with an overview of methodological issues in the assessment of stereotypes, focusing on measures of perceived group variability.

METHODOLOGICAL ISSUES IN THE ASSESSMENT OF STEREOTYPES AND STEREOTYPE ACCURACY

A variety of measures has been used to assess perceived group variability, and the use of different measures has sometimes led researchers to rather different conclusions. In an effort to reconcile some of these conflicting findings, Park and Judd (1990; Park, Judd, & Ryan, 1991) conducted a study that examined the relations among the various measures. Male and female subjects were asked to complete five different tasks in which they judged either men as a group or women as a group. The five tasks included (1) the percentage estimate task, in which subjects estimated the percentage of group members that they believed would possess stereotypic and counterstereotypic attributes (Park & Rothbart, 1982); (2) the distribution task (Judd & Park, 1988; Linville et al., 1986, 1989; Park & Hastie, 1987) in which subjects indicated the distribution of 100 randomly selected group members by placing a number in each of eight boxes spanning a given dimension, with those numbers summing to 100; (3) the dot task (Judd & Park, 1988), in which subjects indicated the distribution of the group as a whole by using one of three sizes of dots to indicate the relative number of group members who fell at each of eight points along a given dimension; (4) the range and mean rating task (Jones et al., 1981), in which subjects rated where on average the group fell on a scale labeled at the end points, and then indicated where the most extreme (highest and lowest) group members would fall; and finally, (5) the similarity rating task (Park & Rothbart, 1982), in which subjects provided a global judgment of how similar group members were to one another, using a 10-point scale.

From these five tasks, Park and Judd (1990) computed 10 measures of perceived group variability. The distribution and dot tasks yielded three measures each: the mean on stereotypic items minus the mean on counterstereotypic items, the standard deviation, and the probability of differentiation, or P_d (see Linville et al., 1986, 1989). The range and mean rating task yielded two measures: the mean on stereotypic items minus the mean on counterstereotypic items, and the extremity difference or range. The percentage estimate task yielded one measure: the percentage on stereotypic items minus the percentage on counterstereotypic items; and finally, the similarity rating task yielded one measure: a simple rating of global similarity.

The pattern of intercorrelations among these measures and a latent variable analysis indicated that the 10 measures assessed two different forms of perceived group variability. Park and Judd (1990) refer to these two forms of perceived variability as stereotypicality and dispersion. The measures of each form of perceived variability and the tasks from which they were derived are given in Table 4.1. Note that 4 of the 10 measures assessed the perceived stereotypicality of a group. Indeed, one of the earliest measures used to assess perceived group variability, the percentage estimation task (Park & Rothbart, 1982), is a measure of perceived stereotypicality. The 3 measures of the difference between the perceived central tendency of the group on stereotypic versus counterstereotypic attribute dimensions also assess perceived stereotypicality. Stereotypicality, then, appears to reflect the extent to which the group as a whole is perceived as fitting the group stereotype. To the extent that subjects perceive most group members to be stereotypic and only a minority to be counterstereotypic, the group is perceived to be more extreme, that is, more stereotypically homogeneous.

Five of the 10 measures assessed the perceived dispersion of a group. These measures include the standard deviation and P_d from the distribution and dot tasks, and the range. Dispersion thus appears to re-

TABLE 4.1. Measures of Perceived Stereotypicality and Dispersion

Task	Stereotypicality	Dispersion
Percentage estimate	Stereotypic items–counterstereotypic items	
Distribution	Stereotypic mean–counterstereotypic mean	Standard deviation P_d
Dot	Stereotypic mean–counterstereotypic mean	Standard deviation P_d
Range and mean rating	Stereotypic mean–counterstereotypic mean	Range
Similarity	Rating	Rating

Note. P_d, probability of differentiation. The similarity task yields one rating that appears to assess both forms of perceived variability although it is not a particularly good measure of either (Judd & Park, 1990).

fer to the extent to which group members are perceived to be tightly clustered or highly dispersed around the mean of the group. The global similarity rating appeared to assess both types of perceived group variability; however, it was not a particularly good measure of either one.

One might expect higher stereotypicality to be associated with lower dispersion. For example, to the extent that one perceives women as a group to be highly stereotypic, one might perceive individual women as being tightly clustered around the group mean, that is, very similar to one another. However, Park and Judd (1990) demonstrated that this need not be the case. That is, these two forms of perceived group variability were essentially orthogonal in their investigation of gender stereotypes. Moreover, the two forms of perceived variability appear to have different effects on judgments of individual group members. For example, some evidence indicates that subjects who perceive a group more stereotypically are more likely to judge individual group members in a stereotype-consistent fashion, whereas subjects who perceive a group to be more dispersed tend to be less confident in their judgments (Ryan et al., in press). Statistically, with highly extreme perceptions of the group (i.e., extreme judgments of central tendency), there is likely to be less perceived dispersion. Nevertheless, we cannot presume that assessing the accuracy of subjects' perceptions of the stereotypicality of the group will necessarily tell us about the accuracy of subjects' perceptions of the dispersion of group members. A comprehensive analysis of stereotype accuracy therefore requires the assessment of both stereotypicality and dispersion.

Three Types of Stereotype Inaccuracy

Current conceptualizations of stereotypes thus enable us to distinguish between the perceived extremity of the central tendency of a group and the perceived dispersion of group members. In addition, stereotypes can be characterized with respect to their perceived valence, that is, the degree to which a group is perceived to be positive versus negative. These three characteristics of stereotypes—perceived central tendency extremity, dispersion, and valence—provide a means of distinguishing among three types of stereotype inaccuracy. First, let us consider stereotypes with respect to the perceived extremity of the group's central tendency on stereotypic versus counterstereotypic dimensions. The traditional notion that stereotypes are exaggerations of "social reality" suggests that stereotypes overestimate the prevalence of stereotypic attributes and underestimate the prevalence of counterstereotypic attributes. In other words, the stereotype is an exaggeration, because the group is perceived to be more stereotypic than is in fact the case. Judd and Park (1993) have referred to this as "stereotypic inaccuracy." Consider, for example, the cultural stereotype of African Americans. Attributes and attitudes that are considered part of this stereotype (Judd, Park, Ryan, Brauer, & Kraus, 1995; Ryan, 1994; Ryan et al., in press) are presented in Table 4.2. To the extent that one's stereotype of African Americans is an exaggeration of social reality, one should overestimate the "actual" central tendency of African Americans on stereotypic dimensions (e.g., streetwise and poor) and underestimate the "actual" central tendency of

TABLE 4.2. Attributes Contained in Cultural Stereotype of African Americans as a Function of Stereotypicality and Valence

Attribute valence	Attribute stereotypicality	
	Stereotypic	Counterstereotypic
Positive	Streetwise	Academically intelligent
	Emotionally expressive	"A kid growing up in the U.S. has unlimited opportunities."
Negative	Poor	Sheltered
	"I've had a lot of run-ins with the police."	"I have usually been given whatever material things I needed or wanted without having to work for them."

African Americans on counterstereotypic dimensions (e.g., academically intelligent and sheltered).

Now consider stereotypes with respect to perceptions of the valence of the group. Traditionally, stereotypes have been conceptualized as inaccurate in their valence. Indeed, traditional approaches generally assume that stereotypes of out-groups are more negative than is in fact the case and are therefore prejudiced. This assumption implies that stereotypes overestimate the prevalence of negative attributes in the group and underestimate the prevalence of positive attributes. Valence inaccuracy may also occur when positive attributes are overestimated and negative attributes are underestimated; in this case, the group would be perceived to be more positive than is in fact the case, a situation that may be more likely to occur for in-group stereotypes. In either case, the examination of valence inaccuracy involves assessing subjects' perceptions of the group's central tendency on positive versus negative attribute dimensions. Consider again the stereotype of African Americans with respect to the attributes in Table 4.2. Valence inaccuracy would occur to the extent that one overestimated the "actual" central tendency of African Americans on negative attributes (e.g., poor and sheltered) and underestimated the "actual" central tendency of African Americans on positive attributes (e.g., streetwise and academically intelligent). In this particular example, one's stereotype would be considered prejudiced. One might expect an out-group member, for example, a White American, to hold a prejudiced stereotype towards this group while also perceiving his or her own group to be relatively more positive than is in fact the case. In this example, then, one's stereotypes would reflect ethnocentrism. Note that, conceptually, stereotypic inaccuracy and valence inaccuracy can be independent of each other; there is no necessary relationship between them. It is possible, for example, to perceive African Americans in a relatively stereotypic manner and yet not feel particularly negative towards them (e.g., one might overestimate both positive and negative stereotypic attributes to the same degree).

Finally, consider stereotypes with respect to perceptions of the dispersion of group members on stereotype relevant attribute dimensions. Stereotypes have often been assumed to be overgeneralizations. This implies inaccuracy in perceptions of the dispersion of group members. More specifically, to the extent that group members are perceived to be more or less dispersed around the central tendency of the group than is in fact the case, there is dispersion inaccuracy. If the inaccuracy is in the direction of perceiving less dispersion among group members than actually exists, the stereotype would be considered an overgeneralization. Consider once again the stereotype of African Americans in Table 4.2.

To the extent that one underestimates the heterogeneity of African Americans on the eight dimensions, one's stereotype may be considered an overgeneralization.

Note that dispersion inaccuracy can occur regardless of one's perceptions of the group's central tendency on these dimensions. As we noted previously, the extent to which a group is perceived to be stereotypic (or negative) need not be related to the degree of dispersion that is perceived to exist among group members (Park & Judd, 1990). This same line of reasoning follows for the assessment of the three forms of stereotype accuracy. Conceptually, it certainly seems possible to perceive African Americans as being quite streetwise and poor (but not academically intelligent or sheltered), on average, and yet perceive that there is a great deal of diversity among individual African Americans. Conversely, one might perceive African Americans to be relatively moderate, on average, with respect to the stereotype and yet fail to perceive much heterogeneity among individual African Americans. One can certainly imagine an individual who does not have an extreme stereotype of African Americans, but who still perceives that "they're all the same to me." It is likely, however, that with more extreme perceptions of the group (i.e., more extreme judgments of central tendency), there may be less perceived dispersion. Again, however, strictly speaking, dispersion inaccuracy need not be related to either stereotypic inaccuracy or valence inaccuracy.

To summarize, stereotypes may be considered inaccurate with respect to three properties: perceived central tendency on stereotypic versus counterstereotypic attribute dimensions (i.e., stereotypic inaccuracy), perceived central tendency on positive versus negative attribute dimensions (i.e., valence inaccuracy), and perceived dispersion of group members on stereotypic and counterstereotypic attribute dimensions (i.e., dispersion inaccuracy). Inasmuch as these forms of stereotype inaccuracy are conceptually unrelated, a comprehensive accuracy analysis requires an assessment of all three types. In previous accuracy research, these distinctions have been ignored so that, for example, stereotypic inaccuracy has been confounded with valence inaccuracy (e.g., La Piere, 1936; McCauley & Stitt, 1978). Moreover, aside from our own recent work (Judd & Park, 1993; Judd et al., 1991), there have been no attempts in previous research to assess the accuracy of stereotypes with respect to the perceived dispersion of group members.

Up to this point, we have discussed two major issues that researchers need to consider in the assessment of stereotype accuracy: methodological problems, including both response language confounds and invalid accuracy criteria; and the assessment of different types of accuracy. We now turn to a discussion of the type of design, that is, the full-accuracy design (Judd & Park, 1993) that will allow more meaningful conclusions than have been possible from past research. The most important characteristic of the full-accuracy design is that it allows the researcher to ask a variety of important questions that are unconfounded with differences in response language. But it is important to keep in mind that the ability to reach more meaningful conclusions rests on the assumption that a reasonably valid accuracy criterion is available.

USING THE FULL-ACCURACY DESIGN TO ASSESS STEREOTYPE ACCURACY

The full-accuracy design requires the collection of data from at least two different subject groups who are asked to judge at least two different target groups with respect to positively valenced and negatively valenced stereotypic and counterstereotypic attributes. Subjects may be asked to make two types of judgments: First, they may be asked to estimate the prevalence of the attributes in the group, for example, by estimating the percentage of group members whom they believe possess particular attributes. Or, they may be asked to indicate their perceptions of the group's central tendency on the attribute dimensions of interest. Either of these judgments allow the researcher to assess both stereotypic and valence inaccuracy. Second, subjects may be asked to indicate their perceptions of the range of individuals in the group, or to generate a frequency distribution of group members from which a standard deviation can be calculated. Both the range and standard deviation measures allow the researcher to assess dispersion inaccuracy. Table 4.3 illustrates the full-accuracy design for a study examining the accuracy of African Americans' and White Americans' stereotypes. If subject and target groups are identical, as in the example given in Table 4.3, the researcher can examine in-group/out-group differences in stereotype accuracy. In any case, the particular attributes that are selected for study should be both stereotypic of one group and counterstereotypic of the other group in order to unconfound target group effects from the effects of attribute stereotypicality. Furthermore, both positively and negatively valenced attributes of each type should be included so that stereotypic inaccuracy and valence inaccuracy can be assessed independently of each other and independently of individual differences in the tendency to give high or low scale ratings.

In principle, the full-accuracy design allows one to assess both the

TABLE 4.3. Example of the Full-Accuracy Design

Attribute type	Subjects		Accuracy criterion
	African Americans	White Americans	
African American target group			
Positive stereotypic	X	X	Y
Negative stereotypic	X	X	Y
Positive counterstereotypic	X	X	Y
Negative counterstereotypic	X	X	Y
White American target group			
Positive stereotypic	X	X	Y
Negative stereotypic	X	X	Y
Positive counterstereotypic	X	X	Y
Negative counterstereotypic	X	X	Y

Note. X's represent subjects' judgments of each target group. These may be prevalence estimates (e.g., judgments of central tendency) or dispersion estimates (e.g., estimates of the range of individuals within the group). Y's represent the target group's "actual" standing on the attribute dimension, that is, the accuracy criterion.

absolute magnitude of inaccuracy as well as relative differences in inaccuracy as a function of, for example, in-group/out-group membership. In practice, however, assessing absolute levels of inaccuracy by examining discrepancies between a judgment and a criterion is highly problematic because of the three types of response language confounds (Cronbach, 1955; Judd & Park, 1993) that we described previously. Obviously, this is a fundamental problem for researchers interested in assessing stereotype accuracy. Traditional assumptions about stereotype accuracy require the examination of discrepancies between subjects' perceptions of the group and the group's "actual" standing on an attribute dimension. But response-language confounds apparently make it impossible to examine these assumptions. What, then, are the kinds of questions that researchers can and should be asking about stereotype accuracy? Actually, the full-accuracy design allows one to ask a number of questions about stereotype accuracy. These questions fall into three main categories: questions concerning relative group differences, within-subject sensitivity correlations, and correlates of stereotype accuracy.

Examining Relative Group Differences

First, one can ask questions concerning *relative group differences* that may exist in stereotypic, valence, and dispersion discrepancy scores. For example, the researcher can compute, for each subject, the difference between that subject's perceived central tendency and the group's actual central tendency on each attribute dimension. These discrepancies can then be analyzed as a function of subject group, target group, and attribute stereotypicality. If identical subject groups and target groups are used (as in Table 4.3), one can then reach meaningful conclusions regarding at least three issues that are likely to be of interest to stereotyping researchers. First, one can examine whether the stereotypes of both in-groups and out-groups are exaggerations by testing for a main effect of attribute stereotypicality; that is, one can examine whether, on average, across target groups and subject groups, stereotypic attributes are overestimated and counterstereotypic attributes underestimated. Second, one can examine whether the stereotype of one target group is exaggerated to a greater extent than the stereotype of the other target group by testing for an attribute stereotypicality by target group interaction. For example, one can ask whether the stereotype of African Americans is exaggerated to a greater degree than the stereotype of White Americans. Third, one can examine whether the out-group stereotype is more exaggerated than the in-group stereotype by testing for an attribute stereotypicality by subject group by target group interaction.

An analysis of the same data as a function of subject group, target group, and attribute valence allows one to ask similar sorts of questions about relative group differences in valence inaccuracy. In this case, the main effect of attribute valence would indicate whether positive attributes are overestimated and negative attributes underestimated, that is, whether there is a general positivity bias. The attribute valence by target group interaction would indicate whether, for example, there is a greater tendency to exaggerate the positivity of White Americans as compared with African Americans. One can also look for evidence of ethnocentrism in the data, that is, whether negative inaccuracies are smaller and positive inaccuracies greater in judgments of the in-group as compared with the out-group (a test of the attribute valence by subject group by target group interaction).

If subjects provide judgments of perceived dispersion and there are measures of actual dispersion in the group, one can similarly examine *relative group differences* in perceived–actual dispersion discrepancies, that is, dispersion inaccuracy. For example, one may wish to analyze perceived–actual discrepancies in group dispersion as a function of subject group and target group, and either attribute stereotypicality or attribute valence. In either case, one is likely to be interested in examining whether subjects underestimate dispersion to a greater extent when judging the out-group as compared with the in-group or, in other words, whether the out-group stereotype is more of an overgeneralization than the in-group stereotype (a test of the subject group by target group interaction). One might also expect a target group main effect indicating, for example, greater dispersion inaccuracy in the stereotype of African Americans than of White Americans; that is, the stereotype of African Americans may be characterized by greater overgeneralization than the stereotype of White Americans.

To illustrate the sorts of problems that arise in the interpretation of results from partial accuracy designs, recall McCauley and Stitt's (1978) study in which White subjects estimated the percentage of Black Americans and Americans in general who possessed demographic attributes that are generally associated with the stereotype of Blacks. Note that McCauley and Stitt's conclusion that White subjects underestimated actual differences between Blacks and Americans in general may have been due to the difference in target groups (i.e., Black Americans vs. Americans in general), the difference in subjects' group membership (i.e., in-group vs. out-group), or the stereotypicality of the attributes (Judd & Park, 1993). Of course, like most of the previous research on stereotype accuracy, there was no attempt to distinguish between stereotypic inaccuracy and valence inaccuracy, nor were subjects asked to provide dispersion estimates.

Other effects may also be of interest when examining stereotypic, valence, and dispersion discrepancy scores; we have pointed out only those that are likely to be of primary interest. The important point is that because of response-language confounds, one can only reach meaningful conclusions about relative group differences in discrepancy scores; conclusions regarding the absolute magnitude of those discrepancies are not possible.

Examining Within-Subject Sensitivity Correlations

Second, one can eliminate the problems associated with discrepancy scores by defining accuracy in terms of subjects' sensitivity to the actual between-attribute differences that exist in a group. Consider, for example, the stereotype that men are aggressive and forceful but not nurturant or passive. A woman's stereotype of men may be accurate in the sense that she accurately detects the extent to which men, as a whole, are aggressive versus passive versus forceful versus nurturant; that is, her perceptions of the group with respect to these four attributes correlate highly with the group's actual location on the four dimensions. This measure of stereotype accuracy is independent of any tendency to under- or overestimate the prevalence of the attributes.

Thus, one can assess stereotype accuracy by examining within-subject sensitivity correlations (e.g., Judd & Park, 1993; Judd et al., 1991) rather than perceived–actual discrepancies. One simply computes, for each subject across attributes, the correlation between a subject's judgments of the group and the group's actual standing on each dimension. Four separate sensitivity correlations can be computed to examine the accuracy of a subject's judgments on stereotypic versus counterstereotypic attributes, and on positively valenced versus negatively valenced attributes. Furthermore, one can compute correlations between the perceived and actual percentage of group members possessing each attribute or, alternatively, between estimates of the perceived and actual central tendency of the group (reflecting sensitivity to between-attribute differences in the preponderance of stereotypic and counterstereotypic attributes). And one can compute correlations between the perceived and actual dispersion of group members (e.g., between the perceived and actual range) across attribute dimensions (reflecting sensitivity to between-attribute differences in dispersion). These correlations can be analyzed in the same manner as discrepancy scores, as a function of target group, subject group, attribute stereotypicality, and attribute valence. Note, however, that sensitivity correlations assess a different kind of stereotype accuracy than perceived–actual discrepancies. Specifically, correlations assess subjects' sensitivity to the actual between-attribute differences of the group. Perceived–actual discrepancies, on the other hand, assess the traditional assumptions concerning stereotype inaccuracy that we described earlier, namely, exaggeration, prejudice, and overgeneralization.

Examining Correlates of Stereotype Accuracy

The third category of questions one can ask concerns the relationship between accuracy, measured either as perceived–actual discrepancies or within-subject sensitivity correlations, and those variables that one might expect to be correlated with stereotype accuracy. At the beginning of this chapter, we noted that a variety of theoretical approaches has guided research on stereotyping and prejudice over the years. These approaches suggest a number of interesting variables that may affect stereotype accuracy. For example, a researcher approaching the problem from an individual differences perspective might want to know whether people who demonstrate an intolerance for ambiguity hold less accurate stereotypes, and whether their stereotypes are particularly less accurate in terms of specific types of inaccuracy. In particular, one might expect intolerance for ambiguity to be associated with the tendency to underestimate perceived dispersion, and a reduced sensitivity to between-attribute differences in the group's actual central tendency or dispersion (i.e., lower sensitivity correlations).

According to social identity theory, perceived threat to a group's well-being ought to increase perceived group differences and ethnocentrism (Tajfel & Turner, 1979). One might expect these sorts of effects in turn to reduce stereotype accuracy and, perhaps, to affect certain types of inaccuracy more than others. It may be, for example, that perceived threat exacerbates in-group/out-group differences in valence inaccuracy such that out-group members overestimate the prevalence of negative attributes and underestimate the prevalence of positive attributes, whereas in-group members overestimate the prevalence of positive attributes and underestimate the prevalence of negative attributes. Individuals may also become more sensitive to between-attribute differences in the out-group's actual location on negative versus positive attributes, and more sensitive to between-attribute differences in the in-group's location on positive versus negative attributes.

One might also wish to examine whether factors such as prejudice and familiarity moderate stereotype accuracy. For example, one could examine whether highly prejudiced individuals demonstrate greater exaggeration or overgeneralization than less prejudiced individuals by examining correlations of prejudice with stereotypic and dispersion discrepancy scores. Similarly, one might wish to examine whether individuals who are more familiar with the group demonstrate greater sensitivity in their judgments of the group from one attribute to another. In this case, one would examine the correlation between familiarity and a within-subject sensitivity correlation reflecting, for example, sensitivity to variations in the group's actual location on stereotypic and counterstereotypic attributes.

Other questions researchers may wish to ask include the following: Do individuals who are more motivated to form accurate judgments of a group demonstrate greater stereotype accuracy? Does the manner in which a stereotype is acquired affect its accuracy? Do members of lower status or less powerful groups show greater sensitivity in their judgments of higher status groups? Do individuals who hold more accurate stereotypes of a group communicate more effectively with representatives of that group? In short, there are a host of interesting questions one could ask about the sorts of factors that play a role in stereotype accuracy. And, for the most part, these sorts of questions have not been examined. We shall return to this issue later in the chapter as we discuss potential causes and consequences of stereotype inaccuracies in more detail.

We have outlined a method for assessing stereotype accuracy that addresses the methodological problems of previous research. We now turn to a more detailed discussion of the findings from our own research on stereotype accuracy, in which we have used a full-accuracy design. Because our accuracy research has been guided largely by work on the perceived variability of social groups, we begin our discussion with an overview of the major issues and findings that have emerged from the perceived group variability literature.

EMPIRICAL RESEARCH ON IN-GROUP AND OUT-GROUP STEREOTYPES AND THEIR ACCURACY

Interest in the perceived variability of social groups was initially motivated by the well-documented out-group homogeneity effect, that is, the tendency to perceive out-groups as less variable than in-groups (Jones et al., 1981; Judd & Park, 1988; Linville et al., 1986, 1989; Park & Judd, 1990; Park & Rothbart, 1982). In an effort to understand this phenomenon, researchers have devoted a great deal of attention to delineating the cognitive processes underlying the acquisition and representation of information about the variability of social categories. This research, which has been strongly influenced by the work of cognitive psychologists studying object categories (e.g., Fried & Holyoak, 1984; Hintzman, 1986; Posner & Keele, 1968, 1970), has resulted in the development of at least three models that attempt to account for the representation of variability information in social categories. Each model provides a different explanation for the development of differences in perceptions of variability, and thus has implications for understanding the accuracy of those perceptions.

Cognitive Representations of Social Categories

The exemplar-based model (Linville et al., 1986, 1989) posits that in-group/out-group differences in perceived variability result from greater familiarity with in-group members. According to this model, people represent category information, primarily in the form of individual instances, or exemplars. When a group variability judgment is needed, a sample of category exemplars is retrieved from memory and from these, a variability judgment is formed. Because people are typically more familiar with the in-group, they tend to have a greater number of in-group than out-group exemplars stored in memory. Assuming that actual variability is equal, and that the same sampling and inference processes occur, groups represented by more instances are expected to be perceived as more variable. Based on this model, Linville and her colleagues (1989) have argued that the out-group homogeneity effect is mediated by greater familiarity with in-group members. Although they have presented a set of studies suggesting that this is indeed the case, none of these studies included measures of familiarity. Furthermore, other research indicates that greater familiarity with the in-group does not mediate the out-group homogeneity effect (Jones et al., 1981; Judd & Park, 1988; Park et al., 1992). In one study, we measured five potential mediators of the out-group homogeneity effect, including familiarity, and then tested the familiarity hypothesis empirically (Park et al., 1992). We found that in-group/out-group differences in familiarity were not related to in-group/out-group differences in perceived variability. Thus, we have argued that greater familiarity with in-group members is not sufficient to account for in-group/out-group differences in perceived variability (Judd & Park, 1988; Kraus, Ryan, Judd, Hastie, & Park, 1993; Park et al., 1991, 1992).[2]

In contrast, proponents of the abstraction-based model (Judd & Park, 1988; Park & Judd, 1990; Park et al., 1991) posit that individuals represent category information in the form of abstractions about the characteristics of the category as a whole, as well as in the form of individual instances. Category-level abstractions include estimates of the perceived central tendency and variability of the group that are formed on-line, as category exemplars are encountered. Individuals are expected to form more highly differentiated representations of in-groups than out-groups as a result of motivational factors (e.g., a veridical representation of the in-group may be considered more useful), encoding processes, and retrieval processes (see Park et al., 1991, for a more detailed overview).

More recently, we have proposed an alternative mechanism of category representation that suggests individuals organize knowledge about groups into subgroups, or subtypes, that are at an intermediate level of generality relative to individual instances and category-level abstractions (Kraus et al., 1993; Park et al., 1992). According to the subgrouping model, we are likely to process information about the in-group at both superordinate and subordinate levels, but we develop less differentiated cognitive structures for the out-group and are therefore more likely to process information about the out-group at a superordinate level of generality (i.e., category-level). Differences in the level at which we process information about in-groups and out-groups lead to differences in perceptions of the variability of group members. One way to assess the degree to which individuals process information at a subordinate level is to ask subjects to generate subgroups for both the in-group and out-group. A larger number of subgroups should reflect a stronger tendency to think about the group at a subgroup level. Consistent with this idea, we have found that people generate a greater number of subgroups for the in-group than for the out-group, and this difference mediates in-group/out-group differences in perceived variability (Park et al., 1992).

The implications of these models for stereotype accuracy have yet to be explored. However, we can speculate on some possibilities. It seems likely that all of these models play a role in the way perceivers mentally represent information about social categories. Perceivers may represent social categories differently depending on such factors as the type of information encountered, the perceiver's relationship to the category, the goal of the perceiver, and the setting in which the information is encountered. Different cognitive representations, then, may lead to greater stereotype accuracy depending on these factors. For example, it seems appropriate that perceivers represent group information in the form of category instances or exemplars early in the process of stereotype development, when there tends to be a relative lack of information on which to base abstractions about the group as a whole. The use of an exemplar-based representation at this stage in the stereotype formation process may result in more accurate perceptions of the group. At some point, however, the amount of information about the group is likely to become rather unwieldy. In order to manage the amount of information, perceivers may form abstractions about the group. Furthermore, depending on how important information about the group is, perceivers may develop relatively complex cognitive structures that include information about various subgroups of the larger group. Recall that we have found that in-group/out-group differences in the generation of subgroups mediates the out-group homogeneity effect for groups having established stereotypes (Park et al., 1992). We have also found that subjects who perceive greater out-group homogeneity are able to make finer discriminations about the in-group's actual location across attribute dimensions, but are unable to make the same sorts of discriminations for the out-group (Judd et al., 1991). Perhaps, then, the organization of information about a group into subgroups leads to more accurate perceptions of the group as a whole at a later stage of the stereotype-development process. Of course, at this point, we can merely speculate. Much more research is needed concerning stereotype accuracy and the conditions under which perceivers are likely to use various types of cognitive structures.

Role of Perceived Group Variability in the Stereotyping Process

Perceived group variability has been the focus of a great deal of research, largely because of its potential for helping us to understand the process of stereotype use; that is, insofar as perceptions of group variability reflect the uncertainty of the stereotype, people who perceive greater diversity among group members should be less likely to use the stereotype (i.e., the central tendency) to make a group-relevant judgment. For example, people who perceive men, as a group, to be highly variable, may be less likely to judge any given individual man they meet in a stereotypic manner. Despite the importance of this implication, however, few studies have directly examined the role of perceived group variability in stereotype use. Using artificial groups in a laboratory setting, Park and Hastie (1987) found that perceived group variability influences the extent to which people generalize from information concerning an individual group member to the group as a whole, as well as the tendency to judge an individual to be a member of a particular social group.

We have recently completed a study that directly examined the role of perceived group variability in the application of stereotypes to individuals whose group membership is known (Ryan et al., in press). We looked at the role of perceived group variability in the use of ethnic group stereotypes, specifically, the stereotypes that Asian Americans are mathematical and that African Americans are mean and threatening. Consistent with the work of Krueger and Rothbart (1988), we found that subjects who perceived a group to be more stereotypic were more likely to judge individual group members in a stereotype-consistent manner. In addition, subjects who perceived a group to be more dispersed were less confident in their trait judgments of individual group members. This research suggests, then, that the two forms of perceived variability identified by Park and Judd (1990) may have different sorts of effects.

The process by which stereotypes influence judgments of individual group members is of critical importance to social scientists as well as society at large. It certainly seems that stereotype accuracy ought to be an important variable influencing the accuracy of judgments of individual group members. However, like defining stereotype accuracy, the process of stereotype use is complex. The relationship between stereotype accuracy and accuracy in judgments of individual group members is thus unlikely to be simple. We will return to this issue at the end of the chapter as we discuss directions for future research on stereotype accuracy.

The Accuracy of Social Stereotypes

More recently, we have begun to examine the extent to which subjects' stereotypes reflect the "actual" variability of in-groups and out-groups, using the full-accuracy design we have described. In one study, we examined the accuracy of in-group and out-group stereotypes in random samples of business and engineering majors at the University of Colorado (Judd & Park, 1993; Judd et al., 1991). Subjects judged both their in-group and their out-group with respect to the same set of eight attributes. Half of the attributes were stereotypic of engineering majors and counterstereotypic of business majors (e.g., analytical); the other half were stereotypic of business majors and counterstereotypic of engineering majors (e.g., extroverted). Subjects completed several tasks to assess perceived stereotypicality and dispersion, including the dot task, the range and mean rating task, and the percentage estimate task that we described earlier. From these tasks, we computed three measures of perceived stereotypicality and three measures of perceived dispersion (see Table 4.1). Subjects also rated themselves on the same set of eight dimensions and from these self-ratings, we computed measures of the groups' "actual" central tendency and variability on each attribute dimension.

First, we examined the data for evidence of out-group homogeneity. The means from the percentage estimate task and the range task are reported in Table 4.4. Note that the stereotypicality means reflect the percentage of group members believed to possess stereotypic attributes minus the percentage of group members believed to possess counterstereotypic attributes. Thus, higher values on the percentage estimate task reflect greater perceived stereotypicality. Higher values on the range task reflect greater perceived dispersion. For both measures, an in-group/out-group difference in perceived variability is indicated by a reliable subject group by target group interaction. Consistent with previous research, these data revealed strong evidence of out-group homogeneity; that is, the out-group was perceived to be both less dispersed and more stereotypic than the in-group. Furthermore, this was true across all of the measures used.

TABLE 4.4. Mean Perceived Stereotypicality and Dispersion

	Target group	
Perceived variability measure	Business	Engineering
Stereotypicality (percentage estimate)		
Business subjects	19.48	39.87
Engineering subjects	34.16	24.02
Dispersion (range)		
Business subjects	15.20	14.42
Engineering subjects	14.23	14.70

Note. Stereotypicality is the percentage of group members perceived to possess stereotypic versus counterstereotypic attributes. Dispersion is the difference between subjects' ratings of the two most extreme (highest and lowest) group members on 21-point scales.

Next we examined stereotype accuracy using both discrepancy scores and sensitivity correlations. For each target group, we computed the actual percentage of subjects who indicated that they possessed each of the eight attributes. We also computed the actual range, that is, the difference between the highest and lowest self-ratings provided by the group members. These were our accuracy criteria. For each subject, we then computed perceived–actual discrepancies by subtracting the actual percentage estimate from the perceived percentage estimate, and the actual range from the perceived range. Thus, positive discrepancies reflect overestimation, and negative discrepancies reflect underestimation of the actual characteristics of the group (i.e., of group members' aggregate self-judgments). Finally, we computed for each subject the correlation between perceived and actual percentage estimates, and between perceived and actual dispersion across the eight attributes. Higher correlations reflect greater sensitivity to between-attribute differences in the group's actual central tendency or actual dispersion. All correlations were transformed to Fisher Z statistics prior to analysis.

Mean discrepancy scores and sensitivity correlations for the percentage estimate measure of stereotypicality are given in Table 4.5. Correlations reported in the tables have been converted back to their original metric. These data revealed consistent in-group/out-group differences in stereotype accuracy. More specifically, discrepancy scores indicated that the stereotype of the out-group was more strongly exaggerated than that of the in-group. And, stereotypicality sensitivity correlations were lower for the out-group than for the in-group, indicating that subjects were less sensitive to between-attribute differences in

TABLE 4.5. Mean Perceived Stereotypicality Discrepancy Scores
and Sensitivity Correlations

	Target group	
Accuracy measure	Business	Engineering
Discrepancy scores		
Business subjects	.74	18.02*
Engineering subjects	8.22*	9.99*
Sensitivity correlations		
Business subjects	.743*	.588*
Engineering subjects	.577*	.709*

Note. Discrepancy scores reflect the extent to which subjects' perceptions of stereotypicality from the percentage estimate task overestimated the group's actual stereotypicality, using the aggregated self-perceptions of group members as the accuracy criterion. Sensitivity correlations are within-subject correlations between the percentage of group members perceived to possess each attribute and the actual percentage of group members indicating that they possessed the attribute.
*$p < .05$.

the out-group's self-reported location on stereotype-relevant dimensions.

Dispersion measures also revealed consistent in-group/out-group differences in accuracy. Mean discrepancy scores and sensitivity correlations for the range measure of perceived dispersion are reported in Table 4.6. The discrepancy scores indicated that overgeneralization (i.e., underestimation of dispersion) was present to a greater degree for the out-group stereotype than for the in-group stereotype, based on our self-report criteria. Furthermore, dispersion sensitivity correlations indicated that stereotype accuracy was somewhat lower for the out-group than the in-group ($p < .08$). Note also that subjects' judgments of dispersion are less sensitive than their judgments of stereotypicality.

A second study assessed stereotypic accuracy for Democrats and Republicans (Judd & Park, 1993), using data from the 1976 National Election Study conducted by the Survey Research Center at the University of Michigan. These data included judgments of Democrats as a group, Republicans as a group, and self-ratings with respect to attitudes towards 10 social policy issues (e.g., school busing). The data also included a measure of each respondent's strength of party affiliation. Data were gathered from a representative sample of voters, so that subjects' self-ratings provided an unbiased estimate of the two groups' actual po-

TABLE 4.6. Mean Perceived Dispersion Discrepancy Scores
and Sensitivity Correlations

	Target group	
Accuracy measure	Business	Engineering
Discrepancy scores		
Business subjects	−.66*	−1.36*
Engineering subjects	−.94*	−1.27*
Sensitivity correlations		
Business subjects	.069	.492*
Engineering subjects	−.080	.518*

Note. Discrepancy scores reflect the extent to which subjects' perceptions of dispersion from the range task overestimated the group's actual range. Sensitivity correlations are within-subject correlations between the perceived range of group members on each attribute dimension and the actual range of group members on that attribute. Both measures use the aggregated self-perceptions of group members as the accuracy criterion.
*$p < .05$

sitions on the policy issues. Note that this accuracy criterion may be less subject to biases that are ordinarily associated with self-ratings. Although it may be that an individual who reports that he or she is analytical is not in fact analytical, it seems more difficult to argue that one who reports that he or she endorses school busing to achieve integration does not in fact hold such an attitude.

As in the previous study, the data indicated that stereotypes of the in-group were more accurate than stereotypes of the out-group; that is, subjects overestimated the stereotypicality of the out-group more than the in-group, and subjects were more sensitive to actual differences among attributes when judging the in-group as compared with the out-group. Finally, recall that in addition to relative group differences in discrepancy scores and within-subject sensitivity correlations, researchers can ask questions about correlates of stereotype accuracy. In this study, Judd and Park (1993) examined strength of party affiliation as a possible moderator of stereotype accuracy among Democrats and Republicans. Interestingly, they found that subjects who were strongly affiliated with their political party were more accurate in their judgments of the in-group and less accurate in their judgments of the out-group than subjects who were weakly affiliated. These results might be seen as inconsistent with the general notion that politically involved individuals are also politically informed in general (e.g., Lusk & Judd, 1988). Rather, it appears that individuals may be more politically informed for the in-group and less so for the out-group. The finding does seem consistent, however, with a social identity theory interpretation. In-group members may be motivated to form more veridical representations of the in-group and to perceive out-group members as more similar to one another. It follows, then, that perceptions of the in-group should be more accurate than perceptions of the out-group (as the previous study also demonstrated), and that this should be more true of individuals who are more strongly identified or affiliated with their group.

To summarize, these studies revealed consistent in-group/out-group differences in stereotype accuracy on a variety of measures. Specifically, stereotypes of out-groups were characterized by greater exaggeration (i.e., overestimation of stereotypic attributes and underestimation of counterstereotypic attributes), and greater overgeneralization (i.e., underestimation of the dispersion of group members), as compared with in-group stereotypes. Furthermore, subjects demonstrated greater sensitivity to actual between-attribute differences in the central tendency and dispersion of in-groups as compared with out-groups. Finally, strength of affiliation with the in-group appears to be one factor that influences stereotypic accuracy.

DIRECTIONS FOR FUTURE RESEARCH: IDENTIFYING THE CAUSES AND CONSEQUENCES OF STEREOTYPE INACCURACIES

We have argued for a more detailed examination of stereotype accuracy than has been possible in past research, noting that stereotype inaccuracy may be manifested in a variety of ways: the tendency to over- or underestimate the actual central tendency (e.g., exaggeration), valence (e.g., ethnocentrism), and dispersion of a group (e.g., overgeneralization), or the relative insensitivity to variations between attributes in these actual values. There is as yet little empirical research concerning the causes and consequences of these different forms of inaccuracy. However, the existing stereotyping literature certainly suggests some interesting possibilities.

First, it certainly seems that group membership should play an important role in both the development of stereotype inaccuracies and in the consequences of these inaccuracies for subsequent group-relevant judgments. Our research indicates that in-group stereotypes are more accurate than out-group stereotypes with respect to both perceived stereotypicality and perceived dispersion. Note, however, that these studies did not investigate in-group/out-group differences in valence accuracy, nor did they investigate stereotype accuracy for groups having strong group loyalties and a history of intense conflict, such as African Americans and Whites. Thus, there remains a need for additional research concerning in-group/out-group differences in the different forms of inaccuracy and the relations among these forms.

In addition to in-group/out-group differences, we believe that investigating the process of induction into a group and its consequences for stereotype accuracy is vitally important to our understanding of the stereotyping process. Group membership is typically treated as a factor that varies only between subjects; subjects are either members or nonmembers of the group. Thus, researchers tend to ignore the fact that an individual's relationship to many groups and social categories (e.g., occupational groups) may be fluid, undergoing change as the individual moves from considering possible group membership to attaining full membership in the group and perhaps ultimately to leaving the group (Moreland & Levine, 1982). The ability to make fine discriminations among group members may be especially important to in-group members, and perceptions of the in-group may therefore be more susceptible to revision in response to new information. We might therefore expect accuracy in perceptions of the dispersion of in-group members to increase as individuals become full-fledged group members. But, at the same time, there may be little change in the accuracy of perceived stereotypicality. We might also expect greater valence *in*accuracy as individuals become more fully identified with their group and are therefore more motivated to perceive it in a positive light. Furthermore, it seems likely that individuals would become increasingly more sensitive to between-attribute differences in the actual characteristics of in-group members, perhaps particularly so on positive attributes. Finally, different types of induction processes may have different sorts of effects on the various forms of stereotype inaccuracies. For example, an induction process that focuses on instilling a sense of positive in-group identity and group cohesiveness may increase valence and dispersion inaccuracy. But an induction process that focuses on the development of certain skills may increase stereotypic inaccuracy and leave valence inaccuracy relatively unaffected.

There are a variety of information-processing factors that seem likely to lead to different types of stereotype inaccuracies. For example, research on illusory correlations suggests that stereotypes develop in part from a tendency to overestimate the frequency of co-occurrence of distinctive stimuli (Hamilton, 1981). Inasmuch as illusory correlations involve the overestimation of the prevalence of distinctive attributes, this information-processing bias seems especially likely to result in stereotype exaggeration. Or, to the extent that the attributes are evaluatively valenced, illusory correlations seem likely to lead to valence inaccuracy. Other research indicates that social perceivers underuse information that disconfirms their stereotypes. For example, individuals may perceive group members who violate the stereotype as exceptions, isolating them into a functionally distinct category (Johnston & Hewstone, 1992; Weber & Crocker, 1983). These subtyped individuals may be seen as unrepresentative of the group and are therefore unlikely to have much effect on the perceiver's stereotype of the group as a whole. Presumably, then, subtyping should result in the underestimation of dispersion and, perhaps, a failure to revise one's perceived central tendency of the group accordingly. A study by Park and Hastie (1987) suggests a means by which stereotypes may become inaccurate with respect to perceived dispersion. Their work indicates that, given identical information, when stereotypes are initially developed based on abstractions about the group rather than on individual instances, the group is perceived to be less variable. Abstraction-based stereotypes, then, seem more likely to lead to the underestimation of dispersion, that is, overgeneralization.

Other work suggests motivational factors that are particularly likely to lead to valence inaccuracy or prejudice. For example, the scapegoating literature suggests that the prevalence of negative attributes will be overestimated in an effort to rationalize one's displaced hostility toward a group (Dollard et al., 1939). In addition, some theories suggest that the derogation of out-groups fulfills a need for self-enhancing social comparisons (e.g., Bettelheim & Janowitz, 1964). More recently, Stangor and Ford (1992) have argued that these sorts of motivations lead the perceiver to adopt an expectancy-confirming orientation to the processing of social information that affects stereotype development. Presumably, such an orientation leads one to develop a stereotype that is inaccurate in some form. Perhaps the type of inaccuracy that develops depends on the particular motivation. For example, self-enhancement motives seem especially likely to lead to valence inaccuracy, whereas an intolerance for ambiguity may be especially likely to lead to stereotype exaggeration and overgeneralization. Stangor and Ford also argued, however, that individuals may often adopt an accuracy orientation in which they attempt to form impressions of social groups that provide important and useful information. Perceivers who adopt such a strategy should form relatively accurate stereotypes, although the degree of accuracy may vary as a function of the characteristics of the social groups about which it is considered most important to be accurate.

In addition to identifying factors that may affect stereotype accuracy, it is also important to investigate the manner in which stereotype accuracy may influence subsequent group-relevant judgments and behaviors. In particular, what role might stereotype accuracy play in trait judgments of individual group members? While it seems that stereotype accuracy should influence the accuracy with which individual group members are judged, this is a complicated issue. The effects of stereotype accuracy will obviously depend on the extent to which the stereotype versus individuating information is used. We know that stereotype use depends on such factors as the strength of the stereotype (Krueger & Rothbart, 1988; Ryan et al., in press), the salience of category information (Beckett & Park, 1995), the diagnosticity of individuating information (Krueger & Rothbart, 1988), the nature of the judgment task (Glick, Zion, & Nelson, 1988), and the social perceiver's goals in a social situation or impression formation task (e.g., Neuberg, 1989). In any case, there appear to be at least two reasons why the stereotype may lead to inaccurate judgments of an individual. First, the stereotype may be too heavily weighted relative to individuating information about the target, and second, the stereotype itself may be inaccurate in a way that is relevant to the particular judgment.

Assuming that the stereotype is activated, and depending on the extent to which it is weighted, our work (Ryan et al., in press) suggests that the different forms of stereotype inaccuracies may affect different sorts of group-relevant judgments. If the stereotypicality of a group is overestimated, it seems likely that an individual member of the group will be judged in a more stereotypic manner than is warranted; that is, stereotype exaggeration should lead one to overestimate the extent to which an individual group member possesses stereotypic versus counterstereotypic traits. Similarly, valence inaccuracy should affect the judged location of an individual group member on trait dimensions. But, it should do so as a function of the valence rather than the stereotypicality of the attribute. For example, a prejudiced stereotype should lead one to overestimate the extent to which an individual group member possesses negative versus positive traits. Finally, dispersion inaccuracy seems likely to affect the confidence with which one judges an individual group member. For example, underestimating the dispersion of a group, that is, overgeneralizing, may lead one to be more confident in judging an individual group member than the evidence warrants.

In addition to trait judgments of individuals, we would expect stereotype inaccuracies to affect social *behaviors* and other sorts of group-relevant judgments, for example, social policy decisions. In general, stereotypic and valence inaccuracies should affect the content of the judgment or behavior, whereas dispersion inaccuracy should affect one's confidence in that judgment. For example, stereotype exaggeration may lead one to overattend to stereotype-consistent information when gathering information about a newly encountered group member (Skov & Sherman, 1986; Snyder & Swann, 1978; Trope & Bassok, 1982). On the other hand, overgeneralization may lead one to terminate the information-gathering phase prematurely. Of course, this type of confirmatory information-gathering strategy is in turn likely to affect stereotype accuracy, resulting in conclusions that the group is more stereotypic and less dispersed than is in fact the case. In the case of social policy decisions, we would expect stereotype exaggeration and prejudice to affect the general content of a social program. But dispersion inaccuracy seems more likely to affect one's confidence that the program will be effective, as well as the degree to which a variety of interventions are deemed necessary to meet the needs of individual group members.

Finally, to the extent that stereotype inaccuracies affect judgments of and behaviors toward the members of a group, it seems likely that they would ultimately affect the behaviors and self-perceptions of the group members themselves. Certainly, there is an extensive literature documenting the existence of a self-fulfilling prophecy in which target group members come to behave or perceive themselves in a manner that is consistent with the stereotypes of others (e.g., Jussim, 1989; Snyder, Tanke, & Berscheid, 1977). Here, we would expect stereotypic and valence inaccuracies to affect the content and affective tone of the target individual's resulting behavior or self-perception. On the other hand, dispersion inaccuracy should affect the strength of the target's resulting behavior and self-perceptions. For example, target individuals may find more opportunities to engage in disconfirming behaviors or may even actively attempt to change an actor's behaviors or perceptions of them if they sense that they are not held with a high degree of confidence. Alternatively, they may give up on their ability to change others' perceptions of them and perhaps even come to believe that the actor's perceptions are indeed correct if the actor's behavior reflects the high degree of confidence that we would expect to result from an extreme underestimation of dispersion.

Clearly, there are unlimited possibilities for additional research; stereotype accuracy seems likely to play a central role in many stereotyping processes. However, because stereotype inaccuracy may take a variety of forms and may have different sorts of effects, our understanding of accuracy and the stereotyping process is likely to be incomplete if research is limited to one group's perceptions of the stereotypicality, or central tendency, of another. The assessment of stereotype accuracy is certainly complex; there are multiple accuracy questions, and they are obviously not easy to address. Nevertheless, we are optimistic about the potential for determining the processes that lead to various forms of stereotype inaccuracy, as well as the processes by which these forms of inaccuracy may influence subsequent group-relevant judgments.

ACKNOWLEDGMENT

This research was supported by National Institute of Mental Health Grant No. R01MH-45049 to Bernadette Park and Charles M. Judd.

NOTES

1. Triandis and Vassiliou (1967) and Vinacke (1949) used similarity of heterostereotypes (i.e., perceptions of an out-group) and autostereotypes (i.e., perceptions that the members of that group have of their group) to indicate that stereotypes contain a kernel of truth. We do not classify these as studies of accuracy, because the assessment of autostereotypes simply provides an indicator of the group members' stereotypes of their own group. Essentially, these studies investigated the content rather than the accuracy of cultural stereotypes.

2. Islam and Hewstone (1993) have demonstrated that amount of contact is positively correlated with greater perceived out-group variability. However, they did not specifically examine either familiarity or the out-group homogeneity effect. Furthermore, as they point out, the process by which amount of contact leads to greater perceived variability is not yet clear.

REFERENCES

Abate, M., & Berrien, F. K. (1967). Validation of stereotypes— Japanese versus American students. *Journal of Personality and Social Psychology, 7,* 435–438.

Adorno, T. W., Frenkel-Brunswik, E., Levinson, D. J., & Sanford, R. N. (1950). *The authoritarian personality.* New York: Harper & Row.

Allport, G. W. (1954). *The nature of prejudice.* Garden City, NY: Doubleday.

Ashmore, R. D., & Del Boca, F. K. (1981). Conceptual approaches to stereotypes and stereotyping. In D. L. Hamilton (Ed.), *Cognitive processes in stereotyping and intergroup behavior* (pp. 1–35). Hillsdale, NJ: Erlbaum.

Beckett, N. E., & Park, B. (1995). Use of category versus individuating information: Making base-rates salient. *Personality and Social Psychology Bulletin, 21,* 21–31.

Bettelheim, B., & Janowitz, M. (1964). *Social change and prejudice.* New York: Free Press.

Cronbach, L. J. (1955). Processes affecting scores on "understanding of others" and "assumed similarity." *Psychological Bulletin, 52,* 177–193.

Dawes, R. M., Singer, D., & Lemons, F. (1972). An experimental analysis of the contrast effect and its implications for intergroup communication and the indirect assessment of attitude. *Journal of Personality and Social Psychology, 21,* 281–295.

Dollard, J., Doob, L., Miller, N. E., Mowrer, O., & Sears, R. (1939). *Frustration and aggression.* New Haven, CT: Yale University Press.

Duckitt, J. (1992). Psychology and prejudice: A historical analysis and integrative framework. *American Psychologist, 47,* 1182–1193.

Fried, L. S., & Holyoak, K. J. (1984). Induction of category distributions: A framework for classification learning. *Journal of Experimental Psychology: Learning, Memory, and Cognition, 10,* 234–257.

Funder, D. C. (1987). Errors and mistakes: Evaluating the accuracy of social judgment. *Psychological Bulletin, 101,* 75–90.

Glick, P., Zion, C., & Nelson, C. (1988). What mediates sex discrimination in hiring decisions? *Journal of Personality and Social Psychology, 55,* 178–186.

Goldberg, P. A., Gottesdeiner, M., & Abramson, P. R. (1975). Another put-down of women? Perceived attractiveness as a function of support for the feminist movement. *Journal of Personality and Social Psychology, 32,* 113–115.

Hamilton, D. L. (1981). *Cognitive processes in stereotyping and intergroup behavior.* Hillsdale, NJ: Erlbaum.

Hamilton, D. L., & Trolier, T. K. (1986). Stereotypes and stereotyping: An overview of the cognitive approach. In J. F. Dovidio & S. L. Gaertner (Eds.), *Prejudice, discrimination, and racism* (pp. 127–163). Orlando, FL: Academic Press.

Hintzman, D. L. (1986). "Schema abstraction" in a multiple-trace memory model. *Psychological Review, 93,* 411–428.

Islam, M. R., & Hewstone, M. (1993). Dimensions of contact as predictors of intergroup anxiety, perceived out-group variability, and out-group attitude: An integrative model. *Personality and Social Psychology Bulletin, 19,* 700–710.

Johnston, L., & Hewstone, M. (1992). Cognitive models of stereotype change (3): Subtyping and the perceived typicality of disconfirming group members. *Journal of Experimental Social Psychology, 28,* 360–386.

Jones, E. E., Wood, G. C., & Quattrone, G. A. (1981). Perceived variability of personal characteristics in in-groups and out-groups: The role of knowledge and evaluation. *Personality and Social Psychology Bulletin, 7,* 523–528.

Judd, C. M., & Park, B. (1988). Out-group homogeneity: Judgments of variability at the individual and group levels. *Journal of Personality and Social Psychology, 54,* 778–788.

Judd, C. M., & Park, B. (1993). Definition and assessment of accuracy in social stereotypes. *Psychological Review, 100,* 109–128.

Judd, C. M., Park, B., Ryan, C. S., Brauer, M., & Kraus, S. (1995). Stereotypes and ethnocentrism: Diverging interethnic perceptions of African American and White American youth. *Journal of Personality and Social Psychology, 69,* 460–481.

Judd, C. M., Ryan, C. S., & Park, B. (1991). Accuracy in the judgments of in-group and out-group variability. *Journal of Personality and Social Psychology, 61,* 366–379.

Jussim, L. (1989). Teacher expectations: Self-fulfilling prophecies, perceptual biases, and accuracy. *Journal of Personality and Social Psychology, 57,* 469–480.

Katz, D., & Braly, K. (1933). Racial stereotypes of one hundred college students. *Journal of Abnormal and Social Psychology, 28,* 280–290.

Kenny, D. A. (1991). A general model of consensus and accuracy in interpersonal perception. *Psychological Review, 98,* 155–163.

Kraus, S., Ryan, C. S., Judd, C. M., Hastie, R., & Park, B. (1993). Use of mental frequency distributions to represent variability information in social categories. *Social Cognition, 11,* 22–43.

Krueger, J., & Rothbart, M. (1988). Use of categorical and individuating information in making inferences about personality. *Journal of Personality and Social Psychology, 55,* 187–195.

Kruglanski, A. W. (1989). The psychology of being "right": The problem of accuracy in social perception and cognition. *Psychological Bulletin, 106,* 395–409.

La Piere, R. T. (1936). Type-rationalizations of group antipathy. *Social Forces, 15,* 232–237.

Linville, P. W., Fischer, G. W., & Salovey, P. (1989). Perceived distributions of the characteristics of in-group and out-group members: Empirical evidence and a computer simulation. *Journal of Personality and Social Psychology, 57,* 165–188.

Linville, P. W., Salovey, P., & Fischer, G. W. (1986). Stereotyping and perceived distributions of social characteristics: An application to in-group–out-group perception. In J. Dovidio & S. Gaertner (Eds.), *Prejudice, discrimination, and racism* (pp. 165–208). New York: Academic Press.

Lusk, C. M., & Judd, C. M. (1988). Political expertise and the structural mediators of candidate evaluations. *Journal of Experimental Social Psychology, 24,* 105–126.

Martin, C. L. (1987). A ratio measure of sex stereotyping. *Journal of Personality and Social Psychology, 52,* 489–499.

McCauley, C., & Stitt, C. L. (1978). An individual and quantitative measure of stereotypes. *Journal of Personality and Social Psychology, 36,* 929–940.

Moreland, R. L., & Levine, J. M. (1982). Socialization in small groups: Temporal changes in individual–group relations. *Advances in Experimental Social Psychology, 15,* 137–192.

Neuberg, S. L. (1989). The goal of forming accurate impressions during social interactions: Attenuating the impact of negative expectancies. *Journal of Personality and Social Psychology, 56*, 374–386.

Nisbett, R. E., & Kunda, Z. (1985). Perceptions of social distributions. *Journal of Personality and Social Psychology, 48*, 297–311.

Nisbett, R. E., & Ross, L. (1980). *Human inference: Strategies and shortcomings of social judgment.* New York: Prentice-Hall.

Park, B., & Hastie, R. (1987). The perception of variability in category development: Instance- versus abstraction-based stereotypes. *Journal of Personality and Social Psychology, 53*, 621–635.

Park, B., & Judd, C. M. (1990). Measures and models of perceived group variability. *Journal of Personality and Social Psychology, 59*, 173–191.

Park, B., Judd, C. M., & Ryan, C. S. (1991). Social categorization and the representation of variability information. In M. Hewstone & W. Stroebe (Eds.), *European review of social psychology* (Vol. 2, pp. 211–245). New York: Wiley.

Park, B., & Rothbart, M. (1982). Perception of out-group homogeneity and levels of social categorization: Memory for the subordinate attributes of in-group and out-group members. *Journal of Personality and Social Psychology, 42*, 1051–1068.

Park, B., Ryan, C. S., & Judd, C. M. (1992). Role of meaningful subgroups in explaining differences in perceived variability for in-groups and out-groups. *Journal of Personality and Social Psychology, 63*, 553–567.

Posner, M. I., & Keele, S. W. (1968). On the genesis of abstract ideas. *Journal of Experimental Psychology, 77*, 353–363.

Posner, M. I., & Keele, S. W. (1970). Retention of abstract ideas. *Journal of Experimental Psychology, 83*, 304–308.

Ryan, C. S. (1994, June). *Stereotype accuracy in a sample of African American and White American college students.* Paper presented at the American Psychological Association Conference on Stereotype Accuracy, Philadelphia.

Ryan, C. S., Judd, C. M., & Park, B. (in press). Effects of racial stereotypes on judgments of individuals: The moderating role of perceived group variability. *Journal of Experimental Psychology.*

Schuman, H. (1966). Social change and the validity of regional stereotypes in East Pakistan. *Sociometry, 29*, 428–440.

Sherif, M., & Sherif, C. W. (1953). *Groups in harmony and tension.* New York: Harper.

Skov, R. B., & Sherman, S. J. (1986). Information-gathering processes: Diagnosticity, hypothesis confirmatory strategies, and perceived hypothesis confirmation. *Journal of Experimental Social Psychology, 22*, 93–121.

Snyder, M., & Swann, W. B., Jr. (1978). Hypothesis testing processes in social interaction. *Journal of Personality and Social Psychology, 36*, 1202–1212.

Snyder, M., Tanke, E. D., & Berscheid, E. (1977). Social perception and interpersonal behavior: On the self-fulfilling nature of social stereotypes. *Journal of Personality and Social Psychology, 35*, 656–666.

Stangor, C., & Ford, T. E. (1992). Accuracy and expectancy-confirming processing orientations and the development of stereotypes and prejudice. In W.

Stroebe & M. Hewstone (Eds.), *European review of social psychology* (Vol. 3, pp. 57–89). New York: Wiley.

Swann, W. B., Jr. (1984). Quest for accuracy in person perception: A matter of pragmatics. *Psychological Review, 91,* 457–477.

Tajfel, H. (1969). Cognitive aspects of prejudice. *Journal of Social Issues, 25,* 79–98.

Tajfel, H. (1970). Experiments in intergroup discrimination. *Scientific American, 223*(2), 96–102.

Tajfel, H., & Turner, J. C. (1979). An integrative theory of intergroup conflict. In W. G. Austin & S. Worchel (Eds.), *The social psychology of intergroup relations* (pp. 33–47). Monterey, CA: Brooks/Cole.

Triandis, H. C., & Vassiliou, V. (1967). Frequency of contact and stereotyping. *Journal of Personality and Social Psychology, 7,* 316–328.

Trope, Y., & Bassok, M. (1982). Confirmatory and diagnosing strategies in social information gathering. *Journal of Personality and Social Psychology, 43,* 22–34.

Vinacke, W. E. (1949). Stereotyping among national–racial groups in Hawaii: A study in ethnocentrism. *Journal of Social Psychology, 30,* 265–291.

Weber, R., & Crocker, J. (1983). Cognitive processes in the revision of stereotypic beliefs. *Journal of Personality and Social Psychology, 45,* 961–977.

III

STEREOTYPE FUNCTION
AND USE

5

Self-Fulfilling Prophecies and the Maintenance of Social Stereotypes: The Role of Dyadic Interactions and Social Forces

LEE JUSSIM
CHRISTOPHER FLEMING

Self-fulfilling prophecies may be particularly pernicious sources of stereotype maintenance, because members of the dominant group can point to the actual behavior of the oppressed group as "evidence" for the "validity" of their stereotypes. A self-fulfilling prophecy occurs when an initially erroneous social belief leads to its own fulfillment. Purely cognitive forms of confirmation involve people interpreting, explaining, or remembering others' behavior as supporting their own beliefs, in the absence of objective evidence of confirmation (e.g., Brewer, Chapter 8, this volume; Darley & Fazio, 1980; Jussim, 1989, 1991; Miller & Turnbull, 1986). In contrast, when a self-fulfilling prophecy occurs, targets actually behave in a manner that confirms the originally erroneous belief.

For example, in the United States in the 19th century, slaves were not allowed to attend school, learn to read, or otherwise receive any sort of formal learning. Slave owners would then point to the ignorance and superstitiousness of the slaves as evidence of their inherent inferiority, and of their need to be "cared for" by "benevolent" slave masters. Similarly, through much of the Middle Ages in many parts of Europe, Jews were not allowed to enter most professions or trades that involved business transactions with Christians, with one notable exception—they were allowed to become money lenders (the canon at the time was that money lending was a sin, so it was prohibited to Christians). Especially when Jews were interested in being repaid for loans, Christians could then point to the sinful, cheap, and grasping nature of Jews as justification for everything from defaulting on loans, to confiscating their property, to pogroms and massacres.

This chapter has several main purposes. Although previous reviews have touched on the role of stereotypes in creating self-fulfilling prophecies (e.g., Darley & Fazio, 1980; Jussim, 1990, 1991; Merton, 1948; Miller & Turnbull, 1986; Snyder, 1984), one unique contribution of this chapter is that it provides the first comprehensive review of existing research in this area. The overwhelming majority of empirical studies of self-fulfilling prophecies have focused on dyadic interactions. Dyadic interactions involve two individuals at a time (teacher–student, employer–employee, etc.). We both describe and critically analyze theoretical and methodological limitations to these studies, and, consequently, their meaning and interpretation. In addition, we discuss some of the factors that may moderate (increase or reduce) dyadic self-fulfilling prophecies. After this review, we draw broad conclusions about the state of, and limitations to, social science knowledge regarding the contribution of dyadic self-fulfilling prophecies to the maintenance of social stereotypes.

Some of the most powerful self-fulfilling prophecies may not occur at the level of interactions between individuals. Instead, they may involve broader societal forces. Our previous examples of slavery in 19th-century America, and Jews in Europe in the Middle Ages did not fundamentally involve dyadic interactions. They involved major political and social factors. Merton's (1948) original article describing the self-fulfilling prophecy emphasized the role of broad sociological forces far more than dyadic interactions. Ironically, however, sociological level self-fulfilling prophecies have received almost no direct empirical attention. Furthermore, many of the specific examples of self-fulfilling prophecies cited in Merton's analysis are no longer relevant today (we will discuss this in more detail later). Therefore, we integrate information from education, social psychology, sociology, anthropology, and current events in an attempt to update Merton's analysis and show how his fundamental ideas are still relevant as we approach the 21st century. First, however, we present a brief historical overview of research and theory on self-fulfilling prophecies.

SELF-FULFILLING PROPHECIES:
HISTORICAL OVERVIEW

The concept of the self-fulfilling prophecy was first proposed by sociologist Robert Merton (1948) who applied the idea to phenomena as diverse as test anxiety and bank failures. However, most of Merton's article focused on understanding the role of self-fulfilling prophecies in creating social problems, such as discrimination against Jews and African Americans. We will return to Merton's analysis in a subsequent section on sociological level self-fulfilling prophecies.

The self-fulfilling prophecy, however, did not receive much empirical attention until Rosenthal's pioneering work on experimenter effects. This research showed that researchers may (intentionally or not) act in such a way as to evoke from their research subjects (animal and human) behavior that confirms their expectations. For example, one study focused on psychology students who were training rats to run a maze (Rosenthal & Lawson, 1964). Half the students were led to believe that their rats were especially smart; the other half were led to believe that their rats were especially dumb. In fact, there were no differences between the rats in the different groups (students were randomly assigned to rats). Nonetheless, it took less time for the rats believed to be smarter to learn to run the maze than it took for the rats believed to be dumber. Students' beliefs about their rats' intelligence were self-fulfilling.

But it was Rosenthal and Jacobson's (1968a) seminal and controversial Pygmalion study that launched self-fulfilling prophecies as a major social and scientific phenomenon. Rosenthal and Jacobson led teachers to believe that some students in their classes were "late bloomers"—students destined to show sudden and dramatic increases in IQ over the course of the school year. In fact, these students had been selected at random. Results showed that, especially in the earlier grade levels, the "late bloomers" gained more in IQ than the other students. Although Rosenthal and Jacobson induced teachers to develop positive expectations, the implications for social problems seemed obvious. The summary of this study, which appeared in *Scientific American* (Rosenthal & Jacobson, 1968b) was titled "Teacher Expectations for the Disadvantaged" presumably because of its (1) relevance to understanding why students from low socioeconomic backgrounds often had difficulties at school, and (2) its potential relevance for alleviating those social problems. Rosenthal and Jacobson suggested that inducing teachers to develop high expectations was at least as effective as programs requiring far more money and effort, such as Head Start.

This study was heavily criticized at the time (e.g., Elashoff & Snow,

1971), and remains controversial today (e.g., Wineburg, 1987). Many critics questioned the very existence of the self-fulfilling prophecy phenomenon (for reviews, see Harris, 1989, and Rosenthal, 1974). Consequently, it sparked numerous attempts at replication and was the prototype for hundreds of follow-up experiments. However, the controversy ended with Rosenthal and Rubin's (1978) meta-analysis of the first 345 studies, which conclusively documented the existence of self-fulfilling prophecies.

With the basic phenomenon firmly established, many researchers began studying the social and psychological processes underlying self-fulfilling prophecies. Virtually all major reviews (e.g., Brophy & Good, 1974; Darley & Fazio, 1980; Jussim, 1986) agree that three main steps are necessary for a self-fulfilling prophecy to occur:

1. Perceivers develop erroneous expectations.
2. Perceivers' expectations influence how they treat targets.
3. Targets react to this treatment with behavior that confirms the expectation.

Abundant evidence documents the role of stereotypes in leading to erroneous expectations for individuals (e.g., Allport, 1954; Hamilton, Sherman, & Ruvolo, 1990). Because the role of stereotypes in leading to expectations for individuals is also addressed in many of the chapters in this book, our review will focus primarily on the latter two steps—evidence showing that stereotype-based expectations lead perceivers to treat targets differently, depending on targets' social group membership; and evidence showing that targets respond to such differential treatment in a manner that confirms the stereotype-based expectation.

The role of self-fulfilling prophecies in contributing to the long-term maintenance of inaccurate social beliefs may now be obvious—Through self-fulfilling prophecies, initially false beliefs become objectively true. Thus, Rosenthal and Lawson's (1964) students' "smart" rats really did run mazes more quickly; and Rosenthal and Jacobson's (1968a, 1968b) "late bloomers" really did obtain higher IQ test scores. Thus, even if a stereotype is initially inaccurate, if the stereotype is self-fulfilling, people can then point to the "evidence" as "support" for their stereotype. Theoretically, therefore, initially inaccurate beliefs may be maintained indefinitely. Consequently, this chapter reviews research that documents how stereotypes may be self-fulfilling and also discusses some of the limitations to the stereotype-maintaining effects of self-fulfilling prophecies. Next, therefore, we review the empirical evidence regarding dyadic self-fulfilling prophecies.

DYADIC SELF-FULFILLING PROPHECIES

Social psychological research has focused extensively and almost exclusively on self-fulfilling prophecies occurring between two individuals. Research has explicitly examined whether and how stereotypes about ethnicity, gender, social class, physical attractiveness, and hyperactivity in children lead to self-fulfilling prophecies.

Ethnicity

The role of self-fulfilling prophecies in contributing to inequalities between ethnic groups may seem "obvious." The dominant ethnic group (Whites) holds negative stereotypes about many ethnic minority groups; Whites treat members of ethnic minority groups less favorably than they treat other Whites, so that members of minority groups receive lower quality education and lower paying jobs (if any).

Undoubtedly, this sequence may sometimes occur. And the desire to understand social sources of inequality may underlie much research on self-fulfilling prophecies. However, we are aware of only a single study implicating self-fulfilling prophecies in ethnic inequalities. In the first of Word, Zanna, and Cooper's (1974) classic experiments, White perceivers interviewed targets for a job. In fact, however, targets were confederates who had been carefully trained to engage in the same set of behaviors with each subject. Half the confederate targets were African Americans and half were White. The main dependent variables were interviewers' nonverbal behavior.

Consistent with a self-fulfilling prophecy, perceivers were colder to African American targets than to White targets. In comparison to White targets, interviewers sat farther away from African American targets, had more speech dysfluencies when talking to them, and conducted shorter interviews.

This, however, only shows that White perceivers treated African American interviewees differently than they treated White interviewees. It does not show that this treatment actually undermined the performance of the African American interviewees. This, however, was the purpose of their second experiment.

In the second experiment, confederates were trained to interview subject–applicants in either of two ways: (1) the cold style comparable to that received by the African American interviewees in Study 1, or (2) the warm style comparable to that received by the White interviewees in Study 2. All subject–applicants in this study were White. Results showed that the applicants who were treated coldly, as were the African American applicants in Study 1, actually performed more poorly in the interview (as rated by independent judges) than did the applicants treated warmly. The type of treatment accorded African American applicants in Study 1 undermined the actual interview performance of White applicants in Study 2. Thus, Whites' stereotypes were fulfilled.

The research on ethnicity and self-fulfilling prophecies is extremely limited in several ways. First, Word et al. (1974) remains the only study examining influences of ethnic stereotypes on target behavior. The study needs replication. Would the pattern hold today, in colleges other than Princeton (where it was conducted), and among nonstudent samples? Our view is that this is an extremely narrow base from which to reach any firm conclusions.

Second, the existence of social and economic inequalities is a phenomenon to be explained. Although it may be consistent with a self-fulfilling prophecy explanation, it does not provide prima facie evidence that all, or even most, ethnic differences result from self-fulfilling prophecies. In fact, one of the few studies to assess empirically the validity of Whites' racial stereotypes found that Whites actually tend to *underestimate* differences between African Americans and other Americans (McCauley & Stitt, 1978). This result suggests that self-fulfilling prophecies would often operate to *reduce* ethnic inequalities.

Third, throughout U.S. history, many ethnic groups (e.g., Asians, Irish, Jews) have been the target of intensely negative stereotypes (and prejudice and discrimination), but have nonetheless attained educational and occupational success comparable to or beyond that of most Whites (Marger, 1991). Thus, although dyadic self-fulfilling prophecies may contribute to ethnic differences, the magnitude of that contribution is probably modest, and they are certainly only one among many contributors.

Fourth, the United States remains highly segregated (e.g., Marger, 1991). This means that many African Americans rarely interact with Whites. Therefore, mistreatment of individual African Americans by individual Whites probably cannot provide a comprehensive account of ethnic inequalities. In the section on group-level, self-fulfilling prophecies, however, we will discuss these issues in more detail.

Gender

Both experimental and naturalistic studies have documented the potentially self-fulfilling nature of gender stereotypes. First we discuss the experiments, and then we review the naturalistic studies.

Experimental Studies

Zanna and Pack (1975) led female students to believe that they would be interacting with either a desirable or undesirable man, who held either traditional or nontraditional gender-role stereotypes. These female students expressed more traditional gender-role attitudes and scored more poorly on an anagrams test when they believed they would interact with a desirable man holding traditional gender-role attitudes (in comparison to when they believed they would interact with either of the undesirable men or with a desirable man holding nontraditional gender-role attitudes). In a follow-up study (von Baeyer, Sherk, & Zanna, 1981), women actually met with a male job interviewer who (they were informed) held either sexist or nonsexist attitudes. When anticipating a sexist interviewer, the women arrived wearing more makeup and accessories, and were less likely to make eye contact. They were also more likely to respond to questions concerning marriage and children in traditionally feminine ways.

These studies show that when women want something from sexist men, they may alter their behavior to confirm traditional stereotypes about women. These studies did not provide evidence that men act on their gender stereotypes in such a way as to evoke stereotype-confirming behavior from women. Providing such evidence, however, was exactly the purpose of the next experiment.

Skrypnek and Snyder (1982) examined the role of men's gender stereotypes in influencing the behavior of women. Because interactants were in different rooms, they could not see one another. Therefore, Skrypnek and Snyder were able to manipulate the target's supposed gender. Male perceivers received a questionnaire allegedly completed by their partner—this provided information to each perceiver about the target's gender.

By using an electronic signaling system, male perceivers negotiated a division of 24 pairs of tasks with female targets. Both individuals simultaneously indicated their first choice. If they both chose the same task, they then engaged in a series of negotiations to decide on the final division. These tasks were rated by independent judges for the degree to which they were masculine or feminine.

Results provided clear evidence of self-fulfilling prophecies. Perceivers initially chose more masculine tasks for themselves when they believed the target was female than when they believed the target was male. In addition, they were more likely to accept the less-preferred task when they believed they were negotiating with a man. These actions clearly influenced the female targets. Those targets labeled "male" ultimately accepted marginally significantly more masculine tasks, and the targets labeled "female" ultimately accepted working on significantly more feminine tasks. Thus, the (female) targets came to behave in a manner consistent with males' beliefs about their gender.

Naturalistic Studies

Naturalistic studies, too, provide evidence of the self-fulfilling nature of gender stereotypes. In one early study, Palardy (1969) separated first grade teachers into two groups: those who believed girls learned how to read more quickly than boys, and those who believed boys and girls learned to read equally quickly. Consistent with the self-fulfilling prophecy hypothesis, by the end of first grade, and even though student IQ was statistically controlled, girls had higher reading achievement test scores than boys, but only in the classes in which teachers believed girls learned to read more quickly.

Another early study (Doyle, Hancock, & Kifer, 1972) focused on three primary predictions:

1. First-grade teachers have higher expectations for girls than boys.
2. These different expectations would be erroneous.
3. Erroneous expectations would be self-fulfilling.

All three predictions were supported. Although there were no differences in boys' and girls' IQ scores (103.0 and 102.8, respectively), teachers estimated that boys had IQ scores of 99.9 and girls had scores of 104.5 (a difference that was statistically significant). Teachers *under-estimated* the IQs of nearly 59% of the boys, and they *overestimated* the IQs of nearly 57% of the girls.

They then divided students into two groups: those whose IQ scores teachers overestimated or underestimated. The main outcome variable, reading achievement scores, was then submitted to a discrepancy (over- vs. underestimated IQ) by sex analysis of covariance (using actual IQ scores as a covariate—this controls for differences between students that existed prior to the assessment of teacher expectations). Results were consistent with a self-fulfilling prophecy: Despite slightly lower IQ scores, girls had higher reading achievement scores, and the effect for discrepancy was highly significant. Students with a mean IQ of 98 (those in the overestimated group) actually outperformed those with a mean IQ of 107 (those in the underestimated group).

Another naturalistic study focused on the self-fulfilling effects of over 1,000 mothers' gender stereotypes on their children's self-perception of ability in math, sports, and social activities (Jacobs & Eccles, 1992). They found that the children's gender interacted with their mothers' gender stereotypes. The children felt they had more ability when their gender corresponded to the gender that their mother believed was generally superior. For example, among mothers who believed that boys were better at math, boys evaluated their math ability more highly than girls evaluated their own math ability (this pattern was reversed among the minority of mothers who felt that girls were better at math).

However, their results also showed that the children were not completely (or even mostly) at the mercy of their mothers' stereotypes. Children's actual skill in these areas was consistently a stronger predictor of self-perceptions than was mothers' stereotypes.

Taken together, the laboratory and naturalistic studies provide clear and strong evidence that gender stereotypes may be self-fulfilling. The experimental studies showed that whether perceivers beliefs about targets' gender or targets' beliefs about perceivers' gender stereotypes were manipulated, self-fulfilling prophecies occurred. These studies provided strong evidence of a possible causal influence of gender stereotypes on targets. However, they suffered the ecological validity typical of most experiments (they were artificial laboratory studies, experimenters deceived subjects, etc.). These limitations, however, were themselves overcome by the naturalistic studies, which showed self-fulfilling effects of gender stereotypes both in classrooms and the home. Gender stereotypes are at least partially self-fulfilling, which serves to maintain those stereotypes.

Social Class

Abundant evidence shows that people hold higher expectations for individuals from middle class backgrounds than from lower class backgrounds (Dusek & Joseph, 1983; Jussim, Coleman, & Lerch, 1987). Nonetheless, we are aware of only two studies that have examined whether these expectations are self-fulfilling.

Perhaps the most dramatic and well-known study of social class-based self-fulfilling prophecies was performed by Rist (1970). Rist observed that by the eighth day of class, a kindergarten teacher had divided her class into three groups—supposedly smart, average, and dumb. Each group sat at its own table (tables 1, 2, and 3, respectively). Furthermore, the main difference between the students was not intelligence—there were no mean differences in IQ scores among the three tables on a test administered at the end of the school year. Instead, the main difference was social class. In comparison to the other students, the students at table 1 came from homes that had greater income, were less likely to be supported by welfare, were more likely to have both parents present, and the children themselves were cleaner and more likely to dress appropriately, and so forth. There were comparable differences between the students at tables 2 and 3. Table 1 was positioned closest to the teacher, and she proceeded to direct nearly all of her time and attention to those students. In addition, she was generally friendlier and warmer to the smart students. Consequently, Rist interpreted his study as documenting strong self-fulfilling prophecies.

The differences Rist (1970) observed in teacher treatment of middle class versus poor students would be inappropriate and unjustified, even if there were real differences in the intelligence of the children at the different tables. Nonetheless, despite Rist's conclusions, the study provided no evidence of self-fulfilling prophecy. Although Rist provided a wealth of observations concerning teacher treatment, he provided few regarding student performance. The only objective performance data that he provided were the IQ tests, which showed that by the end of the school year, there were *no* significant differences among the students at the three tables. Thus, although the teacher may have held very different expectations for middle- versus lower-class students, and even though the teacher may have treated students from different backgrounds very differently, this had no effect on students' IQ scores (see Jussim & Eccles, 1995, for a more detailed critique of this study).

A naturalistic study that included over 10,000 students (Williams, 1976) provided a much more rigorous analysis of the role of social class in educational self-fulfilling prophecies. Williams used path analytic techniques to assess relations among teacher expectations, and students' previous and future achievement and social class. Consistent with most studies examining social class, Williams found that teachers held higher expectations for students from upper socioeconomic backgrounds. However, differences in teacher expectations for middle- and lower-class students evaporated after controlling for students' previous levels of performance. This means that, rather than students' social class biasing teacher expectations, teachers accurately perceived genuine differences in achievement among students from differing socioeconomic backgrounds. Of course, accurate expectations do not create self-fulfilling prophecies.

A colleague once described Rist (1970) as "a real tear jerker" and we cannot help but agree. Nonetheless, the less well-known Williams

(1976) study is much stronger than Rist's study on almost all important scientific grounds: Rist relied primarily on his own subjective and potentially biased observations, whereas Williams relied on school records and questionnaires; Rist focused on 30 students, whereas Williams focused on over 10,000 students; Rist claimed to provide strong evidence of self-fulfilling prophecy but actually provided none, whereas Williams rigorously tested for bias and self-fulfilling prophecy, and failed to find any. We do not doubt that social class may sometimes lead to self-fulfilling prophecies. However, with respect to drawing conclusions about the current state of our knowledge about social class, Williams deserves dramatically more weight than Rist.

Physical Attractiveness

Abundant research shows that many people hold considerably more favorable perceptions of physically attractive individuals than of unattractive individuals (see reviews and meta-analysis by Eagly, Ashmore, Makhijani, & Longo, 1991; Feingold, 1992). As with social class, however, we are aware of only two studies that have empirically examined whether such beliefs may be self-fulfilling.

In a classic study (Snyder, Tanke, & Berscheid, 1977), male perceivers received a photograph indicating that their female interaction partner, who was actually in another room, was either physically attractive or unattractive (this was determined through a pilot test, in which judges rated the women's photographs). In fact, male–female interaction partners were randomly assigned to attractiveness condition. They then had a telephone conversation. The main findings were that male perceivers were warmer and friendlier to female targets whom they (erroneously) believed were more attractive, and these females reciprocated with similarly high levels of warmth and friendliness.

A recent study (Frieze, Olson, & Russell, 1991) focused on the relation between physical attractiveness and income among about 700 MBAs. It is included here because the authors framed their predictions almost entirely in self-fulfilling prophecy terms. On the basis of research such as that of Snyder et al. (1977), Frieze et al. (1991) predicted that attractive MBAs would receive higher starting salaries than unattractive MBAs, and that these differences would increase over time.

Their results partially supported this prediction. Attractive men received significantly higher starting salaries than unattractive men, but attractiveness was not significantly related to the starting salaries of women. More attractive and less overweight men received significantly higher starting salaries, but again there were no effects of attractiveness or weight for women. Physical attractiveness significantly predicted subsequent salaries for both men and women, and the salary differential between attractive and unattractive MBAs increased over time.

Because of certain limitations, however, the relevance of these studies to understanding whether physical attractiveness stereotypes are self-fulfilling is not clear (see Jussim, 1993, and Jussim & Eccles, 1995, for detailed critical analyses of these studies). In short, two factors may limit the generalizability of the Snyder et al. (1977) study:

1. It provided no evidence that perceivers' stereotypes were erroneous—perceivers' only error was in assuming that they were talking to the person in the photograph.
2. An initial interaction held over the phone may hold little relevance for face-to-face interactions involving long-term social relationships.

The Frieze et al. (1991) study has different limitations. First, there was no assessment of employers' expectations for individual employees. Whether the relation between physical attractiveness and income was mediated by employers' physical attractiveness stereotypes, however, is unknowable from their data. Second, their results seemed to provide considerable evidence of accuracy. Work experience consistently predicted income to a greater extent than did attractiveness or weight.

In addition, their analyses likely suffered from at least one important omitted variable. Research consistently shows that physically attractive adults are more socially skilled than less attractive adults (e.g., Goldman & Lewis, 1977; see meta-analysis by Feingold, 1992). It seems likely that more socially skilled MBAs would deserve and actually receive higher salaries than less socially skilled MBAs. Thus, attractiveness may predict MBA's income because it is a proxy for social skill, rather than because of self-fulfilling prophecies.

Although the development of individual differences in social skill is beyond the scope of this article, one may wonder where these differences come from. Is it not possible that self-fulfilling prophecies created a difference where none previously existed? Although it is possible, the mere existence of social skill differences provides neither empirical evidence nor logical justification for supporting a self-fulfilling-prophecy explanation (or any other explanation). There are many plausible alternative explanations for why social skill differences between the attractive and unattractive exist. Further current evidence indicates that the expectancy explanation is one of the *weakest* accounts for those differences (see Feingold's 1992 meta-analysis).

Hyperactive Children

Social scientists commonly emphasize the pernicious effects of applying diagnostic labels (e.g., handicapped, learning disabled, emotionally disturbed, schizophrenic) to people (e.g., Jones, Farina, Hastorf, Markus, Miller, & Scott, 1984; Rist, 1982; Rosenhan, 1973). Diagnostic labels are essentially social stereotypes: categories of psychological and physical infirmities, within which there is considerable variation among individuals. Many complaints about labels focus on their inaccuracy or their tendency to bias evaluations and judgments. Although these issues are beyond the scope of this chapter (for a review, see Jussim, Madon, & Chatman, 1994), researchers often suggest or imply that inaccurate labels create self-fulfilling prophecies. Nonetheless, we are aware of only two highly similar studies that have addressed this issue empirically.

Harris, Milich, Johnston, and Hoover (1990) and Harris, Milich, Corbitt, Hoover, and Brady (1992) both examined the self-fulfilling effects of the ADHD label (attention-deficit/hyperactivity disorder) on peer interactions among elementary school boys. Results from the two studies showed broad effects of the expectancy on both the perceivers and targets. Perceivers "observed" more ADHD-like symptoms, were less friendly, and talked less to targets labeled as ADHD. They also gave ADHD-labeled targets less credit for strong task performance. ADHD-labeled targets enjoyed the interaction less, felt they did less well on the task, accepted less credit for good performance, and felt that their partners were meaner.

The research by Harris et al. (1992), however, also helps put these findings in some context. They used a "balanced-placebo" design: Perceivers' expectations were manipulated orthogonally to targets' actual diagnostic status; that is, targets either were or were not diagnosed as having ADHD. Regardless of their actual ADHD status, however, half the targets were labeled as having ADHD and half were not. Thus, Harris et al. were able to sort out expectancy effects from genuine differences between ADHD and normal targets. In general, for both perceivers and targets, the effects of actually *being normal* versus diagnosed as ADHD were substantially larger than the differences between *being labeled* ADHD or normal. Thus, this study shows that although the label may contribute to a cycle of negative peer interactions for children with ADHD, most differences between ADHD children and their normal peers are genuine and do not exist primarily in the mind of perceivers.

Stereotypes and Dyadic Self-Fulfilling Prophecies: Moderators

Although dyadic self-fulfilling prophecies undoubtedly occur, there is no evidence that they are either particularly large or pervasive (for reviews, see Jussim, 1990, 1993; Jussim & Eccles, 1995). Self-fulfilling-prophecy effects are typically about .1 to .3 (in terms of correlation and regression coefficients—see Brophy, 1983, and Jussim, 1991, for reviews; see Raudenbush, 1984, and Rosenthal & Rubin, 1978, for meta-analyses). However, this does not preclude the possibility that there are conditions under which stereotypes lead to much stronger (and weaker) self-fulfilling prophecies. Therefore, we review three broad classes of factors that may affect expectancy effects: (1) characteristics of the perceiver; (2) characteristics of the target; and (3) situational factors.

Perceiver Characteristics

Perceivers' goals moderate the influence of their expectations on targets. Self-fulfilling prophecies are more likely to occur when perceivers desire to arrive at a stable and predictable impression of a target (Snyder, 1992), and when they are offered an incentive for confirming a belief about a target (Cooper & Hazelrigg, 1988). Self-fulfilling prophecies are less likely when perceivers are motivated to develop an accurate impression of a target (Neuberg, 1989), and when perceivers' main goal is to get along in a friendly manner with targets (Snyder, 1992). These findings lead to the following question: When are perceivers likely to be motivated by accuracy and/or a desire to get along in a friendly manner?

Perceiver prejudice, cognitive rigidity, and belief certainty are all likely to increase self-fulfilling prophecies. Prejudiced individuals are not likely to be motivated by either accuracy concerns or the desire to get along with members of the group they dislike. People high in cognitive rigidity or belief certainty also may not be motivated to consider viewpoints different than their own. Cognitive rigidity, which is usually construed as an individual difference factor (e.g., Adorno, Frenkel-Brunswik, Levinson, & Sanford, 1950; Allport, 1954; Harris, 1989), and belief certainty, which is usually construed as a situational factor (Jussim, 1986; Swann & Ely, 1984), are both similar in that they render people unlikely to alter their beliefs when confronted with disconfirming evidence. Whether the source is prejudice, cognitive rigidity, or belief certainty (which may tend to co-occur within individuals—see Adorno et al., 1950), people who are overconfident in their expectations may be most likely to maintain biased perceptions of individuals and to create self-fulfilling prophecies (Babad, Inbar, & Rosenthal, 1982; Harris, 1989; Swann & Ely, 1984).

Target Characteristics

Self-Concept

When people have unclear self-perceptions, they are more susceptible to all sorts of social influence (Bem, 1970; Festinger, 1954; Markus, 1977), including self-fulfilling prophecies (Jussim, 1986, 1990; Swann & Ely, 1984). In contrast, when targets have clear self-perceptions, they are not only less likely to fulfill others' expectations, but also they often convince perceivers to view them much as they view themselves (Jussim, 1986; Swann & Ely, 1984).

Goals

Targets may become more or less susceptible to self-fulfilling prophecies, depending on their goals. When perceivers' have something targets want (such as a job), and when targets are aware of the perceiver's beliefs, they often confirm those beliefs in order to create a favorable impression (Zanna & Pack, 1975; von Baeyer et al., 1981). Similarly, when targets desire to facilitate smooth social interactions, they are also more likely to confirm perceivers' expectations (Snyder, 1992). These studies suggest a general principle: When targets are in low power positions compared to perceivers, they may be more susceptible to self-fulfilling prophecies. This suggests that people from stigmatized groups may be particularly subject to self-fulfilling prophecies, because they may commonly find themselves in lower power positions (if they consistently found themselves in higher power positions, we suspect that their group would cease to be stigmatized for very long).

However, the outlook may not be quite that grim. When targets believe that perceivers hold a negative belief about them, they often act to disconfirm that belief (Hilton & Darley, 1985). Similarly, when their main goal is to defend a threatened identity, or express their personal attributes, they are also likely to disconfirm perceivers' expectations (Snyder, 1992). Perhaps, therefore, when people belonging to stigmatized groups know that someone holds an inappropriate, negative view of them, they may work particularly hard to dispel that view. Doing so will usually reduce or eliminate self-fulfilling prophecies and lead perceivers to change their views of the target (Jussim, 1986; Swann & Ely, 1984).

Age

Self-fulfilling prophecies were strongest among the youngest students in the original Rosenthal and Jacobson (1968a) study, suggesting that younger children may be more malleable than older children and adults. However, a meta-analysis has shown that the strongest teacher expectation effects occurred in first, second, *and* seventh grade (Raudenbush, 1984). Furthermore, the largest self-fulfilling prophecy effects yet reported were obtained in a study of adults (Israeli military trainees; Eden & Shani, 1982). Although these findings do not deny a moderating role for age, they do suggest that situational factors may also influence targets' susceptibility to self-fulfilling prophecies.

Situational Factors

People may be more susceptible to confirming others' expectations when they enter new situations. Whenever people engage in major life transitions, such as entering a new school or starting a new job, they may be less clear and confident in their self-perceptions. As previously discussed, unclear self-perceptions render targets more susceptible to confirming perceivers' expectations.

This analysis may help explain the seemingly inconsistent findings regarding age. Students in first, second, and seventh grade, and new military inductees, are all in relatively unfamiliar situations. Therefore, all may be more susceptible to self-fulfilling prophecies than are other students or adults in more familiar surroundings.

The potential for increased self-fulfilling prophecies in new situations has particular relevance for the success of affirmative action programs, and, therefore, for stereotype maintenance. One purpose of affirmative action programs is to increase the representation in certain jobs of individuals belonging to groups victimized by discrimination. Often, therefore, affirmative action programs involve hiring new people. However, if adults are highly susceptible to self-fulfilling prophecies when they start new jobs, the initial success of individuals hired through affirmative action programs may be partially dependent on others' expectations. When employers and coworkers believe affirmative action employees are inferior to others, therefore, they may create an environment that undermines the performance of the beneficiaries of such programs (Nacoste, 1987; Pettigrew & Martin, 1987).

Stereotypes and Dyadic Self-Fulfilling Prophecies: Conclusions

Both experimental and laboratory studies converge on several broad conclusions:

1. Social stereotypes leads people to develop expectations for individuals from those groups.
2. At least sometimes, those expectations may be inaccurate.
3. When expectations are inaccurate, they may lead to self-fulfilling prophecies.

Erroneous, stereotype-based expectations influence perceiver behavior toward and judgments regarding targets; they influence targets' self-perceptions and attributions; and they influence targets' interactions with perceivers and performance on tasks. In this manner, self-fulfilling prophecies contribute to the maintenance of social stereotypes.

The literature also suggests that, overall, the role of dyadic self-fulfilling prophecies in maintaining stereotypes is not likely to be large. Only a few of the self-fulfilling prophecy studies have directly compared the self-fulfilling effects of stereotypes to actual differences between individuals comprising the stereotyped groups (Frieze et al., 1991; Harris et al., 1992; Jacobs & Eccles, 1992; Williams, 1976). All, however, have shown that actual differences between targets tend to be larger, and often much larger, than differences resulting from expectancy effects.

Research on social perception in general and interpersonal expectancies in particular has been slowly moving away from an earlier belief that bias, error, and self-fulfilling prophecies pervaded social interaction (e.g., E. E. Jones, 1986; R. A. Jones, 1977; Kahneman & Tversky, 1973; Nisbett & Ross, 1980), and toward the conclusion that people's social beliefs are often reasonably accurate (Brophy, 1983; Funder, 1987; Jussim, 1990, 1991, 1993; Kenny & Albright, 1987). Even the long-standing assumption that stereotypes are necessarily inaccurate has been repeatedly challenged on both conceptual and empirical grounds (e.g., Brigham, 1971; Campbell, 1967; Fox, 1992; Ryan, Park, & Judd, Chapter 4, this volume; Jussim, 1990, 1991; Mackie, 1973; McCauley & Stitt, 1978; McCauley, Stitt, & Segal, 1980).

This is important because, at the dyadic level, interpersonal accuracy represents a major limit on the self-fulfilling power of stereotype-based expectations. By definition, only inaccurate expectations create self-fulfilling prophecies. Even when stereotypes do lead to inaccurate initial expectations, the research discussed thus far shows that people's beliefs about individuals are generally highly influenced by those individuals' actual behaviors, attributes, and accomplishments (for reviews, see also Brophy, 1983; Jussim, 1990, 1991, 1993). This suggests that many errors will be readily corrected through social interaction.

Of course, people are not always accurate. Furthermore, the claim that people are responsive to targets' actual characteristics does not deny the possibility of bias or self-fulfilling prophecy. For example, teachers will generally evaluate students who score one standard deviation above the mean on a standardized test more favorably than students who score at the mean, regardless of their group membership (Jussim, 1989; Jussim & Eccles, 1992). This shows that their beliefs are highly influenced by relevant information about individual students. Nonetheless, they may still evaluate one group more favorably than another among students with similar scores. For example, elementary and junior high school teachers often assign higher math grades to girls than boys, even though teachers' perceptions are usually highly accurate, and even though boys' and girls' similar performance on standardized tests indicates little or no difference in their objective achievement (Kimball, 1989).

When expectations are inaccurate, they may create self-fulfilling prophecies. And even when perceivers are responsive to disconfirming evidence, their expectations may still influence their own judgments and targets' behavior. Therefore, even though accuracy may prevent self-fulfilling prophecies from pervading and dominating dyadic social interactions, stereotype-based expectations may still contribute to group differences where none previously existed (Doyle et al., 1972; Palardy, 1969).

ARE EXPECTANCY EFFECTS UNIMPORTANT?

Although self-fulfilling prophecies may not be as large as once claimed, they are not trivial. A naturally occurring effect of "only" .2 means that, on average, of all targets of high expectations, 10% show substantial improvement; and of all targets of low expectations, 10% show substantial decreases in performance (see Rosenthal, 1984). Most researchers agree that such effects are important (Brophy, 1983; Cooper, 1979; Jussim, 1990; Rosenthal, 1985).

One way to understand how important this might be is to consider the effect as if it were the result of some large-scale social program (Rosenthal & Jacobson, 1968b). A program that led 10% of students who had been performing below average to perform above average probably would be hailed as a major accomplishment; a social policy that undermined students' performance so that 10% of those who had been above-average achievers became below average, probably would be considered an outrage. This is the power of "small" expectancy effects.

Another reason why even effect sizes of .2 may be larger than they seem involves the accumulation of expectancy effects over several years. If, for example, members of one ethnic group reap the benefits of positive expectancy effects every year, and if members of another group are the victims of negative expectancy effects every year, huge self-fulfilling prophecy effects will accumulate over several years. Although both Rist (1970) and Frieze et al. (1991) attempted to address this issue, these studies had so many limitations that they must be viewed only as suggestive. The field experiment by Rosenthal and Jacobson (1968a) and West and Anderson's (1976) naturalistic study, both of which provided clear tests of the accumulation hypothesis, instead found that self-fulfilling prophecies dissipated from the first year to the second year. Whether self-fulfilling prophecy effects accumulate over periods longer than 1 year remains an inadequately addressed empirical question.

SOCIOLOGICAL SELF-FULFILLING PROPHECIES

Although self-fulfilling prophecies clearly occur in dyadic interactions, they may have only limited involvement in many of the deepest and most intractable social problems associated with stereotypes, prejudice, and discrimination. For example, the ghettoization of Jews in Europe, the Hindu caste system, American slavery, and South African apartheid could not have been maintained by the actions of a handful of individuals. In general, one private citizen, no matter how strong the stereotype, cannot single-handedly force another to live in a ghetto, unless there is considerable institutional support for such an action. Similarly, in dyadic interactions, if the target convinces perceivers to adopt a more accurate expectation, the potential for self-fulfilling prophecy is drastically reduced.

Because there has been little empirical research on sociological level self-fulfilling prophecies, this section of our chapter is necessarily more discursive and speculative. However, we suspect that sociological level self-fulfilling prophecies may be much more powerful and have much more lasting effects than dyadic ones. Major institutions (government, business, churches, etc.) often do indeed have the power to "institutionalize" stereotypes. For example, although slavery has been outlawed in the United States for 130 years, its after effects are still readily apparent.

Similarly, there is no longer apartheid in South Africa, but ethnic differences are still a major social problem for the country.

In fact, Merton's (1948) original article primarily discussed self-fulfilling prophecies as explanations for broad sociocultural patterns and social problems. In this section, we will review the limited empirical evidence regarding sociocultural, institutional, and group-level self-fulfilling prophecies. Even in the absence of hard scientific evidence, we attempt to follow in Merton's original groundbreaking footsteps by speculating on the potential involvement of self-fulfilling prophecies in some broad social patterns and problems.

What Do We Mean by a "Sociological or Group" Level of Analysis?

The meaning of dyadic level self-fulfilling prophecies is probably obvious—one person's initially erroneous beliefs lead to interactions with a second person that evoke from that second person behaviors confirming the first' person's expectations. The nature of group-level self-fulfilling prophecies may be less obvious (in this chapter, we use the terms "group" and "sociological" to mean the same thing), especially because, after all, groups are nothing but collections of many individuals. The fundamental difference between the two is that sociological or group-level self-fulfilling prophecies require actions on the part of many people (often in the form of cultural institutions). To help clarify these differences, we next present a few examples of sociological level self-fulfilling prophecies and discuss how they simply cannot be accounted for by dyadic interactions.

Bank Failures

Some self-fulfilling prophecies require interactions between groups of people (or between people and institutions). For example, let us assume that Mary decides that the Last National Bank is having financial problems, when, in fact, the bank is perfectly solvent. Mary then removes all her money (about $5,000) from Last National and places it in Suburban Bank of America. Because both these banks are huge and have assets in the billions, this one person's action has no effect on the solvency or profitability of either bank.

Now consider Merton's (1948) classic example of bank runs during the Great Depression. Somehow a false rumor starts that Small Town Bank is teetering on the brink of insolvency. Half of the depositors in Small Town then rush to remove their savings. Of course, like most profitable banks, Small Town does not keep half of its assets liquid. When the run starts, the bank is no longer able to pay its depositors. It becomes insolvent. Note, however, that self-fulfilling this originally false rumor requires interaction between a mass of people and an institution.

Exclusion of African Americans from Unions

Consider another example—one closer to the focus of this chapter. Merton (1948) documented how, in the early part of this century, most labor unions barred African Americans from membership. Union members often claimed that African Americans were strikebreakers and could not be trusted (this, of course, was a stereotype). This severely limited African Americans' job opportunities. When faced with a strike, companies often offered jobs to all takers, and African Americans often jumped at the chance for work. Thus, the union's beliefs about African Americans were confirmed. It is important to note, however, that if an individual union member, acting alone, held this stereotype of African Americans, it would have had no effect whatsoever on reducing African Americans' job opportunities.

Merton's (1948) examples involving bank failures and exclusion of African Americans from unions nicely illustrate the nature of sociological self-fulfilling prophecies, but they have little direct relevance to American society in the late 20th century. Do sociological self-fulfilling prophecies still contribute to social problems and the maintenance of social stereotypes? Unfortunately, the empirical research addressing group-level self-fulfilling prophecies is extremely limited. Nonetheless, in the next section, we attempt to integrate research and theory from psychology, education, sociology, and history in order to suggest that sociological self-fulfilling prophecies may be a powerful force in the maintenance of some social stereotypes.

School Tracking as a Mechanism for Undermining Positive Effects of Desegregation

School tracking refers to the policy of segregating students into different classes according to their ability. For example, smart students may be assigned to one class, average students to another, and slow students to yet another. Tracking may be intended as a prosocial intervention. By putting students with similar capacities together, teachers have the opportunity to tailor their lessons in such a way as to maximize those students' learning and achievement. Undoubtedly, this actually happens, at least sometimes. However, we next describe how tracking may also lead to a self-fulfilling prophecy that helps sustain negative stereotypes regarding African Americans.

Teachers with negative attitudes toward desegregation are most likely to track students by ability level (Epstein, 1985). People opposed to desegregation are more prejudiced than those favoring desegregation (Weigel & Howes, 1985). Thus, teachers more likely to track are probably often more prejudiced than those who do not track. Why may prejudiced teachers be more likely to track? Prejudiced teachers may contribute to African Americans' underachievement by assigning them to lower tracks. This "works" because once assigned to a lower track, students rarely move up (Brophy & Good, 1974; Epstein, 1985). Among prejudiced teachers, such practices may result from an intentional desire to harm African American students, or from a belief in the intellectual inferiority of African American students. Regardless, the ultimate impact may be to undermine the achievement of some African American students, thereby confirming negative stereotypes of African Americans.

"We Have Met the Enemy and They Is Us": Self-Fulfilling Prophecies in the Ivory Tower

This quote from the comic strip *Pogo* may aptly capture the existence of stereotype-maintaining self-fulfilling prophecies among academics. The terms "self-fulfilling prophecy" and "stereotype" are often used by academics as accusations against laypeople's allegedly flawed, biased, and error-prone social–perceptual processes (see, e.g., Brigham, 1971; Jussim, McCauley, & Lee, in press). Ironically, however, academia is one of the few places for which there is empirical evidence of institutional level self-fulfilling prophecies being involved in stereotype maintenance. We discuss this next.

Academic institutional prestige may be self-fulfilling. University reputation and prestige may be conceptualized as a type of social stereotype. Receiving a degree from Oxford is both an accomplishment, and an occurrence that marks one as a member of a group (graduates from Oxford). Even without knowing much about an individual's actual course work, training, or experiences, people may assume something very different about a person who received a college degree from Harvard, than one who received one from Slippery Rock State College (when academics know little about a particular college or program, they may often assume its quality is something less than top-notch). Just as beliefs about African Americans, poor people, or handicapped children may be accurate or inaccurate, so may beliefs about the scientific competence and training of people receiving degrees from Cambridge, Mississippi State, and Philadelphia Textiles College.

In general, it seems likely that many academics hold higher expectations and more favorable impressions of individuals associated with prestigious institutions. If so, these individuals may then receive better jobs, more access to resources, more grants, and they may publish more, thereby confirming the "validity" of the belief in the quality of that institution. Thus, just as "classic" stereotypes may lead to injustices and inequalities partially through self-fulfilling prophecies, stereotypes associated with institutional prestige also may be self-sustaining.

For example, Rodgers and Maranto (1989) tested several models of relations between individual academics' ability, their graduate program quality, the quality of their first job, and their publication quality and quantity. The best-fitting model indicated that graduate program prestige directly influenced the quality of one's first academic job. Furthermore, this effect was independent of all indicators of competence and performance—neither general intellectual ability, nor even pre-Ph.D. productivity (quality and quantity of articles published) had any influence on the quality of one's first academic job. In other words, Mary, who received her Ph.D. from Elite Private University (EPU) and has no publications, will likely begin her career with a better academic job than Louise, who received her degree from Smalltown State University, even though she has five publications. This alone constitutes a stereotype-maintaining institutional level self-fulfilling prophecy. EPU can then point to its "stellar" track record of placing its students at top jobs as justification for deserving its prestigious reputation!

It turns out, however, that the self-fulfilling nature of academic institutional stereotypes ("reputations") are even more self-fulfilling. All models that Rodgers and Maranto (1989) assessed showed that quality of first job influenced publication quality and quantity (better job, more and better publications). This, then, confirms the "appropriateness" of ascribing higher prestige to their Ph.D.-granting institution (after all, their students really did become more productive).

Another study showed that a similar prestige-based bias influences acceptance of manuscripts submitted for publication in peer-reviewed psychology journals. Peters and Ceci (1982) first selected 12 papers published by researchers at prestigious institutions. They then transcribed these papers back into manuscript form, and made a few other minor and cosmetic changes. Next, they changed the names of all authors to fictitious persons, and changed institution names to convey dubious-sounding reputations. For example, a prestigious university might have been changed to "Tri-Valley Center for Human Potential." Three of the articles were detected as resubmissions, leaving nine to continue the review process to completion.

Results showed that eight of these nine previously published manuscripts were rejected. Sixteen of the 18 referees recommended rejection, and the editors agreed. One seemingly viable alternative to bias was simply that there is a lot of random noise in the process. The strongest version of this alternative (i.e., that journal acceptance is purely random) predicts that these resubmitted papers would have been accepted at the base-rate for acceptance at those journals. However, Peters and Ceci (1982) showed that the rejection rates they obtained significantly exceeded even the normal rejection rates for their sample of journals.

Their results, especially when coupled with those of Rodgers and Maranto (1989), strongly suggest operation of a prestige-maintaining, self-fulfilling prophecy in academics. By virtue of getting better first jobs, individuals from prestigious institutions received more access to resources (grant support, graduate assistants, low teaching loads, prestigious colleagues), even when neither their ability nor their performance exceeded that of individuals from less prestigious institutions. Once they have their first job, even when their research is of no higher quality than their colleagues at less prestigious institutions, journals are more likely to accept their articles for publication. Higher publication productivity (and probably grant-getting productivity, too) then fulfills (and "validates") the stereotype of quality and competence associated with prestigious universities. Self-fulfilling prophecies may play no small role in success in the ivory tower.

Social Class and Funding of Public Education

In many states throughout the United States, public schools are funded through local property taxes. This policy often leads to greater spending per pupil in upper middle-class and wealthy areas than in working-class and poor areas (e.g., Sullivan, 1994). Increased spending improves schools in several ways: It reduces the ratio of students to teachers; it allows schools to hire more highly qualified teachers; and it increases the number of professional support staff available to teachers and students, such as psychologists, counselors, social workers (Bidwell & Kasarda, 1975). When the ratio of teachers to students is lower, and when teachers' qualifications are higher, students actually score higher on standardized achievement tests (Bidwell & Kasarda, 1975). It seems, therefore, that funding schools through property taxes creates a socioeconomic self-fulfilling prophecy at the sociological level: Students from poor areas receive an education inferior to that received by students from middle-class areas. The lower standardized test scores that result from lower spending will reduce the chances of students from lower socioeconomic backgrounds being accepted into high quality colleges. This, in turn, will reduce their occupational opportunities, thereby perpetuating their lower socioeconomic status.

The Los Angeles Riots of 1992

On April 30, 1992, Los Angeles was home to one of the most destructive civil disturbances of this century. The Los Angeles riots are often considered to be a response to the perceived injustice of the "not guilty" verdicts returned in the case against the police officers who beat Rodney King, an African American motorist. Although surely the consequence of the complex interplay of many social forces, the causes and results of the Los Angeles riots may be illuminated by a three-step self-fulfilling prophecy analysis.

This analysis begins with Whites' negative stereotypes about minority groups. Whites have historically held, and continue to hold, negative stereotypes about many minority groups (see reviews by Allport, 1954; Marger, 1991). For example, the Los Angeles County Social Survey (described in Wallace, 1992) was conducted before and after the Rodney King verdict. Among the findings: About 45% of the non-Black sample rated Blacks as lower in intelligence; about 63% rated Blacks as more likely to prefer living on welfare; and about 49% rated Blacks as being hard to get along with. Many Whites continue to view African Americans as lacking motivation or ambition and as hostile and violent (Devine, 1989; Marger, 1991; Wallace, 1992).

These beliefs probably contribute to the second step: discrimination. In the last 20 years, Whites seem to have become less sympathetic to social programs, such as school desegregation and affirmative action, that are designed to provide greater educational and occupational opportunities to minorities (Marger, 1991). Through blatant and subtle forms of discrimination, many Whites continue to limit and undermine the quality of life for many minority groups.

Discrimination may contribute to a self-fulfilling prophecy in several ways. First, it may create a festering resentment among many minority group members—a resentment that the "right" social conditions may trigger into riotous behavior. Second, it probably reduces support for and investment in the general social structure. For example, many African American teenagers may not vigorously pursue high educational achievement for either of two reasons: (1) High achievement may be seen as "acting White" and as rejecting one's own ethnic group (e.g., Fordham & Ogbu, 1986; Steele, 1992), or (2) because of later job discrimination, education is seen as producing little or no economic payoff. Regardless, people who are not heavily invested in the social system may be considerably more likely to "take what they can get" when a "golden opportunity," such as a riot, appears. Thus, even when the rioters were inspired more by self-interest than by abstract political agendas, discrimination probably played an important role. This type of violent, antisocial behavior, of course, confirms for many Whites the validity of their negative beliefs about minorities.

Our analysis of the Los Angeles riots was presented in the spirit of Merton's (1948) original paper and was similarly speculative. We cannot prove that self-fulfilling prophecies actually contributed to the Los Angeles riots. Merton himself acknowledged this problem: He felt that the only way to know whether a certain social problem reflected a self-fulfilling prophecy was with time. It was only after unions dropped their exclusion of minorities that one could determine conclusively whether minorities were intrinsically strikebreakers or whether union policies had led them to become strikebreakers.

Similarly, it will only be possible to tell whether self-fulfilling prophecies contributed to the Los Angeles riots when discrimination is drastically reduced. Highly suggestive, however, is the fact that middle class African Americans did not riot, even though their anger at the Rodney King verdict may have been just as great as that of lower class African Americans. Riots by African Americans and other minorities probably will continue until there is greater perceived equality in educational and economic opportunity.

CONCLUSIONS

In this chapter, we have identified some of the ways that self-fulfilling prophecies may help maintain erroneous social stereotypes. Most social psychological research has focused on dyadic self-fulfilling prophecies—interactions between two individuals. This research has examined self-fulfilling effects of a wide variety of social stereotypes, including ethnicity, gender, social class, physical attractiveness, and hyperactivity in children. Thus, perceivers may find "objective evidence" to support their erroneous stereotypes when they evoke from targets behavior that confirms their stereotypes.

Nonetheless, we have also identified several important limitations to the role of dyadic self-fulfilling prophecies in maintaining social stereotypes. First, with the exception of gender, there has not been much empirical research on the self-fulfilling nature of specific social stereotypes. Because individual studies invariably have important limitations, only one or two studies have investigated particular stereotypes, and because whether most stereotypes regularly lead to self-fulfilling prophecies remains largely unknown.

Second, most of the naturalistic studies show that the self-fulfilling effect of stereotype-based expectations tends to be relatively small (about .2 or less, in terms of correlation and regression coefficients). Especially in conjunction with the considerable evidence showing that, in general, perceivers judge targets far more on the basis of their personal characteristics than on the basis of their membership in social groups (for reviews, see Jussim, 1990, 1991), this suggests that the extent to which dyadic self-fulfilling prophecies sustain erroneous social stereotypes is probably modest at best. The long-term maintenance of erroneous social stereotypes probably involves factors considerably more powerful than dyadic self-fulfilling prophecies.

Sociological level self-fulfilling prophecies may be one such factor. Self-fulfilling prophecies involving political and institutional policies, and broad-based oppression of social groups, may influence the educational and occupational opportunities of large numbers of people. We have suggested that school tracking may contribute to ethnic self-fulfilling prophecies; that funding schools through property taxes may contribute to social class self-fulfilling prophecies; that allocation of academic rewards (jobs, article acceptances, etc.) are characterized by self-fulfilling prophecies based on institutional prestige; and that a self-fulfilling prophecy analysis might contribute to understanding the 1992 Los Angeles riots.

Of course, empirical research on these types of sociological self-fulfilling prophecies is considerably more difficult than research on dyadic self-fulfilling prophecies. Consequently, the extent to which they contribute to the maintenance of erroneous social stereotypes is unknowable. However, we suspect that at least sometimes, such effects may be fairly powerful.

REFERENCES

Adorno, T., Frenkel-Brunswik, E., Levinson, D., & Sanford, R. N. (1950). *The authoritarian personality.* New York: Harper.

Allport, G. (1954). *The nature of prejudice.* Cambridge, UK: Addison-Wesley.

Ashmore, R. D., & Del Boca, F. K. (1981). Conceptual approaches to stereotypes and stereotyping. In D. L. Hamilton (Ed.), *Cognitive processes in stereotyping and intergroup behavior* (pp. 1–35). Hillsdale, NJ: Erlbaum.

Babad, E., Inbar, J., & Rosenthal, R. (1982). Pygmalion, Galatea, and the Golem: Investigations of biased and unbiased teachers. *Journal of Educational Psychology, 74*, 459–474.

Bem, D. (1970). *Beliefs, attitudes, and human affairs.* Monterey, CA: Brooks/Cole.

Bidwell, C. E., & Kasarda, J. D. (1975). School district organization and student achievement. *American Sociological Review, 40*, 55–70.

Brigham, J. C. (1971). Ethnic stereotypes. *Psychological Bulletin, 76*, 15–38.

Brophy, J. (1983). Research on the self-fulfilling prophecy and teacher expectations. *Journal of Educational Psychology, 75*, 631–661.

Brophy, J., & Good, T. (1974). *Teacher–student relationships: Causes and consequences.* New York: Holt, Rinehart & Winston.

Campbell, D. (1967). Stereotypes and the perception of group differences. *American Psychologist, 22*, 817–829.

Cooper, H. (1979). Pygmalion grows up: A model for teacher expectation communication, and performance influence. *Review of Educational Research, 49*, 389–410.

Cooper, H., & Hazelrigg, P. (1988). Personality moderators of interpersonal expectancy effects: An integrative research review. *Journal of Personality and Social Psychology, 55*, 937–949.

Darley, J. M., & Fazio, R. H. (1980). Expectancy-confirmation processes arising in the social interaction sequence. *American Psychologist, 35*, 867–881.

Devine, P. (1989). Stereotypes and prejudice: Their automatic and controlled components. *Journal of Personality and Social Psychology, 56*, 5–18.

Doyle, W. J., Hancock, G., & Kifer, E. (1972). Teachers' perceptions: Do they make a difference? *Journal of the Association for the Study of Perception, 7*, 21–30.

Dusek, J., & Joseph, G. (1983). The bases of teacher expectancies: A meta-analysis. *Journal of Educational Psychology, 75*, 327–346.

Eagly, A. H., Ashmore, R. D., Makhijani, M. G., & Longo, L. C. (1991). What is beautiful is good, but . . . : A meta-analysis of research on the physical attractiveness stereotype. *Psychological Bulletin, 110*, 109–128.

Eden, D., & Shani, A. B. (1982). Pygmalion goes to boot camp: Expectancy, leadership, and trainee performance. *Journal of Applied Psychology, 67*, 194–199.

Elashoff, J. D., & Snow, R. E. (1971). *Pygmalion reconsidered.* Worthington, OH: Charles A. Jones.

Epstein, J. L. (1985). After the bus arrives: Resegregation in desegregated schools. *Journal of Social Issues, 41*, 23–44.

Feingold, A. (1992). Good-looking people are not what we think. *Psychological Bulletin, 111*, 304–341.

Festinger, L. (1954). A theory of social comparison processes. *Human Relations, 7*, 117–140.

Fordham, S., & Ogbu, J. U. (1986). Black students' school success: Coping with the burden of "acting White." *Urban Review, 18,* 176–206.

Fox, R. (1992). Prejudice and the unfinished mind: A new look at an old failing. *Psychological Inquiry, 3,* 137–152.

Frieze, I. H., Olson, J. E., & Russell, J. (1991). Attractiveness and income for men and women in management. *Journal of Applied Social Psychology, 21,* 1039–1057.

Funder, D. C. (1987). Errors and mistakes: Evaluating the accuracy of social judgment. *Psychological Bulletin, 101,* 75–90.

Goldman, W., & Lewis, P. (1977). Beautiful is good: Evidence that the physically attractive are more socially skilled. *Journal of Experimental Social Psychology, 13,* 125–130.

Hamilton, D. L., Sherman, S. J., & Ruvolo, C. M. (1990). Stereotype-based expectancies: Effects on information processing and social behavior. *Journal of Social Issues, 46,* 35–60.

Harris, M. J. (1989). Personality moderators of expectancy effects: Replication of Harris and Rosenthal (1986). *Journal of Research in Personality, 23,* 381–387.

Harris, M. J., Milich, R., Corbitt, E. M., Hoover, D. W., & Brady, M. (1992). Self-fulfilling effects of stigmatizing information on children's social interactions. *Journal of Personality and Social Psychology, 63,* 41–50.

Harris, M. J., Milich, R., Johnston, E. M., & Hoover, D. W. (1990). Effects of expectancies on children's social interactions. *Journal of Experimental Social Psychology, 26,* 1–12.

Hilton, J., & Darley, J. (1985). Constucting other persons: A limit on the effect. *Journal of Experimental Social Psychology, 21,* 1–18.

Jacobs, J. E., & Eccles, J. S. (1992). The impact of mothers' gender-role stereotypic beliefs on mothers' and children's ability perceptions. *Journal of Personality and Social Psychology, 63,* 932–944.

Jones, E. E. (1986). Interpreting interpersonal behavior: The effects of expectancies. *Science, 234,* 41–46.

Jones, E. E. (1990). *Interpersonal perception.* New York: Freeman.

Jones, E. E., Farina, A., Hastorf, A. H., Markus, H., Miller, D. T., & Scott, R. (1984). *Social stigma: The psychology of marked relationships.* New York: Freeman.

Jones, R. A. (1977). *Self-fulfilling prophecies: Social, psychological and physiological effects of expectancies.* Hillsdale, NJ: Erlbaum.

Jussim, L. (1993). Accuracy in interpersonal expectations: A reflection–construction analysis of current and classic research. *Journal of Personality, 61,* 637–668.

Jussim, L. (1991). Social perception and social reality: A reflection–construction model. *Psychological Review, 98,* 54–73.

Jussim, L. (1990). Social reality and social problems: The role of expectancies. *Journal of Social Issues, 46,* 9–34.

Jussim, L. (1989). Teacher expectations: Self-fulfilling prophecies, perceptual biases, and accuracy. *Journal of Personality and Social Psychology, 57,* 469–480.

Jussim, L. (1986). Self-fulfilling prophecies: A theoretical and integrative review. *Psychological Review, 93,* 429–445.

Jussim, L., Coleman, L. M., & Lerch, L. (1987). The nature of stereotypes: A comparison and integration of three theories. *Journal of Personality and Social Psychology, 52,* 536–546.

Jussim, L., & Eccles, J. (1995). Naturalistic studies of interpersonal expectancies. *Review of Personality and Social Psychology, 15,* 74–108.

Jussim, L., Madon, S., & Chatman, C. (1994). Teacher expectations and student achievement: Self-fulfilling prophecies, biases, and accuracy. In L. Heath, F. Bryant, J. Edwards, E. Henderson, J. Myers, E. Posavac, Y. Suarez-Balcazar, & R. S. Tinsdale (Eds.), *Applications of heuristics and biases to social issues* (pp. 303–334). New York: Plenum Press.

Jussim, L., McCauley, C. R., & Lee, Y. T. (1995). Why study stereotype accuracy and inaccuracy? In Y. T. Lee, L. Jussim, & C. R. McCauley (Eds.), *Stereotype accuracy: Toward appreciating group differences* (pp. 3–27). Washington, D.C.: American Psychological Association.

Kahneman, D., & Tversky, A. (1973). On the psychology of prediction. *Psychological Review, 80,* 237–251.

Kenny, D. A., & Albright, L. (1987). Accuracy in interpersonal perception: A social relations analysis. *Psychological Bulletin, 102,* 390–402.

Kimball, M. M. (1989). A new perspective on women's math achievement. *Psychological Bulletin, 105,* 198–214.

Mackie, M. (1973). Arriving at "truth" by definition: The case of stereotype inaccuracy. *Social Problems, 20,* 431–447.

Markus, H. (1977). Self-schemata and processing information about the self. *Journal of Experimental Social Psychology, 21,* 1–18.

Marger, M. N. (1991). *Race and ethnic relations* (2nd ed.). Belmont, CA: Wadsworth.

McCauley, C., & Stitt, C. L. (1978). An individual and quantitative measure of stereotypes. *Journal of Personality and Social Psychology, 36,* 929–940.

McCauley, C., Stitt, C. L., & Segal, M. (1980). Stereotyping: From prejudice to prediction. *Psychological Bulletin, 87,* 195–208.

Merton, R. K. (1948). The self-fulfilling prophecy. *Antioch Review, 8,* 193–210.

Miller, D. T., & Turnbull, W. (1986). Expectancies and interpersonal processes. *Annual Review of Psychology, 37,* 233–256.

Nacoste, R. (1987). Social psychology and affirmative action: The importance of process in policy analysis. *Journal of Social Issues, 43,* 127–132.

Neuberg, S. L. (1989). The goal of forming accurate impressions during social interactions: Attenuating the impact of negative expectancies. *Journal of Personality and Social Psychology, 56,* 374–386.

Nisbett, R., & Ross, L. (1980). *Human inference: Strategies and shortcomings of social judgment.* Englewood Cliffs, NJ: Prentice-Hall.

Palardy, J. (1969). What teachers believe—What students achieve. *Elementary School Journal, 69,* 370–374.

Peters, D. P., & Ceci, S. J. (1982). Peer review practices of psychological journals: The fate of published articles, submitted again. *Behavioral and Brain Sciences, 5,* 187–255.

Pettigrew, T., & Martin, J. (1987). Shaping the organizational context for Black American inclusion. *Journal of Social Issues, 43,* 41–78.

Raudenbush, S. W. (1984). Magnitude of teacher expectancy effects on pupil IQ as a function of the credibility of expectancy inductions: A synthesis of findings from 18 experiments. *Journal of Educational Psychology, 76,* 85–97.

Rist, R. (1970). Student social class and teacher expectations: The self-fulfilling prophecy in ghetto education. *Harvard Educational Review, 40,* 411–451.

Rist, R. C., & Harrell, J. E. (1982). Labeling the learning disabled child: The social ecology of educational practice. *American Journal of Orthopsychiatry, 52,* 146–160.

Rodgers, R. C., & Maranto, C. L. (1989). Causal models of publishing productivity in psychology. *Journal of Applied Psychology, 74,* 636–649.

Rosenhan, D. L. (1973). On being sane in insane places. *Science, 179,* 250–258.

Rosenthal, R. (1974). *On the social psychology of the self-fulfilling prophecy: Further evidence for Pygmalion effects and their mediating mechanisms.* New York: MSS Modular.

Rosenthal, R. (1984). *Meta-analytic prodedures for the social research.* Beverly Hills: Sage.

Rosenthal, R. (1985). From unconscious experimenter bias to teacher expectancy effects. In J. Dusek (Ed.), *Teacher expectancies* (pp. 38–65). Hillsdale, NJ: Erlbaum.

Rosenthal, R., & Jacobson, L. (1968a). *Pygmalion in the classroom: Teacher expectations and student intellectual development.* New York: Holt, Rinehart & Winston.

Rosenthal, R., & Jacobson, L.F. (1968b). Teacher expectations for the disadvantaged. *Scientific American, 218,* 19–23.

Rosenthal, R., & Lawson, R. (1964). A longitudinal study of the effects of experimenter bias on the operant conditioning of laboratory rats. *Journal of Psychiatric Research, 2,* 61–72.

Rosenthal, R., & Rubin, D. B. (1978). Interpersonal expectancy effects: The first 345 studies. *Behavioral and Brain Sciences, 3,* 377–386.

Skrypnek, B. J., & Snyder, M. (1982). On the self-perpetuating nature of stereotypes about women and men. *Journal of Experimental Social Psychology, 18,* 277–291.

Snyder, M. (1984). When belief creates reality. *Advances in Experimental Social Psychology, 18,* 247–305.

Snyder, M. (1992). Motivational foundations of behavioral confirmation. *Advances in Experimental Social Psychology, 25,* 67–114.

Snyder, M., Tanke, E. D., & Berscheid, E. (1977). Social perception and interpersonal behavior: On the self-fulfilling nature of social stereotypes. *Journal of Personality and Social Psychology, 35,* 656–666.

Steele, C. (1992, April). Race and the schooling of Black Americans. *Atlantic Monthly*, pp. 68–78.

Sullivan, J. F. (1994, July 13). Top Jersey court orders new plan for school funds. *New York Times*, pp. A1, B6.

Swann, W. B., Jr., & Ely, R. J. (1984). A battle of wills: Self-verification versus behavioral confirmation. *Journal of Personality and Social Psychology, 46,* 1287–1302.

von Baeyer, C. L., Sherk, D. L., & Zanna, M. P. (1981). Impression management in the job interview: When the female applicant meets the male (chauvinist) interviewer. *Personality and Social Psychology Bulletin, 7,* 45–51.

Wallace, A. (1992, September 3). Riots changed few attitudes, poll finds. *Los Angeles Times*, pp. B1, B8.

Weigel, R. H., & Howes, P. W. (1985). Conceptions of racial prejudice: Symbolic racism reconsidered. *Journal of Social Issues, 41*(3), 117–138.

West, C., & Anderson, T. (1976). The question of preponderant causation in teacher expectancy research. *Review of Educational Research, 46,* 613–630.

Williams, T. (1976). Teacher prophecies and the inheritance of inequality. *Sociology of Education, 49,* 223–236.

Wineburg, S. S. (1987). The self-fulfillment of the self-fulfilling prophecy. *Educational Researcher, 16,* 28–37.

Word, C. O., Zanna, M. P., & Cooper, J. (1974). The nonverbal mediation of self-fulfilling prophecies in interracial interaction. *Journal of Experimental Social Psychology, 10,* 109–120.

Zanna, M. P., & Pack, S. J. (1975). On the self-fulfilling nature of apparent sex differences in behavior. *Journal of Experimental Social Psychology, 11,* 583–591.

6

Language and Stereotyping

ANNE MAASS
LUCIANO ARCURI

Although stereotypes may take very different—verbal and nonverbal—forms, language is probably the dominant means by which they are defined, communicated, and assessed. Some authors have even proposed an intrinsic link between stereotypes and language such that there are no alinguistic stereotypes (Mininni, 1982). Even those who do not share such a radical view probably agree that stereotypic beliefs are transmitted in interpersonal discourse, in textbooks, in mass communication (Van Dijk, 1984, 1987,1988), and that it is language that provides the key tool for communicating prejudice interpersonally and cross-generationally.

Despite the central role of language in stereotype transmission and maintenance, social psychologists have paid relatively little attention to this issue until recently (see Graumann & Wintermantel, 1989, and Hamilton, Gibbons, Stroessner, & Sherman, 1992, as examples for the recent interest in the language–stereotyping link). Initially, language was mainly interesting to stereotype researchers as a way of identifying the *content* of national, ethnic, and racial stereotypes such as in Katz and Braly's (1933) classic work employing a trait checklist referring to various nationalities. Since then, the measurement procedure has been refined considerably (e.g., Brigham, 1971; Linville, Fischer, & Salovey, 1989; McCauley & Stitt, 1978; Park & Judd, 1990), but the idea of measuring stereotypic beliefs through trait ascriptors has remained widely accepted.

Although the focus on stereotype content has never faded completely, it was soon complemented by an increasing interest in *function*. Allport (1954) noticed that linguistic terms may not only define content but also serve as organizing principles and as evaluative references. Following this tradition, the present chapter will be organized by different functions that language fulfills in intergroup contexts. We will try to show that language plays an important role in (1) stereotype transmission, (2) cognitive organization, (3) stereotype maintenance, and (4) expression of stereotypic identities.

STEREOTYPE TRANSMISSION

The first, and most obvious function of language is the *transmission of culturally shared stereotypes* from person to person and from generation to generation. Because language is culturally shared, it provides an ideal means of collectively defining and preserving stereotypic beliefs.

Language-mediated transmission of stereotypes can be studied at different levels of analysis. On the most general level, culturally shared beliefs are wired into the *vocabulary* of a given language. A child growing up at a given time in a given culture acquires a lexicon that reflects these stereotypic beliefs. To give just few examples, depending on the decade in which an American grew up, he or she learned to refer to dark-skinned citizens as "niggers," "Negroes," "Blacks," or "Afro-Americans"—terms that imply very different qualities and evoke very different images and associations (we will discuss the implications of such different terms in the next section on "organizing function"). Another example are sex-specific vocabularies. Overall, the current English vocabulary has many more words referring to males than to females, although this turns around for specific areas of content; for example, there are about 10 times as many expressions to describe promiscuous females as promiscuous males (Ng, 1990). Along the same line, children learn a great number of sayings that associate ethnic or social groups with particular and predominantly negative behaviors or traits and that are quite common in numerous languages, such as "to smoke like a Turk", "*Arabo mentitore*" (Arabian liar), "*promessa da marinaio*" (the sailor's promise—the equivalent to the Gambler's oath in English) or "fare il Portoghese" ("to act like a Portuguese"—the equivalent of "gate crasher" in English).[1] In other words, embedded in the lexicon of any language at any given moment in history are social beliefs about groups that are automatically "absorbed" during language acquisition (we will discuss the implications of such different vocabularies in the next section on "Organizing Function").

Although the lexicon does provide interesting information about potential stereotypes embedded therein, it does not, by itself, provide any information about the frequency and the contexts in which these words are actually used in everyday discourse. To understand language-mediated stereotype transmission in concrete contexts, it is therefore important to analyze group-related (e.g., agist, sexist, racist) talk at the level of mass and interpersonal communication.

As far as *mass communication* is concerned, discourse analysts have argued very forcefully for the hypothesis that prejudice is acquired and transmitted through discursive communication (e.g.,Van Dijk, 1984, 1987, 1988). Analyzing the content of written and spoken material, they have shown that ethnic, racial, and gender stereotypes are (re)produced in news reports, in textbooks, and in talk. To cite just two examples from this rich literature, first Kruse, Weimer, and Wagner (1988), analyzed interaction sequences between males and females verbalized in media texts sampled from a large number of German magazines. Their analysis shows that representations of gender-role relationships in media texts continue to follow traditional clichés, with males occurring more frequently in the role of the logical subject and being portrayed as more active, whereas women are depicted as more passive, more emotional, and frequently as engaging in helpless and/or victim roles. Ironically, stereotypic conceptions of males and females in the mass media do not die easily considering that they even emerge heavily in obituaries, as indicated by the second example, Kirchler. Kirchler (1992) analyzed obituaries concerning deceased male and female managers published in major daily newspapers in Austria, Switzerland, and Germany during the 1970s and 1980s. He found a very different terminology to describe male versus female managers, with men being described as highly knowledgeable and intelligent experts, and women being described as adorable, likable, and highly committed colleagues. Although this difference attenuated somewhat during the 1980s, it is still quite strong. Taken together, these and numerous other content analyses demonstrate that the mass media do indeed contribute in a significant way to the transmission of stereotypic beliefs.

Finally, one may analyze the role of language in stereotype transmission at the *interpersonal level*, such as parent–child or teacher–student interactions. It is evident that interpersonal communication (just like mass communication) uses both linguistic and nonverbal devices for the transmission of stereotypes. For example, children may develop a negative attitude toward Blacks either by observing that their parents are avoiding contact with Black people, or by listening to their parents' conversations in which they may label Blacks as "lazy" or "aggressive."

Although both verbal and nonverbal information may be important and necessary for the transmission of stereotypic beliefs, the two levels of communication may not be used interchangeably. Observing the avoidance behavior or negative nonverbal cues of a parent may be sufficient to learn that certain categories (Blacks, Jews) are seen as less valuable. Yet, it seems unlikely that the *specific content* of a stereotype (Germans are efficient and authoritarian, women are dependent and other-directed, Italians are hospitable and lazy) can be transmitted without linguistic labels. In other words, nonverbal behaviors, on the one hand, may provide rich information about the overall evaluation of a given category and also about what reaction is appropriate in interaction with that category. Verbal labels, such as trait descriptions, on the other hand, provide detailed information about which characteristics are associated with a given category.

One way to test the acquisition of stereotypes through interpersonal communication is to observe adult–child interactions and to study their impact on children's stereotype knowledge. If children do learn stereotypic beliefs about social categories through communication with their parents and teachers, then they should acquire these beliefs faster and to a greater degree the more prejudiced their parents or teachers are. One area in which this was observed is gender stereotyping. For example, work by Fagot, Leinbach, and colleagues (Fagot & Leinbach, 1989; Fagot, Leinbach, & O'Boyle, 1992; Leinbach & Fagot, 1992) shows that children of parents with traditional sex-role attitudes and more conservative attitudes toward women acquire sex category labels (man–woman, boy–girl) earlier and have better knowledge of gender stereotypes than children with less traditional parents (see also Weinraub, Clements, Sockloff, Ethridge, Gracely, & Myers, 1984).

Taken together, this suggests that the learning of category labels and the qualities associated with them are the multiple function of the general lexicon of a given language and of the specific content transmitted in mass communications and interpersonal discourse.

ORGANIZING FUNCTION

Language also fulfills an important *organizing function* by providing key terms around which information is organized. As Allport (1954) argued four decades ago, there are linguistic terms such as social category labels (Jew, Black, Islam, communists) that are unusually potent both as cognitive organizing principles and as evaluative reference points. Indeed, such linguistic anchors seem to be a necessary prerequisite for social categorisation and stereotyping to occur. As a case in point, the enemy image of "communists"—according to Allport—became effective only at the moment when the label "communist" became widely known and was consistently applied to the out-group category. This suggests that linguistic terms, such as category labels (Blacks) or category-related concepts (ghetto), provide the necessary point of reference around which stereotypic information is organized.

This organizing function has been stressed in both psycholinguistic and social psychological writings. According to the Whorfian hypothesis on linguistic relativity (see Whorf, 1956; for an excellent recent discussion of the relation between language and thought, see Hunt & Agnoli, 1991), the lexicon of a given language shapes our thought processes by providing a specific repertory of cognitive schemata. Hoffman, Lau, and Johnson (1986) have provided a particularly interesting example of how language-specific vocabularies affect social information processing. They provided Chinese–English bilinguals with social information for which an economical personality label existed either only in English or only in Chinese. Subjects worked on the impression formation task either in Chinese or in the English language. Results showed that the existence of economic linguistic labels in a given language to describe a given personality type facilitates schematic information processing (going beyond the information given, erroneously recalling schema-congruent information that had not been contained in the personality description, etc.).

Recent social psychology has addressed the link between category labels and thought processes in a somewhat different way by focusing on the organizing function of linguistic labels within a given language rather than studying differences across languages. According to current thinking, personality traits and behavioral information are associated with the relevant category label through associative networks in memory (Stangor & Lange, 1993). Any activation of the label—even if unconscious—spreads through the entire network, thereby increasing the accessibility of the information that is associated with the category. The strongest evidence for the organizing function of semantic networks derives from priming studies using social category labels as primes (e.g., Devine, 1989; Stangor & Lange, 1993; for related research see also Bargh & Pietromonaco, 1982; Greenwald, Klinger, & Liu, 1989; Higgins, King, & Mavin, 1982). Such priming tends to activate the entire semantic network (e.g., personality traits, behavioral tendencies, physical characteristics) associated with this particular group. For example, if we ask subjects to perform a lexical decision task (e.g., is the stimulus that appears on the screen of the computer a "legal" word or not?), their performance will be better (fewer errors, faster decision times) if they were primed by a social category label related to the words used as stimuli in the lexical decision phase (cf. Neely, 1990).

Interestingly, this is not only true for labels referring to specific social categories such as Blacks, Jews, or Italians, but also for common collective pronouns referring, more generally to in-groups and out-groups (e.g., "we," "us," "ours" or "they," "them," "theirs"). Perdue, Dovidio, Gurtman, and Tyler (1990, Exp. 2 and 3) used a semantic priming procedure in which in-group or out-group designators were presented briefly and then visually masked by positive or negative trait adjectives. Subjects either had to decide whether the trait was positive or negative (Exp. 2), or whether the characteristic could or could not describe a person (Exp. 3). As hypothesized, the priming of in-group pronouns strongly facilitated the recognition and categorization of positive traits, as evidenced by considerably reduced decision time, whereas negative traits were more accessible after the priming of out-group pronouns (in Exp. 2 only). Thus, in-group or out-group-related words such as "us" or "them" seem to carry an evaluative connotation that is activated automatically when such words are primed.

Importantly, the activation of category-related concepts, traits, and so forth, tends to occur in a largely *automatic* fashion (unless people are cognitively so busy that the activation of stereotypes is inhibited, see Gilbert & Hixon, 1991). Support for this idea comes from two lines of research: On one side, there is evidence that people encounter great difficulty in ignoring social-category information, suggesting that such information is processed automatically. For example, subjects asked to make decisions regarding one category (e.g., young vs. old age, sad vs. happy mood) are unable to ignore additional dimensions (e.g., sex of target) that are copresent but irrelevant to the execution of the task. As a case in point, a study by Boca, Arcuri, and Zuffi (1994) showed that subjects took considerably longer to discover that two targets expressed the same emotion when these targets were of different rather than of same sex, suggesting that the category information not involved in the task (sex) was automatically activated. On the other side, there is evidence that once the category label is activated, activation will automatically spread through the entire network. As demonstrated by Devine (1989), the subliminal presentation of a social category (e.g., Blacks) activates related concepts (e.g., aggressive) even in those subjects who do not personally endorse it. Hence, most people, regardless of their tendency to refuse or to hide negative attributions to the target group, will automatically activate the association between the category label of the target group and the traits belonging to its social representation. Taken together, these and related studies suggest that social category information is processed automatically, and that there is very little conscious control over spreading activation throughout the cognitive network once the category label has been activated.

This has interesting implications for the link between language and mental representations of social categories. For most social groups, there are numerous labels describing the same category, including both neutral descriptors and ethnophaulisms (see Allen, 1983; Mullen & Johnson, 1993). For example, Americans with African ancestors may be referred to as *Blacks, Afro-Americans, darkies* or *niggers,* and people with preference for same-sex partners may be labeled *gays, homosexuals, fags,* or *queers.* Although these terms refer to the same categories, they are clearly not equivalent, as they evoke very different associations. The semantic network activated by the word "gay" will be distinct from (although partially overlapping with) that activated by the word "fag." This implies that linguistic choices have a great impact on how social groups are perceived. Moreover, if derogatory category labels do activate the associated network automatically, the use of such labels will evoke negative associations and negative evaluations of the target group, even in those persons who do not consciously endorse the stereotype.

The importance of linguistic category labels has long been recognized by minority groups, which have often created new labels that activate neutral or positive associations. The best-known example is the introduction of the term "gay," but there are many other examples. In Italy, the associations for the blind have recently proposed to substitute the term "blind" by "not-seeing" (*non vedente*) because the word "blind" has acquired a secondary and predominantly negative meaning that is unrelated to the fact that somebody lacks eyesight (trusting somebody blindly, being blind as to the consequences of . . . , etc.). Along the same line, the seats for handicapped people on Italian trains or buses are now reserved for the "non-deambulating," a rather complicated, but evaluatively neutral term.

Whereas minorities have long been aware of the differential implications of category labels, social psychologists have paid relatively little attention to the link between language and mental representations of social groups until recently. Yet, there are at least two lines of research that illustrate the power of linguistic choices in intergroup perception, namely, work on racial and ethnic slurs, and work on sexist language use.

Ethnic/Racial Slurs

Greenberg, Pyszczynski and colleagues have investigated the impact of racial or ethnic slurs on the evaluation of minority targets and others associated with the target. Although "ethnophaulisms," or derogatory ethnic labels, are rarely used in the presence of people belonging to the target group in question, they are quite frequently used during interaction with other in-group members. Greenberg and Pyszczynski (1985) have argued that the overhearing of such derogatory labels will automatically activate negative feelings and beliefs associated with that group, and that this will happen even among relatively egalitarian people. To test this hypothesis, they staged a debate between a Black and a White debator in which the Black either won or lost. Subsequently, White subjects overheard a comment from a White confederate criticizing the Black debator either in an ethnically derogatory ("There's no way that nigger won the debate") or in an ethnically neutral manner ("There's no way that pro debator won the debate"). As predicted, the Black was evaluated as less skilled when subjects had overheard the ethnic slur, but only when he lost the debate. In contrast, the ethnically neutral criticism did not affect the evaluation of the target. Thus, the derogatory ethnic label apparently activated negative beliefs that seemed to have guided the evaluation of the target—unless his performance was clearly incoherent with the schema activated by the derogatory label.

In a subsequent experiment, Kirkland, Greenberg, and Pyszczynski (1987) attempted to assess whether this finding would generalize to the evaluation of others associated with the target person. Subjects read the transcript of a jury trial, in which the defendant was always White, whereas the defense attorney was either Black or White. When the defense attorney was Black, a confederate posing as a subject criticized the defense attorney in either an ethnically derogatory manner ("God, Mike, I don't believe it. That *nigger* doesn't know shit") or in a derogatory but ethnically neutral manner ("God, Mike, I don't believe it. That *shyster* doesn't know shit"). The derogatory ethnic label (but not the ethnically neutral label) led to a negative evaluation of the Black defense attorney; more important, the White defendant was perceived more negatively as well and received harsher verdicts when defended by a Black attorney who was the target of the racial slur. Interestingly, unsystematic observations also suggest that many subjects seemed outwardly disturbed by the confederate's ethnic slur but still evaluated both defendant and defense attorney in a way that was consistent with the derogatory label. This suggests that derogatory ethnic labels may, indeed, have a strong and largely automatic effect on the perception of minority members.

Sexist Language: The Case of the Generic Masculine

Convergent evidence for the powerful effect of language on cognitive processes comes from studies on sexist-language use, and in particular on the generic masculine. In many languages, there are specific forms to describe female (e.g., women) or male members of a given category (e.g., men), but the masculine form is usually applied when referring to sex-indefinite humans (e.g., men, primitive men). The same is true for pronouns, when *she, her,* and so forth, refer to females only, whereas he, his, and so forth, can be used either in a male-specific or in a generic sense.

In other languages, this problem is further aggravated by the fact that nouns are gender bound. In German and Italian, for example, the term *Studentin* or *Studentessa* describes a female student, whereas *Student* or *studente* refers to a male student. When describing students in a general, sex-unspecified way, it is the masculine rather than feminine plural that is used (*Studenten* or *studenti,* respectively). There are extreme cases in which the grammatically masculine term is used even when referring exclusively to females. This is particularly likely to occur when describing women in predominantly male, high-status professions. For example, a woman Secretary of State in Italy is referred to as *ministro* rather than *ministra,* a woman surgeon is labeled *chirurgo* rather than *chirurga,* and a woman Deputy Director of Public Prosecutions is called *sostituto* rather than *sostituta,* despite the general rule prescribing the feminine form for female protagonists. Interestingly, no such reversals occur for males entering traditionally female professions (e.g., nurse, midwife, or kindergarten teacher); to our knowledge, there is no single case in either Italian or German in which the grammatically feminine term generalizes to males occupying female professions. In other words, women may be subsumed under masculine labels but not vice versa.

Psychologically, the generic masculine has a number of interesting although worrisome implications: If generics apply with equal likelihood to male and female exemplars, no particular problems arise. However, if the masculine form is primarily linked to males in people's mental representations, and if the use of the masculine form activates predominantly traits, behaviors, and images associated with male exemplars, then the use of the masculine form in a sex-indefinite sense may easily be misinterpreted to be male-specific, even when intended in a general sense. There is, indeed, evidence that the male-specific meaning is acquired earlier than the generic meaning during language acquisition (Hyde, 1984; Nilson, 1977) and that generics are generally interpreted as being male-specific (Kidd, 1971; MacKay, 1980; MacKay & Fulkerson, 1979; Moulton, Robinson, & Elias, 1978; Murdock & Forsyth, 1985) and evoke predominantly male images (Harrison, 1975; Schneider & Hacker, 1973); also, ambiguous visual images (presented at subthreshold speed, such that the viewer can "see" a face but not recognize its gender) are for the most part interpreted as males when paired with a masculine-generic stimulus sentence (Wilson & Ng, 1988).

One of the most powerful demonstrations for the fact that generic words are more easily assimilated into the masculine than into the feminine category comes from a study by Ng (1990) utilizing a procedure derived from research on "proactive inhibition." Studies have generally shown that memory for words deteriorates over time when new words on the list belong to the same category as the previous ones (e.g., a male personal name following a list of all male personal names). When words from a new category are introduced (e.g., female personal name), however, the recall rate improves relative to the last trial, due to a release from proactive inhibition. Ng's argument is as follows: If masculine generic terms such as "man" or "his" apply with equal likelihood to the male and female category, then recall for these words should be comparable whether they are presented after a list of words comprised of masculine words (e.g., "king," "Ivan") or after one comprised of feminine words (e.g., "queen," "Linda"). If, however, generics are androcentric and therefore more closely related to the male than to the female category, then recall for such generics should be much better if presented after a list of feminine items. The results do, indeed, support this latter interpretation, suggesting that the memory code for generics such as "men" is primarily masculine, and that a sentence containing such generics is spontaneously processed as referring to males only. Taken together, these studies demonstrate a striking contradiction in the language–cognition link: Formally, masculine generics represent the grammatically correct form for including both sexes. In reality, organization of information in memory appears to be such that generics are almost exclusively associated with the male category in people's minds. Not only is the male-specific meaning primary with respect to the sex-indefinite meaning, but generics even seem to inhibit the assimilation of female exemplars.

If the generic masculine is, indeed, as androcentric as these and other studies suggest, then its use in everyday discourse may, at the very least, decrease the salience of women. Stahlberg, Sczesny, Otto, Rudolph, and Sorgenfrey (1994) have recently tested this possibility by presenting a alleged newspaper article about a conference in which scientists from either a typically male (geophysics) or a typically female area (nutrition science) proposed ways to improve the public image of their field. Conference participants were either referred to by explicit reference to both males and females (*Wissenschaftlerinnen und Wissenschaftler*), by neutral forms (*die wissenschaftlich Taetigen*—those active in science), or by masculine generics (*Wissenschaftler*). The main dependent variable was the estimate of the percentage of female scientists participating at the conference. For the typically male field (geophysics), there was a linear decline, such that the percentage of women was estimated greatest when the article referred explicitly to both males and females, intermediate when it used the neutral form, and lowest for the masculine-generic form supporting the idea that sexist language use leads people to underestimate the presence of women. Results were less clear for the condition in which subjects a priori assumed a predominance of women (nutrition science): Here the neutral form led to lower estimates than the remaining language forms. These results provide first tentative evidence that linguistic choices may, indeed, affect the salience of women and that the generic masculine form may lead to an underestimation of women, especially in those areas where they objectively constitute a minority group. Masculine generics may not only affect the perceived presence of women, but also may have concrete practical consequences, as shown by Bem and Bem's (1973) study in which women tended to respond less frequently to a job add when it was formulated in the (generic) masculine form.

Politically, these and other studies underline the need for developing alternatives to the generic masculine. In the United States, the introduction of "she or he" or "s/he" is now widely accepted and many professional organizations (including the American Psychological Association) have long included nonsexist language use among their rules. Feminization of language has been considerably slower and less successful in other countries (see Stahlberg et al., 1994, for examples of nonsexist language forms in German speaking countries).

From a psychological point of view, the afore mentioned studies on racist and sexist language are largely in line with social cognitive theorizing, according to which semantic labels automatically activate information associated with the label. Applying this general framework, three interesting implications emerge: First, the linguistic choices made by the speaker (such as the use of ethnophaulisms or masculine generics) will bias the cognitive processes of the listener—which is exactly what has emerged from the research reported earlier (e.g., Greenberg & Pyszczynski, 1985; Ng, 1990; Stahlberg et al., 1994). Second, this will occur in an automatic fashion, such that the listener is neither completely aware of the activating potential of the semantic label nor does he or she exert control over it. Although there is little explicit evidence for this proposition, some of the unsystematic observations (e.g., Kirkland et al., 1987) do suggest that the stereotypes are, indeed, activated by corresponding labels (e.g., racial slur), even in unprejudiced people who do not endorse the stereotype, and who may even be appalled by it. Third, carrying this argument one step further, one may venture the hypothesis that the speaker's linguistic choices may affect the speaker's own thinking in much the same fashion as it affects the listener. Although we are unaware of any stereotype research investigating this possibility, some indirect evidence comes from the attitude literature. For example Eiser (1975; Eiser & Ross, 1977) have shown that speakers required to use partisan language subsequently expressed attitudes consistent with these labels.

Taken together, research on the language–cognition link does suggest that social category labels fulfill an important organizing function and that such labels exert a powerful impact on stereotype-related cognitive processing. However, such evidence ought to be interpreted with caution considering that only a small portion of this work was conducted from a social cognitive perspective. Although interpretable within such framework, the majority of these studies are of sociolinguistic orientation and were not specifically designed to test the functioning of cognitive networks organized around racist/sexist versus nonracist/nonsexist labels; we do hope that future studies will be better suited to test specific hypotheses about the exact processes underlying the language–stereotype link.

STEREOTYPE-MAINTAINING FUNCTION

The third and possibly less obvious function of language lies in its subtle contribution to *stereotype maintenance*. Language is frequently used in such a way as to defend existing stereotypes against disconfirmation. Three aspects of biased language use that have received particular attention in recent years are (1) the degree of *confirmability/disconfirmability* of attributes contained in common stereotypes, (2) the *generality or breadth* of such trait descriptions, and (3) the degree of *abstraction* used to describe behaviors that are congruent versus incongruent with existing stereotypic beliefs (so-called "linguistic intergroup bias"). We will review evidence for each of these tendencies that, together, seem to provide a language-based defense strategy protecting stereotypes against disconfirmation.

Confirmability and Disconfirmability of Stereotypic Attributes

Considering the well-established ethnocentric tendencies in most human groups, it is not surprising that stereotypic beliefs about one's own group tend to be more favorable than those about out-groups. With some exceptions (such as groups of "legitimately" lower status), group members tend to assign fewer positive and more negative trait concepts to the out-group than to the in-group (e.g., Howard & Rothbart, 1980), especially when such traits are important to the group's self-definition (Mummendey & Simon, 1989). But in-group and out-group descriptions differ not only in evaluative content, but also in their robustness, that is, the ease with which they can be disproven. Following Rothbart and Park (1986), it is exactly the negative traits typically contained in out-group stereotypes that are easiest to acquire and most difficult to lose. For these traits, much disconfirming evidence is needed before they will be revised.

Rothbart and Park (1986) presented subjects with a list of trait adjectives varying in favorability and asked them to rate (1) how easily they could imagine behaviors confirming/disconfirming each trait, (2) how frequently occasions arise in the course of normal social interaction that allow for confirming/disconfirming behaviors to occur, and (3) how many confirming/disconfirming behaviors would be required before the trait can be considered confirmed/disproven. The most important result emerging from this study is that unfavorable traits require fewer instances of confirmation before they can be considered confirmed, but more disconfirming instances before they can be repudiated. As Rothbart and Park put it, "Unfavorable traits are easier to acquire and harder to lose than unfavorable traits" (p. 135).

Arcuri and Cadinu (1992) have recently argued that Rothbart and Park's (1986) findings may, at least in part, be a function of the lexical properties of the adjectives used in this type of research. Their argument is based on the Clark's (cf. Clark & Clark, 1977) principle of lexical marking, according to which, in the case of antinoms, we may observe that the pole denoting the judgment dimension, the unmarked one (*proud* → *pride*), can be neutralized, becoming a term able to denote a broad range of objects, situations, or events on the considered dimension. The other pole, the marked one (*humble*, referring to the previous example) implies only a contrastive use, (i.e., the negation of the pole naming the dimension). In other words, the unmarked term can be used in two different ways: broad (degree of *pride*) or contrastive (*proud* rather than *humble*). In contrast, the marked term is used in one sense only: contrastive (*humble* rather than *proud*). Since the majority of evaluatively negative trait adjectives tend to act as marked terms in everyday language (and in research material such as that used in Rothbart and Park's study), they may require less confirming and more disconfirming evidence, not because they are negative, but because they are marked and as such, cover a smaller range of behaviors.

To test the independent effects of marking versus valence, Arcuri and Cadinu (1992) generated a list of personality traits in such a way that the marked–unmarked dimension was diagonal to the positive–negative dimension: (1) positive marked traits, such as *relaxed*; (2) positive unmarked traits, such as *interesting*; (3) negative marked traits, such as *boring*; (4) negative unmarked traits, such as *aggressive*. The series of studies utilizing this material shows that, regardless of valence, marked traits cover a smaller range of events and are much more diagnostic than unmarked traits.

Arcuri and Cadinu's studies (Exp. 5), provide an indirect but powerful test of the diagnosticity of the traits according to their lexical properties. Subjects were presented with sentences in which the behavior performed by an actor was described (e.g., "In a difficult situation, John is behaving as a *courageous* person") using traits belonging to the four categories (i.e., positive marked traits, positive unmarked traits, negative marked traits, negative unmarked traits). Subjects were required to judge whether the behavior was the result of a permanent disposition of the actor or whether it was due to the situation using a rating scale ranging from 0 (*Maximum of Dispositional Attribution*) to 10 (*Maximum of Situational Attribution*). The Park and Rothbart model might predict that the negative traits have a greater informative value and therefore should produce attributional judgments that are more polarized towards the actor's disposition. On the contrary, the model proposed by Arcuri and Cadinu assumes a greater informative value for the marked terms, independent of the evaluative dimension of the traits used. Therefore, the judgments based on these terms would lead subjects to the greatest dispositional attributions. The analysis carried out on the attributional judgments showed a weak effect for valence and a very strong effect for markedness, showing that marked terms are considered more diagnostic about the permanent disposition of the actor than unmarked terms (see Table 6.1).

This suggests that the greater informative value of negative trait adjectives and their greater resistance to change observed in previous research may derive, not from their valence per se, but from their lexical properties, that is, their tendency to be marked rather than unmarked terms. This also implies that the informational advantage of negative

TABLE 6.1. Causal Attributions as a Function of Valence and Markedness

Valence of traits	Markedness		
	Marked	Unmarked	Average
Positive	4.17	5.85	5.01
Negative	3.50	5.35	4.42
Average	3.83	5.60	4.71

Note. Data from Arcuri and Cadinu (1992 , Exp. 5).

traits may be limited to those that are marked, and that a subgroup of positive traits, namely the marked ones, will share this advantage.

Whatever the exact reasons why negative traits are judged to require little behavioral confirmation but considerable disconfirming evidence, there are interesting implications of this finding for stereotype research. First, because out-group stereotypes are predominantly negative, they should be particularly resistant to change because they require more evidence to be disconfirmed and less evidence to be confirmed. Second, considering that there is a wide range of confirmability even within positive and within negative trait adjectives, one may speculate that stereotypes about out-groups will tend to contain exactly those negative terms that are easiest to confirm and most difficult to lose. The logic behind this is simple: If stereotypes are nonveridical, then they should be able to survive over time only if their disconfirmation is relatively difficult.

To test this possibility, Maass, Montalcini, and Paglionico (1995) have recently conducted a study intended to identify the most stereotypic (positive and negative) traits that Italian subjects assigned to the in-group (Italians) and to two out-groups (Jews, Germans). Following Rothbart and Park (1986), an independent sample of subjects then rated how many behavioral instances would be required to confirm or disconfirm the trait.

The results revealed no bias for the in-group stereotype: Positive and negative traits contained in the in-group stereotype were rated as requiring an equal amount of confirming or disconfirming evidence to be accepted or rejected, respectively. Results were quite different for the out-group stereotypes (Jews, Germans). Here, positive traits were rated as requiring much more evidence to be confirmed than to be disconfirmed, whereas negative traits were rated as requiring much evidence to be repudiated but very little to be considered confirmed (see Table 6.2).

TABLE 6.2. Number of Confirming and Disconfirming Behaviors Required in Order to Consider the Trait Confirmed or Disconfirmed, Respectively

Category	Desirability of trait	Number of confirming behaviors	Number of disconfirming behaviors
Italians	Desirable	4.99	4.71
(in-group)	Undesirable	4.58	4.58
Germans	Desirable	5.04	4.56
(out-group)	Undesirable	3.96	4.99
Jews	Desirable	5.50	4.79
(out-group)	Undesirable	4.28	4.98

Note. Data from Maass, Montalcini, and Paglionico (1995).

If these first results hold up in future research, then one may suspect that negative out-group perceptions are intrinsically resistant to change.[2] Although stereotypes about out-groups may contain both positive (*musical*) and negative (*devious*) trait adjectives, these may differ greatly in their resistance to change. Negative beliefs about the out-group seem to require much more disconfirming evidence before they will be revised. This suggests that the functioning of stereotypes cannot be fully understood without analyzing the specific linguistic characteristics of those traits that comprise in-group and out-group stereotypes.

Breadth of Stereotypic Trait Descriptors

Closely related to, but not redundant with the concept of trait confirmability is the idea that traits may differ in breadth. Some traits describe very general, broad characteristics (e.g., *responsible*), whereas others refer to more specific, narrower characteristics (e.g., *punctual*; see Hampson, Goldberg, & John, 1987; Hampson, John, & Goldberg, 1986).

Hamilton et al. (1992) have argued that positive characteristics of liked groups and negative characteristics of disliked groups tend to be expressed by broad traits, whereas negative characteristics of liked groups and positive characteristics of disliked groups tend to be expressed by narrow trait descriptors. Hamilton et al. reanalyzed data by Eagly and Kite (1987) in which American students rated different nationalities on various rating scales and found that positive traits assigned to liked nationalities tended to be broad rather than narrow, whereas undesirable traits ascribed to these nationalities tended to be narrow rather than broad. The opposite tendency was found for disliked nationalities. This argues for the differential use of narrow versus broad trait descriptors in judgments about liked versus disliked social categories. Considering that broad traits have a much wider range of application and are more difficult to disconfirm, this research provides further evidence that the linguistic properties of the traits contained in stereotypes may well contribute to the preservation of perceived intergroup differences.

Language Abstraction

A third mechanism by which language may contribute to stereotype maintenance concerns the way in which people describe specific behavioral episodes. At times, such descriptions imply that the behavior is representative of a more general characteristic or psychological state of the actor. Jones and Nisbett (1972, p. 90) pointed out that language seems to facilitate dispositional inferences from observed acts: "Once we have labelled an action as hostile, it is very easy to move to the inference that the perpetrator is a hostile person. Our language allows the same term to be applied to behavior and to the underlying disposition it reflects."

Although many languages (including English, German, and Italian) facilitate a unit formation of actor and act, this is by no means universal (see, e.g., an interesting series of studies by Miller, 1984, comparing American and Hindu subjects). Even in languages that facilitate correspondent inferences, not all descriptions imply that the act reflects some stable, underlying characteristic or tendency of the actor. At times, dispositional inferences are carefully avoided and the act is described in a very concrete way (*A hit B*), suggesting that the behavioral episode is an isolated event that is not linked to the actor's general characteristics. At times, the same behavior is interpreted as reflecting a more enduring behavioral tendency of the actor (*A is aggressive*).

Linguistic Intergroup Bias

The question then arises when the behavioral episode will be described in ways that link the act to the actor and when it will be described so as to minimize inferences from act to actor. According to the linguistic intergroup bias model (Maass, Salvi, Arcuri, & Semin, 1989) positive in-group and negative out-group behaviors tend to be described in relatively abstract terms, implying that the specific episode is related to more general characteristics of the actor. On the contrary, negative in-group and positive out-group behaviors tend to be described in relatively concrete terms that allow little generalization beyond the specific be-havior.

The degree of language abstractness refers to Semin and Fiedler's (1988, 1992) linguistic category model that in its original version distin-guishes four levels of abstraction in interpersonal terms. The most con-crete terms are descriptive action verbs (DAVs) such as "*A hits B*" that provide an objective description of a specific, observable event. Interpre-tive action verbs (IAVs) are slightly more abstract as they describe a larger class of behaviors ("*A hurts B*") although they maintain a clear reference to a specific behavior in a specific situation. The third level is represented by state verbs (SVs), such as "*A hates B,*" that describe en-during psychological states that generalize beyond specific situations and behaviors but refer to a specific object (person B). Finally, the most abstract terms are adjectives describing a general disposition that gener-alizes across situations, behaviors, and objects ("*A is aggressive*"; for extensions and applications of the linguistic category model see Semin & Fiedler, 1992). Applying this model to the intergroup situation, the linguistic intergroup bias predicts that positive behaviors are communi-cated in more abstract terms when performed by an in-group member than when performed by an out-group member. The opposite holds for negative behaviors, which are described more concretely when per-formed by an in-group member than when performed by an out-group member. For example, the in-group member offering help to a needy person may be described as "helpful" or "altruistic," whereas an out-group member engaging in exactly the same behavior may be described as "helping." In the case of aggressive behaviors, the in-group member may be described as "hurting somebody," whereas the out-group mem-ber may be described as being "aggressive."

Although these different descriptions may be equally accurate and pertinent, their meaning varies greatly. Moving from the concrete to the abstract pole of the continuum, the amount of information provided about the protagonist increases, the implicit stability and typicality of the act increases, as does the likelihood that the same act will be repeated in the future (Maass et al., 1989; Semin & Fiedler, 1988, 1992). Because ab-stract terms such as "state" verbs and adjectives imply great temporal and cross-situational stability, as well as a high likelihood of repetition in the future, this differential language use may indeed bolster existing stereotypic beliefs. Behaviors that confirm negative expectations about the out-group are communicated in an abstract way, suggesting that the observed act reflects a stable characteristic or psychological state of the actor. In contrast, an unexpectedly positive behavior from an out-group member is described in concrete terms, without generalizing beyond the specific context, thereby leaving the stereotype intact.

A yearly horse race competition in an Italian town served as setting for the first test of the linguistic intergroup bias model (Maass et al., 1989). Participants from competing teams were approached and asked to provide verbal descriptions of cartoon scenes in which the protagonists (either belonging to the subject's own team or to an opposing team) engaged in socially desirable or undesirable behaviors. As expected, subjects used highly abstract terms when describing desirable in-group and undesirable out-group episodes, but shifted their language toward the concrete end of the continuum when describing positive out-group and negative in-group behaviors (see Table 6.3).

Since then, the linguistic intergroup bias has consistently been demonstrated in a wide range of experiments conducted in different linguistic and cultural contexts. The linguistic intergroup bias has been shown to operate in political parties (Rubini & Semin, 1994), in interest groups (Maass, Ceccarelli, & Rudin, 1995), between sexes (Fiedler, Semin, & Finkenauer, 1993), competing schools, sport teams, and nations (Arcuri, Maass, & Portelli, 1993; for an overview see Maass & Arcuri, 1992). Importantly, the bias is not confined to controlled experiments. It has also emerged in content analyses of naturally occurring mass communication, such as news reports in both press and television (Maass, Corvino, & Arcuri, 1994). In one of these studies, we analyzed newspaper reports of an anti-Semitic episode that had occurred in Italy a few years ago. During a basketball game between an Italian and an Israeli team, right-wing groups had exposed banners depicting swastikas and anti-Semitic slogans. We found that this episode was described quite differently in Jewish and non-Jewish newspapers in Italy. Although both described the neofascist protagonists in clearly negative terms, they differed greatly in language abstraction. Compared to their Jewish colleagues, non-Jewish journalists used much more concrete language to

TABLE 6.3. Language Abstraction as a Function of Group Membership and Social Desirability

Membership of protagonist	Desirability of behavior	
	Desirable	Undesirable
In-group	2.69	2.51
Out-group	2.47	2.8

Note. From Maass, Salvi, Arcuri, and Semin (1989). Copyright 1989 by the American Psychological Association. Reprinted by permission.

describe the anti-Semitic acts. Although they condemned the aggressive behavior of anti-Semitic groups, they tended to report on such behavior almost exclusively in concrete terms, whereas their Jewish colleagues were much more likely to use abstract terms that generalize beyond the specific event. Another study analyzed evening news broadcasted by Italian TV during and after the Gulf War. Looking separately at phrases referring to the in-group (Allied Forces or leaders) and to the out-group (Iraqi forces or leaders), a clear pattern emerges: The more negative the statements were about Iraq, the more abstract they tended to be. Interestingly, this bias disappeared quickly after the war. For the in-group, no reliable correlation between abstraction and positivity/negativity was observed either during or after the war, indicating a clear bias in mass communication. Similar biases in journalists' language use have also been observed by Ng and Tait (1994) analyzing sports reports in New Zealand. Taken together, these studies provide evidence that the linguistic intergroup bias is operating in mass communication and that the way journalists use language in intergroup contexts constitutes a subtle but powerful source of bias.

Finally, there is now evidence that biased language use consistent with the linguistic intergroup bias is not limited to abstractness across verb types but may even occur within a single linguistic category, namely, adjectives. Semin and Fiedler (1991) have suggested that adjectives may differ in abstractness depending on their derivation.[3] Some adjectives, such as "pushy," are derived from DAVs; others, such as "aggressive" or " helpful," are derived from IAVs; and others, such as "hateful" or "adorable," from SVs. Others, again, are not derived from any verb (e.g., "introverted" or "hostile"). Using this distinction in derivation, Franco and Maass (1995) analyzed those adjectives that basketball fans had ascribed to their in-group and to a competing club (out-group). As expected, negative characteristics of the out-group and positive characteristics of the in-group were described by adjectives derived from relatively abstract verbs or without verb derivation, whereas positive out-group and negative in-group characteristics were described by adjectives with relatively concrete derivation, suggesting that a subtle bias in language use may operate even when people rely exclusively on adjectives to describe in-groups and out-groups.

Taken together, these studies suggest that the linguistic intergroup bias is widespread and robust. At the same time, it is very subtle, making it unlikely that speakers or listeners are fully aware of this bias. Although there is little doubt about the prevalence of the bias, it is not entirely clear which *mechanisms* sustain such differential language use in intergroup contexts.

Cognitive versus Motivational Accounts of Linguistic Intergroup Bias

There are at least two competing explanations for this phenomenon: one cognitive, the other motivational. According to the cognitive interpretation, the linguistic intergroup bias may derive from differential expectancies. One may argue that any expectancy-congruent behavior is described in abstract terms exactly because it is considered a stable and typical behavior tendency of the actor. If I expect Germans to be formal, then any formal behavior of a German actor should be described in abstract terms. In contrast, unexpected or surprising behaviors are considered short-lived and atypical, and as such ought to be described in concrete terms. The linguistic intergroup bias simply derives from the fact that members of a given group usually expect more desirable and fewer undesirable acts from in-group than from out-group members (see Howard & Rothbart, 1980).

Evidence for the role of differential expectancies comes from various studies (Maass, Milesi, Zabbini, & Stahlberg, 1995). In the first experiment, an intergroup setting was chosen in which stereotypes were shared by competing social groups. Northern and southern Italians converge, at least in part, in their beliefs about typically southern and typically northern characteristics. For example, both groups agree that southern Italians tend to be *hospitable* and *warm*, but also *sexist* and *intrusive,* whereas northern Italians are believed to be *industrious* and *emancipated* but also *materialistic* and *intolerant.* Subjects, coming either from the Veneto region in northern Italy or from Sicily, viewed cartoons in which the protagonist (allegedly of northern or southern origin) displayed behaviors indicative of these characteristics. Regardless of the protagonist's category membership (north or south), half of the acts were socially desirable, half were undesirable, and half were typically northern, half typically southern. The subject's task was to select one of four descriptors of the scene, corresponding to the four levels of abstraction in Semin and Fiedler's model. In line with the differential expectancy view, subjects—regardless of their own category membership—described typically northern behaviors of northern protagonists and typically southern behaviors of southern protagonists in abstract terms *regardless* of valence of the act. In contrast, atypical, out-of-role behaviors were described more concretely (see Table 6.4). These first results confirm the role of differential expectancies, suggesting that behaviors that are typical of the protagonist's group are described more abstractly than atypical or unexpected behaviors.

In a second experiment, the differential expectancy view was sub-

TABLE 6.4. Language Abstraction as a Function of the Protagonist's Category Membership and Typicality of the Act

	Typicality	
Protagonist	Northern	Southern
Northern	3.05	2.83
Southern	2.99	3.14

Note. From Maass, Milesi, Zabbini, and Stahlberg (1995). Copyright 1995 by the American Psychological Association. Reprinted by permission.

jected to a stricter test by running an experiment in which the protagonist's membership had no personal relevance at all to the subject, and in which expectations were induced experimentally. Following a procedure developed by Rothbart, Evans, and Fulero (1979), expectations were created by telling subjects that the target person had been described by friends, parents, and teachers as having a given characteristic. Depending on the condition, the person was either described as "sociable," "intelligent," "unsociable," or "unintelligent." Subsequently, subjects received a cartoon showing the target person behaving in a way that either confirmed or disconfirmed the expectancy. Again, subjects had to select one of four descriptions corresponding to the four levels of abstraction. The results showed that regardless of the specific expectancy induced, expectancy-congruent behaviors were described more abstractly than expectancy-incongruent behaviors.

What is most important for our argument is the fact that biased language use consistent with the differential expectancy view occurs even in the complete absence of social-category membership. Even observers not personally involved in the intergroup setting use abstract terms such as state verbs and adjectives to describe behaviors that confirm their expectancies, but shift their language toward the concrete pole of the continuum when describing behavioral episodes that contradict their expectations. This suggests a purely cognitive and rather rational process.

Yet, there is a second, but no less plausible explanation based on motivational principles. According to this viewpoint, one might suspect that the linguistic intergroup bias is driven by *in-group-protective motives*. This hypothesis is loosely based on social identity theory (Tajfel & Turner, 1986; Taylor & Moghaddam, 1987) and assumes that the linguistic intergroup bias serves to enhance or protect one's social identity. Assuming that concrete descriptions dissociate the actor from the act, whereas abstract descriptions imply that the behavior reflects a stable and enduring property of the actor, one may argue that the linguistic intergroup bias helps to portray the in-group in a favorable light while derogating the out-group. In other words, people may show the linguistic intergroup bias as one possible way of maintaining a positive image of their own group which, in turn, enhances their self-esteem. Thus, this bias may have the same function as the many strategies of in-group favoritism that have been observed in social identity research (e.g., discriminatory responses on reward allocation matrices in the minimal group paradigm).

Contrary to the expectancy-based explanation, the in-group-protection hypothesis predicts abstract language use for positive in-group and negative out-group behaviors regardless of stereotypic expectancy. Although the results of the previously cited studies by Maass, Milesi, et al. (1995) suggest that differential expectancies are *sufficient* to produce the linguistic intergroup bias and that motivational processes are unnecessary, this does not prove that in-group-protective motives are necessarily and always irrelevant. Note that the previously mentioned studies did not investigate highly competitive or openly hostile intergroup relations. One may argue that in-group-protective motivations may become the driving force of biased language use in highly competitive intergroup settings.

In order to investigate this possibility, a recent study by Maass, Ceccarelli, and Rudin (1995, Exp. 1) took advantage of an intergroup setting that was known from previous research to be highly conflictual and in which group members generally hold very negative views about the out-group, namely, hunters versus environmentalists. Most important, the degree of intergroup competition was varied experimentally by either reinforcing the existing antagonism between the groups or suggesting that the moment had come to overcome traditional boundaries and to collaborate for the solution of environmental problems. It was hypothesised that the linguistic intergroup bias would be considerably stronger under high rather than low competition. As in previous research (Maass et al., 1989), single-frame cartoons were used in which hunters or environmentalists displayed positive or negative behaviors, and language abstraction was assessed.

The results show that both groups use language in a way that clearly favors the in-group, but this bias is considerably more pronounced under high competition. Parallel findings were obtained for a second measure that gave subjects the opportunity to distribute public funds to hunting versus environmentalist organizations using the traditional matrices employed in social identity research. Just like the linguistic intergroup bias, the matrix measure indicated that difference in favor of the in-group increased under competition. Thus, the same factors that increase in-group favoritism on matrices also increased the magnitude of the linguistic intergroup bias. Most important, there was evidence that the linguistic intergroup bias may, indeed, be a successful strategy in protecting one's personal and collective self-esteem. The greater the bias under high competition, the greater the subsequent self-esteem, whereas language use and self-esteem were unrelated under low competition.

An Integration

Although these studies are only the first attempts to identify the psychological processes underlying the linguistic intergroup bias, we believe that they provide at least a tentative answer to the question of whether this bias is driven by differential expectancies or in-group protective motives. The answer to the question is that both mechanisms may contribute. Differential expectancies seem to be sufficient to produce differential language use in intergroup settings and probably in a wide range of additional situations. The link between cognition and language abstraction may be such that any a priori expectancy (not only stereotypes) determines language abstraction that in turn "protects" existing beliefs against disconfirmation.

At the same time, our data also suggest that the linguistic intergroup bias is not insensitive to motivational needs. In situations in which intergroup competition is salient, the linguistic intergroup bias may have much the same in-group-protective function as other forms of in-group favoritism and out-group discrimination. Although the exact interaction between cognitive and motivational factors has yet to be investigated, it appears likely that language use is the function of both differential expectancies and in-group protective motives. This suggests an interesting link between stereotypes, in-group favoritism, and language. Although stereotypes and in-group favoritism are not completely independent (stereotypes tend to favor the in-group), they may have partially independent effects on language in intergroup contexts. In the absence of in-group threatening factors, stereotypic beliefs tend to determine language use that in turn contributes to the confirmation of such beliefs, thereby feeding into a self-fulfilling cycle. When in-group-protective motivations become very strong, they tend to override stereotypes and exert a direct impact on language use, which then fulfills an in-group-favoring (rather than expectancy-confirming) function.

Considering the findings on trait confirmability, trait breadth, and abstraction together, an interesting pattern emerges: It becomes clear that descriptions of the out-group do not represent a representative sample of negative attributes drawn in a random fashion from the entire vocabulary of a given language. Rather, it is a particular type of negative attribute that is most likely to become part of the negative out-group stereotype, namely those (1) that require most evidence to be disconfirmed, (2) that represent very general, broad traits, and (3) that are highly abstract. To this point, the relation between abstractness, breadth, and confirmability is still largely unexplored, and it remains unclear whether these three characteristics are distinct or partially overlapping features of linguistic expressions contained in negative out-group perceptions. What is evident, however, is that they all share the same function, namely to protect existing beliefs against disconfirmation.

IDENTITY-EXPRESSIVE FUNCTION

Finally, language fulfills an identity-expressive function that has in particular been studied by Giles and colleagues in the framework of "speech accommodation theory" (for an extended review, see Giles, Mulac, Bradac, & Johnson 1987, as well as Giles & Johnson, 1987). The main idea here is that intergroup situations tend to activate sociolinguistic stereotypes, such as those associated with male versus female speech, or Black versus White speech, which in turn induce divergent or convergent shifts in language use. Depending on the type of intergroup relation and the strength of ethnolinguistic identity, people will tend to shift their speech pattern either toward or away from that of the person being addressed. For example, mixed-sex interactions will activate gender-stereotypes, which in turn will induce language shifts such that a male speaker may either accentuate "male" speech or shift toward what he believes to be a typically "female" speech style. Thus, both convergence and divergence are driven by stereotypic beliefs about how in-group and out-group members typically talk but the direction of this speech shift (either toward or away from out-group speech) will depend on a number of factors specified by speech accommodation theory (Giles et al., 1987).

According to this model, *convergence* toward the stereotypic characteristics of the addressee are predicted whenever speakers (1) desire a high level of communicational efficiency, (2) strive for the recipient's social approval, (3) desire a group presentation shared by the recipient, or (4) when the recipient's speech is positively evaluated (for additional predictors of convergence, see Giles et al., 1987).

An example of the convergence toward the stereotypic characteristic of the recipient, driven by beliefs about communicational efficiency, comes from studies on the communication process during caregiver–patient interaction. There is considerable evidence that health-care professionals hold specific stereotypes about different patient groups. The simple fact that an individual is occupying a bed in the hospital may lead health-care providers to assume that the person is dependent and anxious (DeVellis, Wallston, & Wallston, 1980; see also Morimoto, 1955), and some patient groups, such as the elderly, are particularly likely to become the object of stereotypic beliefs. Ashburn and Gordon (1981) compared specific formal and functional characteristics of caregivers' and volunteers' speech among themselves and toward elderly residents in a nursing home. They found that more questions and repetitions were used by staff and volunteers in speaking to elderly people than in speaking to their peers. Other studies (e.g., Caporael, 1981) illustrate the use of "secondary baby talk" by caregivers in speaking to the institutionalized elderly. The secondary baby talk, defined as a specific set of prosodic configurations, was found to be frequent in caregivers' talk to residents and to be indistinguishable from the talk actually addressed to children. Caregivers apparently use such speech because they believe that communication will be more efficient; they reported that residents with low functional activity would like to be spoken to with "secondary baby talk," and felt that the normal speech would be ineffective for interacting with them (Caporael, Lucaszewski, & Culberston, 1983)

Convergence effects have also been observed between social classes, although the convergence of high class speakers toward low-class speakers appears to be motivated by efficiency needs, whereas the convergence of low class speakers seems to reflect the speakers' desire for social integration or approval. For instance, Thakerar, Giles, and Cheshire (1982) presented data indicating that high-status speakers converge to lower status participants by means of slowing down their speech rates and nonstardardizing their accents for "cognitive" reasons, that is, to facilitate recipients' understanding of the message. In contrast, the latter quicken their speech rates and standardize their accents in order to enhance their perceived competence in the eyes of the former.

As predicted by speech accommodation theory, convergence is most likely to occur when out-group speech reflects high status or high social desirability. Research on linguistic assimilation of immigrants in dominant cultures shows that language shifts are typically unilateral with subordinate groups converging to the dominant group in their use of language far more than vice versa (Giles, 1977). For example, Wolfram and Fasold (1974) reported that both Puerto Ricans and Blacks in New York at the beginning of the 1970s considered the latter to be superior in power and prestige, and that Puerto Ricans assimilated the dialect of Blacks far more than vice versa. In terms of Tajfel and Turner's (1979) social identity theory, convergent language shifts have been considered a tactic for achieving a positive self-image. Seeking social approval is the main element of the individual mobility strategy that may be adopted by certain members of subordinate groups who perceive their in-group's social position as legitimate and immutable.

Interestingly however, convergence toward the out-group is not the only linguistic strategy in intergroup contacts. Often speakers *diverge* from the recipient's speech, in an attempt to stress their own social identity (for additional factors motivating divergence, see Giles et al., 1987). For example, Hogg (1985) found that males were judged to sound more "masculine" (by an independent group of observers) when talking to females when gender was made salient than when it was not; in other words, they appeared to be diverging vocally from their opposite-sex interlocutors. Along the same line, Giles and Byrne (1982) have pointed out that as out-group members begin to learn the speech style of the in-group, in-group members tend to diverge in some way so as to maintain linguistic distinctiveness. Taken together, this research suggests that people accentuate their psycholinguistic group membership when social categorization becomes salient, or when there is a threat to their social identity. Interestingly, when such accentuation is undermined, people will attempt to maintain their social identity through other channels. Yang and Bond (1980) asked bilingual Chinese students to respond to a questionnaire on social values either in English or Cantonese. Students forced to respond in English compensated for this fact by expressing attitudes that were much closer to the traditional Chinese values than the comparison group responding in Cantonese. Together, these findings support the idea of ethnolinguistic identity theory that language serves to affirm the speakers ethnic identity.

These results are largely in line with Tajfel and Turner's (1979) social identity perspective, suggesting that people may react to others not so much as individuals but as representatives of different social groups. The more they consider membership in the out-group as prestigious and advantageous, and the more they believe group boundaries to be permeable, the more they tend to adopt the out-group speech. On the contrary, they will tend to accentuate in-group speech whenever intergroup mobility is either not feasible or not desirable, or when in-group identity is threatened.

CONCLUSIONS

The literature on language and stereotyping reviewed here allows a few general, although necessarily tentative conclusions. First of all, it becomes evident from this review that stereotypes are closely—if not inseparably—linked to language. Indeed, it is difficult to imagine language-free stereotyping. This suggests that our knowledge of stereotypes will remain incomplete without an analysis of the language that defines a given stereotype. Fortunately, this review also demonstrates that there has recently been increasing interest in the role of language in stereotyping, although there is not yet any general theory in sight that would link language to stereotyping in a systematic and integrative fashion. Despite the lack of a general theoretical model, there is ample converging research evidence that language fulfills multiple functions, ranging from stereotype transmission to the maintenance of existing stereotypic beliefs. Interestingly, language often seems to fulfill these functions in such a subtle way that it may easily escape conscious control of both speaker and listener. In other words, language seems to play a powerful role, but it is not easy to become fully aware of its impact. It is exactly this feature that renders language analysis such an interesting (and largely unobtrusive) methodological tool, allowing access to the more subtle, less controlled processes of stereotyping.

NOTES

1. According to one explanation, this saying can be traced back to an episode when the Portuguese government sponsored a play in Rome under the condition that Portuguese citizens living in Rome would be allowed to attend for free. Apparently, that night everybody claimed to be Portuguese. The saying therefore derives from an episode in which the Romans cheated and the Portuguese acted legitimately, but ironically the expression "*fare il Portoghese*" implies the opposite meaning.

2. Because the majority of traits indicated by subjects in this study were not classifiable in *marked* versus *unmarked* terms, it was impossible to identify the relative contribution of valence and markedness in this study.

3. Note, however, that Semin and Fiedler (1991) have argued that IAV-derived adjectives are more abstract that SV-derived adjectives, thus proposing an abstractness hierarchy for adjectives that differs from their original verb category model. In contrast, our data were analyzed according to the original model, assuming a linear increase in abstractness from DAV, IAV, SV up to nonderived adjectives.

REFERENCES

Allen, I. L. (1983). *The language of ethnic conflict: Social organization and lexical culture.* New York: Columbia University Press.

Allport, G. (1954). *The nature of prejudice.* Reading, MA: Addison-Wesley.

Arcuri, L., & Cadinu, M. R. (1992). Asymmetries in the attributional processes: The role of linguistic mediators. In L. Arcuri & C. Serino (Eds.), *Asymmetry phenomena in interpersonal comparison: Cognitive and social issues* (pp. 87–100). Napoli: Liguori.

Arcuri, L., Maass, A., & Portelli, G. (1993). Linguistic intergroup bias and implicit attributions. *British Journal of Social Psychology, 32,* 277–285.

Ashburn, G., & Gordon, A. (1981). Features of a simplified register in speech to elderly conversationalists. *International Journal of Psycholinguistics, 8,* 7–31.

Bargh, J. A., & Pietromonaco, P. (1982). Automatic information processing and social perception: The influence of trait information presented outside of conscious awareness on impression formation. *Journal of Personality and Social Psychology, 43,* 437–449.

Bem, S. L., & Bem, D. J. (1973). Does sex-biased advertising "aid and abet" sex discrimination? *Journal of Applied Social Psychology, 3,* 6–18.

Boca, S., Zuffi, M., & Arcuri, L. (1994). *Automatic processes in categorisation of social stimuli: Evidence from an interference task.* Report No. 62, Dipartimento di Psicologia dello Sviluppo e della Socializzazione, University of Padua, Padua, Italy.

Brigham, J. C. (1971). Ethnic stereotypes. *Psychological Bulletin, 76,* 15–38.

Caporael, L. (1981). The paralanguage of caregiving: Baby talk to the institutionalized aged. *Journal of Personality and Social Psychology, 40,* 876–884.

Caporael, L., Lucasziewski, M. P., & Culbertson, G. H. (1983). Secondary babytalk: Judgments by institutionalized elderly and their caregivers. *Journal of Personality and Social Psychology, 44,* 746–754.

Clark, H. H., & Clark, E. U. (1977). *Psychology and language.* New York: Harcourt Brace Jovanovich.

De Vellis, B. M., Wallston, B. S., & Wallston, K. A. (1980). Stereotyping: A threat to individualized patient care. In M. H. Miller & B. Flynn (Eds.), *Current perspectives in nursing: Social issues and trends* (Vol. 2). St. Louis: Mosby.

Devine, P. G. (1989). Stereotypes and prejudice: Their automatic and controlled components. *Journal of Personality and Social Psychology, 56,* 5–18.

Eagly, A. H., & Kite, M. E. (1987). Are stereotypes of nationalities applied to both women and men? *Journal of Personality and Social Psychology, 53,* 451–462.

Eiser, J. R. (1975). Attitudes and the use of evaluative language: A two-way process. *Journal of the Theory of Social Behavior, 5,* 235–248.

Eiser, J. R., & Ross, M. D. (1977). Partisan language, immediacy, and attitude change. *European Journal of Social Psychology, 7,* 477–489.

Fagot, B. I., & Leinbach, M. D. (1989). The young child's gender schema: Environmental input, internal organization. *Child Development, 60,* 663–672.

Fagot, B. I., Leinbach, M. D., & O'Boyle, C. (1992). Gender labeling, gender stereotyping, and parenting behaviors. *Developmental Psychology, 28,* 225–230.

Fianco, F. M., & Maass, A. (1995). *Implicit vs. explicit strategies of outgroup discrimination: The role of intentional control in biased language use and reward allocation.* Unpublished manuscript, University of Padua, Padua, Italy.

Fiedler, K., Semin, G. R., & Kinkenauer, C. (1993). The battle of words between gender groups: A language-based approach to intergroup processes. *Human Communication Research, 19,* 409–441.

Gilbert, D. T., & Hixon, J. G. (1991). The trouble of thinking: Activation and application of stereotypic beliefs. *Journal of Personality and Social Psychology, 60,* 509–517.

Giles, H. (1977). *Language, ethnicity and intergroup relations.* New York: Academic Press.

Giles, H., & Byrne, J. L. (1982). An intergroup approach to second language acquisition. *Journal of Multilingual and Multicultural Development, 1,* 17–40.

Giles, H., & Johnson, P. (1987). Ethnolinguistic identity theory: A social psychological approach to language maintenance. *International Journal of the Sociology of Language, 68,* 69–99.

Giles, H., Mulac, A., Bradac, J., & Johnson, P. (1987). Speech accomodation theory: The first decade and beyond. *Communication Yearbook, 10,* 13–48.

Graumann, C. F., & Wintermantel, M. (1989). Discriminatory speech acts. In D. Bar-Tal, C. F. Graumann, A. W. Kruglanski, & W. Stroebe (Eds.), *Stereotyping and prejudice: Changing conceptions* (pp. 183–204). New York: Springer Verlag.

Greenberg, J., & Pyszczynsky, T. (1985). The effect of an overheard ethnic slur on evaluations of the target: How to spread a social disease. *Journal of Experimental Social Psychology, 21,* 61–72.

Greenwald, A. G., Klinger, M. R., & Liu, T. J. (1989). Unconscious processing of dichoptically masked words. *Memory and Cognition, 17 ,* 35–47.

Hamilton, D. L., Gibbons, P. A., Stroessner, S. J., & Sherman, J. W. (1992). Language, intergroup relations and stereotypes. In G. R. Semin & K. Fiedler (Eds.), *Language, interaction and social cognition* (pp. 102–128). London: Sage.

Hampson, S. E., Goldberg, L. R., & John, O. P. (1987). Category breadth and social-desirability values for 573 personality terms. *European Journal of Personality, 1,* 241–258.

Hampson, S. E., John, O. P., & Goldberg, L. R. (1986). Category breadth and hierarchical structure in personality: Studies of asymmetries in judgments of trait implications. *Journal of Personality and Social Psychology, 51,* 37–54.

Harrison, L. (1975). Cro-Magnon woman—in eclipse. *The Science Teacher, 42,* 8–11.

Higgins, E. T., King, G. A., & Mavin, G. H. (1982). Individual construct accessibility and subjective impressions and recall. *Journal of Personality and Social Psychology, 43,* 35–47.

Hoffman, C., Lau, I., & Johnson, D. R. (1986). The linguistic relativity of person cognition: An English–Chinese comparison. *Journal of Personality and Social Psychology, 51,* 1097–1105.

Hogg, M. A. (1985). Masculine and feminine speech in dyads and groups: A study of speech style and gender salience. *Journal of Language and Social Psychology, 4,* 99–112.

Howard, J., & Rothbart, M. (1980). Social categorization and memory for in-group and out-group behavior. *Journal of Personality and Social Psychology, 38,* 301–310.

Hunt, E., & Agnoli, F. (1991). The Whorfian hypothesis: A cognitive psychology perspective. *Psychological Review, 98,* 377–389.

Hyde, J. S. (1984). Children's understanding of sexist language. *Developmental Psychology, 20,* 697–706.

Jones, E. E., & Nisbett, R. E. (1972). The actor and the observer: Divergent perceptions of the causes of behavior. In E. E. Jones, D. Kanouse, H. H. Kelley, R. E. Nisbett, S. Valins, & B. Weiner (Eds.), *Attribution: Perceiving the causes of behavior* (pp. 79–94). Morristown, NJ: General Learning Press.

Katz, D., & Braly, K. W. (1933). Racial stereotypes of 100 college students. *Journal of Abnormal and Social Psychology, 28,* 280–290.

Kidd, V. (1971). A study of the images perceived through the use of the male pronoun as the generic. *Movements in Contemporary Rhetoric and Communication, 1,* 25–29.

Kirchler, E. (1992). Adorable women, expert man: Changing gender images of women and men in management. *European Journal of Social Psychology, 22,* 363–373.

Kirkland, S. L., Greenberg, J., & Pyszczynski, T. (1987). Further evidence of the deleterious effects of overheard derogatory ethnic labels: Derogation beyond the target. *Personality and Social Psychology Bulletin, 13,* 216–227.

Kruse, L., Weimer, E., & Wagner, F. (1988). What men and women are said to be: Social representation and language. *Journal of Language and Social Psychology, 7,* 243–262.

Leinbach, M. D., & Fagot, B. I. (1992). Acquisition of gender labeling: A test of toddlers. *Sex Roles, 15,* 655–666.

Linville, P. W., Fischer, G. W., & Salovey, P. (1989). Perceived distributions of the characteristics of in-group and out-group members: Empirical evidence and a computer simulation. *Journal of Personality and Social Psychology, 57,* 165–188.

Maass, A., & Arcuri, L. (1992). The role of language in the persistence of stereotypes. In G. Semin & K. Fiedler (Eds.), *Language, interaction and social cognition* (pp. 129–143). Newbury Park, CA: Sage.

Maass, A., Ceccarelli, B., & Rudin, S. (1995). *The linguistic intergroup bias: Ev-*

idence for ingroup-protective motivation. Unpublished manuscript, University of Padua, Padua, Italy.

Maass, A., Corvino, P., & Arcuri, L. (1994). Linguistic intergroup bias and the mass media. *Revue de Internationale Psychologie Sociale, 1,* 31–43.

Maass, A., Milesi, A., Zabbini, S., & Stahlberg, D. (1995). The linguistic intergroup bias: Differential expectancies or in-group-protection? *Journal of Personality and Social Psychology, 68,* 116–126.

Maass, A., Montalcini, F., & Paglionico, N. (1995). *On the (dis-)confirmability of stereotypic attributes.* Unpublished manuscript, Dipartimento di Psicologia dello Sviluppo e della Socializzazione, University of Padua, Padua, Italy.

Maass, A., Salvi, D., Arcuri, L., & Semin, G. R. (1989). Language use in intergroup contexts: The linguistic intergroup bias. *Journal of Personality and Social Psychology, 57,* 981–993.

MacKay, D. G. (1980). Psychology, prescriptive grammar and the pronoun problem. *American Psychologist, 33,* 68–72.

MacKay, D. G., & Fulkerson, D. C. (1979). On the comprehension and production of pronouns. *Journal of Verbal Learning and Verbal Behavior, 18,* 661–673.

McCauley, C., & Stitt, C. L. (1978). An individual and quantitative measure of stereotypes. *Journal of Personality and Social Psychology, 36,* 929–940.

Miller, J. G. (1984). Culture and the development of everyday social explanation. *Journal of Personality and Social Psychology, 46,* 961–978.

Mininni, G. (1982). *Psicosemiotica.* Bari, Italy: Adriatica Editrice.

Morimoto, F. R. (1955). Favoritism in personnel–patient interactions. *Nursing Research, 3,* 109–112.

Moulton, J., Robinson, G. M., & Elias, C. (1978). Sex bias in language use: Neutral pronouns that aren't. *American Psychologist, 33,* 1032–1036.

Mullen, B., & Johnson, C. (1993). Cognitive representation in ethnophaulisms as a function of group size: The phenomenology of being in a group. *Personality and Social Psychology Bulletin, 19,* 296–304.

Mummendey, A., & Simon, B. (1989). Better or different? III: The impact of importance of comparison dimension and relative group size upon intergroup discrimination. *British Journal of Social Psychology, 28,* 1–16.

Murdock, N. L., & Forsyth, D. R. (1985). Is gender-biased language sexist? A perceptual approach. *Psychology of Women Quarterly, 9,* 39–49.

Neely, J. H. (1990). Semantic priming effects in visual word recognition: A selective review of current findings and theories. In D. Bresner & G. Humphreys (Eds.), *Basic processes in reading and visual word recognition.* Hillsdale, NJ: Erlbaum.

Ng, S. H. (1990). The androcentric coding of *man* and *his* in memory by language users. *Journal of Experimental Social Psychology, 26,* 455–464.

Ng, S. H., & Tait, J. (1994). *Biases of journalists' linguistic representation of intergroup events.* Unpublished manuscript, Victoria University of Wellington, New Zealand.

Nilson, A. P. (1977). Sexism in children's books and elementary teaching materials. In A. P. Nilson, H. Bosmajian, H. L. Gershung, & J. P. Stanley

(Eds.), *Sexism and language.* Urbana, IL: National Council of Teachers of English.

Park, B., & Judd, C. M. (1990). Measures and models of perceived group variability. *Journal of Personality and Social Psychology, 59,* 173–191.

Perdue, C. W., Dovidio, J. F., Gurtman, M. B., & Tyler, R. B. (1990). Us and them: Categorization and the process of intergroup bias. *Journal of Personality and Social Psychology, 59,* 475–486.

Rothbart, M., Evans, M., & Fulero, S. (1979). Recall for confirming events: Memory processes and the maintenance of social stereotypes. *Journal of Experimental Social Psychology, 15,* 343–355.

Rothbart, M., & Park, B. (1986). On the confirmability and disconfirmability of trait concepts. *Journal of Personality and Social Psychology, 50,* 131–142.

Rubin, M., & Semin, G. R. (1994). Language use in the context of congruent and incongruent ingroup behaviours. *British Journal of Social Psychology, 33,* 355–362.

Schneider, J. W., & Hacker, S. L. (1973). Sex role imagery and use of the generic "man" in introductory texts: A case in the sociology of sociology. *American Sociologist, 8,* 12–18.

Semin, G. R., & Fiedler, K. (1988). The cognitive functions of linguistic categories in describing persons: Social cognition and language. *Journal of Personality and Social Psychology, 54,* 558–568.

Semin, G. R., & Fiedler, K. (1991). The linguistic category model, its bases, applications and range. In. W. Stroebe & M. Hewstone (Eds.), *European Review of Social Psychology* (Vol. 2, pp.1–50). Chichester, UK: Wiley.

Semin, G. R., & Fiedler, K. (1992). The inferential properties of interpersonal verbs. In G. Semin & K. Fiedler (Eds.), *Language, interaction and social cognition* (pp. 58–78). Newbury Park, CA: Sage.

Stahlberg, D., Sczensky, S., Otto, C., Rudolph, H., & Sorgenfrey, S. (1994). Sexismus in der Sprache: Das generische Maschulinum und die Sichtbarkeit von Frauen. Unpublished manuscript, University of Kiel, Kiel, Germany.

Stangor, C., & Lange, J. (1993). Mental representations of social groups: Advances in understanding stereotypes and stereotyping. *Advances in Experimental Social Psychology, 26,* 357–416.

Tajfel, H., & Turner, J. C. (1979). An integrative theory of intergroup conflict. In W. Austin & S. Worchel (Eds.), *The social psychology of intergroup relations* (pp. 33–47). Monterey, CA: Brooks/Cole.

Tajfel, H., & Turner, J. C. (1986). The social identity theory of intergroup behavior. In S. Worchel & W. G. Austin (Eds.), *Psychology of intergroup relations* (pp. 7–24). Chicago: Nelson-Hall.

Taylor, D. M., & Moghaddam, F. M. (1987). Social identity theory. In D. M. Taylor & F. M Moghaddam (Eds.), *Theories of intergroup relations: International social psychological perspectives* (pp. 59–84). New York: Praeger.

Thakerar, J. N., Giles, H., & Cheshire, J. (1982) Psychological and linguistic parameters of speech accomodation theory. In C. Fraser & K. R. Scherer

(Eds.), *Advances in the social psychology of language* (pp. 205–255). Cambridge, UK: Cambridge University Press.

Van Dijk, T. A. (1984). *Prejudice and discourse: An analysis of ethnic prejudice in cognition and conversation*. Amsterdam: Benjamins.

Van Dijk, T. A. (1987). *Communicating racism: Ethnic prejudice in thought and talk*. Newbury Park, CA: Sage.

Van Dijk, T. A. (1988). *News analysis. Case studies of international and national news in the press*. Hilldale, NJ: Erlbaum.

Weinraub, M., Clements, L. P., Sockloff, A., Ethridge, T., Gracely, E., & Myers, B. (1984). The development of sex role stereotypes in the third year: Relationships to gender labeling, gender identity, sex-typed toy preferences. *Child Development, 55*, 1493–1503.

Wilson, E., & Ng, S. H. (1988). Sex bias in visual images evoked by generics: A New Zealand study. *Sex Roles, 18*, 159–169.

Wolfram, W., & Fasold, R.W. (1974). *The study of social dialects in American English*. Englewood Cliffs, NJ: Prentice Hall.

Yang, K. S., & Bond, M. H. (1980). Ethnic affirmation in Chinese bilinguals. *Journal of Cross-Cultural Psychology, 11*, 411–425.

7

The Self-Regulation of Intergroup Perception: Mechanisms and Consequences of Stereotype Suppression

GALEN V. BODENHAUSEN
C. NEIL MACRAE

> An individual human being starts life with a
> problem: learning how to control himself or
> herself. As in all problems, one starts in a certain
> position with certain limited resources, and must
> then bootstrap those resources somehow into a
> solution.
> —DENNETT (1984, p. 83)

One of the key insights of social psychological analyses of human behavior has been a recognition of the active construction of meaning that
perceivers undertake in mentally representing the social world in which
they live and function (Fiske & Taylor, 1991; Ross & Nisbett, 1991;
Wyer & Srull, 1989). In navigating the complex relationships and interactions that constitute everyday life, people make behavioral choices on
the basis of their subjective interpretations of the people and situations
they encounter. Although our perceptions of the world are ultimately
constrained to some degree by the objective qualities of social stimuli,

our construals do not invariably correspond to actual properties of the entities in question. One important potential source of divergence between subjective impressions and objective "truths" is the operation of inferential processes that use detectable characteristics of social stimuli to derive assumed characteristics that are not readily apparent in the initial perceptual experience. Stereotyping represents a classic case of this process. The detection of group memberships such as sex, race, or age is often trivially easy, but detecting personality traits, interests, and attitudes requires more of an investment of mental resources. As noted throughout this volume, perceivers approach social situations with extensive sets of assumptions about the traits, interests, behavioral proclivities, and other characteristics of social groups that they can use to shape their impressions of individual group members (see Brewer, Chapter 8, this volume).

The process of stereotyping has undeniable appeal for social perceivers, making it possible to form articulated representations of others efficiently and relatively effortlessly (for a review, see Hamilton & Sherman, 1994). In spite of these benefits to the perceiver, however, recent decades have been characterized by a growing realization of, and concern about, the potential costs of stereotyping for the targets of this process. Because stereotypes about out-groups are often negative, stereotypic impressions may lead persons who are members of stereotyped groups to experience systematic disadvantages in important contexts, such as personnel selection, legal decision making, and countless others. Such concerns have led many people to the conclusion that stereotyping others is inappropriate and to be avoided. In this chapter, we explore the prospects for successfully avoiding stereotypic thinking. In particular, we review research documenting the motivational basis for attempts to regulate one's impressions in order to avoid the influence of stereotypes, we consider current models of cognitive self-control, and we summarize the available evidence about the often ironic consequences of attempting to suppress stereotypic modes of thought.

THE WELL-INTENTIONED COGNITIVE MISER: MENTAL DILEMMAS OF MULTICULTURAL SOCIETIES

The demographic and political trends of the 20th century have resulted in the creation of increasingly multicultural societies around the world. Certainly in virtually any urban setting, one can routinely expect to encounter people who differ in terms of their ethnicity, religious affiliation, sexual orientation, and nationality. Even those individuals who live in relatively homogeneous social environments are likely to be frequently exposed to a wide variety of different social groups via the mass media (see Greenberg & Brand, 1994; Harris, 1994). The density and diversity of the modern social landscape give rise to a set of conflicting concerns and interests. On one hand, it may be immensely appealing to the social perceiver to rely on stereotypes in constructing orderly and well-structured representations from the complex array of social stimuli. On the other hand, for many individuals, the notion of relying on stereotypes to judge others has developed decidedly unpleasant connotations. In this section, we outline the roots of this dilemma and explore the motivational impulses to which it gives rise.

The appeal of engaging in stereotyping is clearly multifaceted (Allport, 1954). Social perceivers can satisfy several important motivations by viewing the members of other groups in stereotypic terms. By developing comparatively unfavorable impressions of out-groups, individuals can construct a superior image of their own social groups, and by extension, feel better about themselves (Tajfel & Turner, 1986). Members of advantaged groups can feel more comfortable with social inequities by developing specific beliefs about disadvantaged groups that appear to explain and justify the existence of unequal resource distributions between groups (Jost & Banaji, 1994; Sidanius & Pratto, 1993). The act of stereotyping also appeals to the basic motivation of most social perceivers to conserve mental resources (Macrae, Milne, & Bodenhausen, 1994) while still producing coherent and structured social impressions. The metaphor of the "cognitive miser" (Fiske & Taylor, 1991) aptly captures the human tendency to "satisfice" rather than optimize (Simon, 1957) by engaging only in the amount of thought necessary to produce an apparently adequate understanding of others. Making group-based inferences is typically easily accomplished and bypasses the much more effortful task of detecting and integrating the unique constellation of characteristics possessed by a given individual. Unless there is a pressing motivational impetus for accuracy, stereotyping may be the preferred path to a social impression for most perceivers (Fiske & Neuberg, 1990; Pendry & Macrae, 1994). Moreover, imposing a relatively simple categorical structure on the world may be highly satisfying to many perceivers because it confers a greater sense of predictability and orderliness on a complex social world (Kruglanski, 1989; Tajfel, 1969).

Because of the many needs they fulfill, stereotypes may be called upon very frequently in forming impressions of others. As a result, the process of stereotyping comes to occur in largely automatic ways (Brewer, 1988; Devine, 1989; Gilbert & Hixon, 1991). There are several related criteria for determining whether a mental process can be character-ized as "automatic" (Bargh, 1994). Cognitive processes are said to be automatic when they occur without the perceiver's conscious intent or awareness of them, without the perceiver's ability to control them, or with an efficiency that requires little investment of the perceiver's limit-ed cognitive resources. Once automatized, stereotypes may spring to mind in the presence of out-group members whether they are desired or not, and the perceiver may be powerless to control or prevent this initial activation. In a highly influential paper, Devine (1989) provided evi-dence that stereotypic associations can indeed be activated in an auto-matic fashion. Specifically, she found that even individuals who do not personally subscribe to stereotypic beliefs about African Americans were affected by these stereotypes when they had been "primed" by the presentation of group labels (see also Dovidio, Evans, & Tyler, 1986). Hence, the stereotypes had unintended effects that perceivers were seemingly unable to prevent. Automatic effects are not limited to racial stereotypes. For example, Macrae, Milne, and Bodenhausen (1994) showed that occupational labels can affect information processing with-out the perceiver's awareness by demonstrating their impact when they were activated subliminally. Because, by definition, people are not con-sciously aware of the content of subliminally presented stimuli, the fact that stereotypic labels can affect social perception even under these pres-entation conditions documents another aspect of the automatization of stereotype activation: It can occur without awareness.

The studies we have described so far all used verbal labels to acti-vate stereotypes. It is also important, of course, to know whether the mere presence of an unlabeled but potentially categorizable target is suf-ficient to produce stereotype activation (cf. Gilbert & Hixon, 1991), as many theorists believe. A small but growing body of literature shows that the activation of social categories does indeed occur spontaneously, and its nature is affected by a number of psychological factors. For in-stance, if a person's membership in a particular social category is con-textually salient (e.g., being the only African American in a discussion group), the person is likely to be spontaneously categorized on the basis of this salient group membership (Biernat & Vescio, 1993; Taylor, Fiske, Etcoff, & Ruderman, 1978). Characteristics of the perceiver also affect the stereotype activation process. Personal prejudices (e.g., racial preju-dice) may make certain bases for social categorization chronically salient, so when members of these targeted categories are encountered, they tend to be categorized routinely in terms of this particular group membership rather than other equally applicable categories (Stangor, Lynch, Duan, & Glass, 1992). Do these spontaneous social categorizations result in stereotyping of the target? Research by Zárate and Smith (1990) confirms that they do. In their experiments, they were able to demonstrate that those people who most readily categorize others in terms of their race are also the most likely to draw stereotypic inferences about them. Thus, although there may be some conditions that interfere with the spontaneous activation of stereotypes (see Gilbert & Hixon, 1991), there is good reason to suspect that stereotypic notions can creep automatically into perceivers' thoughts. Because of the ubiquity with which stereotypic ideas are expressed in a culture, they are likely to be well learned even by those who eventually renounce them (Devine, 1989; see Katz, 1976). Although stereotyping may have origins in any of several motivational forces, it tends to develop into an automatic mental habit, even if the perceiver's motivations change.

The habitual nature of stereotyping is probably reinforced by the systematic information-processing biases that contribute to the creation of an illusory mental database supporting stereotypic beliefs. Although little is known about the accuracy of most social stereotypes (cf. Judd & Park, 1993; Jussim, 1991), a great deal of research shows that once stereotypic expectations are formed, they tend to bias subsequent information processing in a confirmatory manner (for an encyclopedic review, see Hamilton & Sherman, 1994). Stereotype-confirming information tends to be processed more extensively and better remembered, whereas inconsistent information is often neglected (e.g., Bodenhausen, 1988; Hamilton & Rose, 1980). This memory bias is stronger with well-developed stereotypes (such as sex and race-related stereotypes; for a review, see Fyock & Stangor, 1994). Inherently ambiguous information tends to be construed as stereotype-confirming (e.g., Duncan, 1976; Sagar & Schofield, 1980). Stereotypic conjectures and fantasies tend to be misremembered as facts (Slusher & Anderson, 1987). Attributions for the behavior of stereotyped targets tend to perpetuate stereotypic ideas, such that when a woman succeeds in a traditionally masculine task, for example, her performance is seen as stemming from luck rather than skill (Deaux & Emswiller, 1974; for overviews, see Hewstone, 1990; Pettigrew, 1979). Finally, perceivers may react to stereotyped targets in ways that elicit stereotype-confirming behavior (i.e., a self-fulfilling prophecy; Darley & Fazio, 1980; Word, Zanna, & Cooper, 1974; for a review, see Snyder, 1984). All of these processes tend to produce a database of knowledge that seems to confirm the original stereotypic expectancies held by the perceiver, although in each case the evidence has been tainted by often unconscious biases and distortions. Even when perceivers encounter individuals who clearly and unambiguously disconfirm their stereotypes, they may be skilled at finding ways to view such cases merely as exceptions to a generally valid rule. By identifying these disconfirming cases as a special subtype of the category, perceivers can cling to their original stereotypic worldview (Weber & Crocker, 1983; for a review of the latest work in this area, see Hewstone, 1994). Because, as previously noted, these stereotypic biases can disadvantage the members of stigmatized social groups in important ways, identifying the mechanisms that produce and maintain the apparent validity of stereotypes in the minds of social perceivers has been an important scientific accomplishment.

Just as social scientists have become increasingly more aware of the biasing effects of stereotypes on social judgment, the general public has also gained an increasing awareness of these important issues. Events of recent decades have given rise to a new level of consciousness about the nature of stereotyping and its association with social injustice. Whereas the cognitive misers of bygone eras might stereotype others quite unselfconsciously, the contemporary perceiver is much more likely to view stereotyping as an unsavory practice to be avoided or concealed. One of the most dramatic and clear-cut trends in American public opinion over the century has been the increasing endorsement of egalitarian standards asserting that members of different ethnic groups are entitled to equal opportunities and equal access to social institutions (Schuman, Steeh, & Bobo, 1985). It is clear that many people have developed explicit egalitarian values that they want to embody in their thought and action, yet they have been socialized to hold stereotypic views and prejudiced feelings toward many minority groups. This fundamental ambivalence has assumed a prominent place in many important analyses of race relations (Gaertner & Dovidio, 1986; Katz, Hass, & Wackenhut, 1986; Myrdal, 1944).

The social perceiver is not likely to feel comfortable with ambivalent reactions to out-groups (Bodenhausen & Macrae, 1994). Individuals who have internalized egalitarian and nonprejudiced standards may be especially uncomfortable with the stereotypic ideas that may automatically arise in intergroup contexts. Devine, Monteith, and their associates (Devine & Monteith, 1993; Devine, Monteith, Zuwerink, & Elliot, 1991; Monteith, 1993; Monteith, Devine, & Zuwerink, 1993) have conducted several fascinating investigations into exactly this state of affairs. Monteith (1993), for example, has examined the determinants and consequences of personal effort toward prejudice reduction. She argued that when people are committed to egalitarian, nonprejudiced standards and their thoughts, feelings, or behavior seem to violate these standards, they tend to become self-focused and direct effort at reducing this discrepancy. Looking specifically at prejudice toward gays, she found that when low-prejudice people become aware of personal discrepancies between how they believe they should versus how they actually do react to gays, they subsequently become more likely to effectively inhibit prejudiced responses to antigay jokes. This work makes clear the fact that low-prejudice persons feel bad when their reactions to out-group members contravene their own nonprejudiced standards, so they are motivated to avoid reacting in stereotypic or prejudiced ways. Even those who have not internalized nonprejudiced standards may be motivated to avoid the expression of stereotypic reactions because of the social disapprobation such expressions can elicit. Clearly, the salience of social norms (and in some contexts, laws) proscribing open expression of stereotypic ideas gives most social perceivers the motivation to inhibit or suppress these ideas.

For many people, then, there is a fundamental mental dilemma associated with intergroup perception. On one hand, there are motivational incentives and well-learned habits of thought that produce, quite automatically, the activation of stereotypic notions in the presence of out-group members. At the same time, such thoughts are often unwanted and considered undesirable. This situation is likely to give rise to a motivation to suppress the unacceptable, intrusive stereotypes. Whereas the stereotyping process may occur quite automatically, successfully overriding this process undoubtedly requires some degree of controlled, conscious effort (Devine, 1989; Fiske, 1989; see also Bargh, 1989, 1994; Hasher & Zacks, 1979). In the remainder of this chapter, we consider the processes that are involved in stereotype suppression and the (often unexpected) consequences that such efforts produce.

GOVERNING THE SOCIETY OF MIND: SELF-REGULATION OF MENTAL PROCESSES

There has recently been a virtual explosion of interest in the topic of cognitive self-regulation among psychologists of several different specializations (see Wegner & Pennebaker, 1993, for a representative sampling of the panorama of intriguing research being conducted in this area). As Baumeister and Newman (1994) have argued, cognitive self-regulation can be accomplished in a variety of ways, some of which may involve a considerable degree of self-deception. Drawing on the metaphor of the human as intuitive lawyer (Fincham & Jaspars, 1980), Baumeister and Newman reviewed evidence showing that when a person prefers a specific conclusion, he or she tends to process information in a biased way that permits exactly this conclusion to be drawn

(Kruglanski, 1989; Kunda, 1990). This process may involve selectively attending to the most preferred evidence (Frey, 1986), setting differential evidential criteria for preferred versus nonpreferred conclusions (Ditto & Lopez, 1992), and many other mechanisms that are automatic, at least in the sense that they are not consciously intended. As a result, the intuitive lawyer may be largely unaware that any "massaging" of the evidence has occurred and may believe his or her judgments to be quite objective. As previously noted, exactly these sorts of mechanisms have been proposed to underlie the insidious intrusion of stereotypes into everyday cognition.

What happens when people become cognizant of the potential for stereotypic bias and attempt to avoid such untoward influences? In this situation, effortful, controlled processes are set in motion in order to counter the effects of automatic ones. One possible strategy is simply to make direct adjustments to one's judgments and conclusions in the direction opposite to the presumed bias (Baumeister & Newman, 1994; Strack, 1992; Wilson & Brekke, 1994). When judging a minority applicant for graduate school, for example, one can simply correct for presumed antiminority biases by adjusting one's evaluation in a positive direction. It is of course an open question whether such adjustments will be sufficient to compensate for unwanted biases or perhaps might even overcompensate for them (e.g., Hatvany & Strack, 1980). More ambitious perceivers might actively attempt to prevent the stereotypic biases from ever entering into their deliberations. In other words, they may attempt to suppress their stereotypes.

Mechanisms of thought suppression have been the focus of an extensive research program conducted by Wegner and his colleagues (for reviews, see Wegner, 1994; Wegner & Erber, 1993). From an impressive base of empirical evidence, these researchers have developed a dual-process model of thought control. The model starts with the realization that for any control process to be effective, it must be able both to test the status of the environment and to operate on the environment when the test process yields less than satisfactory results (Carver & Scheier, 1981; Miller, Galanter, & Pribram, 1960). In the case of mental control, there must be a process to monitor mental contents and a process to operate on mental contents when an undesired thought is detected by the monitoring process.

When the social perceiver resolves to suppress stereotypic reactions to an out-group member, this goal sets in motion a monitoring process that iteratively scans the mind for any sign of the unwanted stereotypic concepts. This process can occur in largely automatic ways (goal-dependent automaticity; see Bargh, 1989) and can involve the detection of stereotypic notions that are receiving mental activation at levels that are not yet sufficient to surpass the threshold of consciousness. When unwanted thoughts threaten to (or actually do) impinge on consciousness, the monitoring process triggers the instigation of the operating process in order to prevent the unwanted intrusion. In the case of thought suppression, a principal strategy of the operating process is to identify mental distracters that will move attention (or mental activation) away from the unwanted thoughts. Whereas the monitoring process is thought to be largely automatic and unconscious, the operating process is considered to be effortful, and at least some aspects of the process are available to consciousness. Perhaps the most important implication of this distinction is that the operating process is resource-dependent, and can only work effectively when the perceiver has sufficient attentional resources to devote to the task. In contrast, the monitoring process, because of its automaticity, can occur unimpeded by constraints on mental resources. In the next section, we will consider some of the important implications of this assumption for the success of attempts to control effectively the expression of stereotypic thoughts.

Evidence for the validity of this model of mental control has been provided from numerous domains of practical importance. For example, Wegner (1994) reviews evidence from studies of (1) attempts to concentrate, (2) attempts to control one's mood, (3) attempts to relax, (4) attempts to control pain, (5) attempts to fall asleep, and many others. Perhaps the most provocative implication of the model is the fact that the very nature of the processes involved in mental control make it likely that attempts at cognitive self-regulation will not only fail under many circumstances, but also they will produce exactly the counterintentional outcome. In the case of stereotype suppression, such an outcome would arise if the attempt to inhibit the expression of stereotypic views subsequently resulted in even greater stereotypic bias. We turn now to a consideration of how the mental system produces such perverse outcomes, and what their implications are for stereotype suppression in particular.

THE BEST-LAID PLANS OF MISERS AND MEN: IRONIES OF COGNITIVE SELF-CONTROL

People are often fairly successful in exercising mental control. Mischel and his colleagues, for example, have elegantly documented the development (across childhood) of the ability to delay gratification, largely accomplished by learning to avoid thoughts of desired objects (e.g., Mischel & Patterson, 1976; Mischel, Shoda, & Rodriguez, 1989). On the other hand, certain aspects of the dual processes involved in mental control make it possible for efforts at cognitive self-regulation to fail, sometimes rather spectacularly. In Wegner's (1994) model of ironic mental processes, a key factor that sets the stage for these ironic failures is the effortfulness of the operating process that strategically directs attention away from unwanted thoughts to any acceptable distracter. Because of the resource-consuming nature of the operating process, efforts at mental control are likely to fail unless cognitive resources are sufficiently plentiful to support the search for distracters. Anything that constrains the availability of free resources will also constrain the prospects for successful thought suppression. Time pressure, distraction and preoccupation, affective states, and even alcohol are factors that may impair thought control by reducing the availability of attentional resources needed to inhibit unwanted thoughts (e.g., Gilbert, 1991; Steele & Josephs, 1990; for a summary, see Wegner, 1994). Perversely, it is precisely these sorts of factors that make it more likely for perceivers to rely on stereotypes in their construals of others (e.g., Bodenhausen, 1990, 1993; Macrae, Hewstone, & Griffiths, 1993; Pratto & Bargh, 1991; Stangor & Duan, 1991). Because of the social perceiver's miserly tendencies, the possibility of effortful processes overriding the "quick and easy" alternative of stereotyping may be particularly diminished when processing resources are in short supply. Unfortunately, many real-life contexts are filled with distractions, stressors, emotions, and other factors that can constrain attentional resources significantly.

Although mentally taxing circumstances are likely to interfere with the effortful operating process that is involved in thought suppression, these factors are not likely to interrupt the automatic monitoring process, which is relatively resource-independent. The process of monitoring working memory for any sign of the unwanted thought, however, does have an unintended consequence. The monitoring process has to "know" what it is looking for, and this paradoxically requires the continuous, albeit low-level activation of a relevant stereotype criterion. If processing resources are in ample supply, this low-level activation of stereotypic search criteria works well, because it allows the potentially intrusive unwanted thoughts to be identified and triggers the operating process, which then activates a distracter. If the operating process is short-circuited, however, then the continuing operation of the monitoring process may simply result in repeated priming of stereotypic concepts that are ultimately not replaced by distracters. As Wegner (1994) notes, this problem may be exacerbated by the fact that, under conditions of thought suppression, the monitoring process is engaged in a feature-positive search (i.e., detecting the presence of a specific feature, in this case, a stereotypic notion) while the operating process is engaged in a feature-negative search (i.e., finding an appropriate distracter, which must be devoid of stereotypic content in order to be suitable). Thus, the monitoring process is looking for the presence of a feature, while the operating process is looking for the absence of a feature. Because feature-positive searches are considered to be easier than feature-negative ones (Newman, Wolff, & Hearst, 1980; Richardson & Massel, 1982; cf. Fiedler, Eckert, & Poysiak, 1989), the monitoring process is executed with greater ease than the operating process in this case. As a consequence, the very act of suppressing a thought can ironically result in its becoming hyperaccessible in memory (Wegner & Erber, 1992).

A study by Wegner, Erber, and Zanakos (1993) provides an interesting demonstration of the hyperaccessibility phenomenon in the domain of mood control. Participants were asked to recall emotional life experiences. Some were instructed to try *not* to take on the mood of the earlier experience, some were instructed to indeed take on that mood, and others received no particular instruction. Half of all participants were also given the additional task of remembering a nine-digit number while performing the other task. It was expected that the digit rehearsal task would interfere with the effortful operating process but not the automatic monitoring process. Those who did not have to remember the digit string were successfully able to control their moods, but those who had the concomitant mental load not only were not successful in mood control, but also their moods actually moved significantly in the unintended direction. These results, as well as many others, demonstrate that as long as the operating process is in place and functioning, mental control can often be successfully accomplished, but if the effortful operating process is impeded, suspended, or abandoned, the unchecked monitoring process can produce hyperaccessibility of unwanted mental contents, setting the stage for counterintentional reactions.

The impressive catalog of ironic effects documented by Wegner and colleagues raises serious questions about the ability of the well-intentioned cognitive miser to avoid the habit of stereotyping others via the suppression of stereotypic concepts in intergroup contexts. Indeed, a study by Wegner, Erber, and Bowman (cited in Wegner, 1994) provides initial evidence that stereotype suppressers are quite prone to engaging in perversely counterintentional behavior. In this study, participants were given the task of completing sentence stems, some of which were taken from the Attitudes Toward Women Scale (Spence & Helmreich, 1972). The sentences were selected so that it was possible to complete them either in relatively sexist or relatively nonsexist ways. Some participants were instructed to try not to be sexist in completing the sentence stems, while others were given no special instructions about sexism. Crossed with this manipulation, half of the participants were placed under high time pressure (respond immediately), while others were not (respond within 10 seconds). The time-pressure manipulation was expected to short-circuit the execution of the effortful operating process, setting the stage for greater sexism among those who were actively striving not to be sexist. This pattern is precisely what occurred. Although people with ample cognitive resources who were trying not to be sexist produced fewer sexist sentence completions than people who were not engaging in thought suppression, people with constrained processing resources who were trying not to be sexist produced more sexist sentence completions than the control participants.

Recent evidence suggests that the intention to suppress stereotypes can backfire even in the absence of any appreciable cognitive load. Whereas a cognitive load directly interferes with the execution of the operating process, this process can also be suspended for other reasons. For instance, the intention to inhibit the stereotype may simply dissipate over time. Because thought suppression is an active, effortful process, the cognitive miser may sometimes be hard pressed to maintain the motivation necessary to support ongoing suppression efforts. Once the suppression motivation is relaxed, the operating process may quickly abate, creating the potential for a rebound effect. A rebound effect is said to occur when once-suppressed thoughts return to exert an impact on thought and behavior that is often greater than would have been the case if the thoughts had never been suppressed in the first place. This effect is likely to occur when unwanted thoughts have been rendered hyperaccessible by the monitoring process, but the operating process (which would ordinarily keep them in check by directing attention to distracters) has been suspended.

Studies conducted by Macrae, Bodenhausen, Milne, and Jetten (1994) documented rebound effects of this sort. In one experiment (Macrae, Bodenhausen, Milne, & Jetten, 1994, Exp. 1), participants were asked to write a prose passage describing what they imagined to be a typical day in the life of a person portrayed in a photograph. The photograph contained visual cues that clearly identified the target as a member of a stereotyped social group, namely skinheads. Half of the participants were admonished not to rely on stereotypes in constructing their passages, while the others were given no special instructions vis-à-vis stereotyping. After completing this passage, participants were given a second target photograph about which to write a projective passage (a different skinhead), but this time participants received no instructions to inhibit stereotypes. Independent raters coded the prose passages in terms of their stereotypicality. For the first prose passage, while the suppression instructions were salient, we expected that stereotype suppressors would be able to successfully exorcise stereotypic content from their impressions of the target, and this was indeed the case. Stereotype suppressors produced significantly less stereotypic initial passages. However, after the suppression motivation was relaxed (in the case of the second passage), the lingering hyperaccessibility (resulting from the earlier monitoring process) was expected to result in a rebound effect. Indeed, participants who had previously been suppressing stereotypes produced markedly more stereotypic second passages than did their no-suppression counterparts.

Another experiment (Macrae, Bodenhausen, Milne, & Jetten, 1994, Exp. 2) pursued this rebound phenomenon in the domain of intergroup behavior. As in the first study, participants wrote projective passages about a skinhead and half did so while actively suppressing stereotypes about this group. As before, the stereotype suppressors produced significantly less stereotypic passages while actively engaging in suppression. After completing the passage construction task, the participants were told that they would next be engaging in a get-acquainted interaction with the person about whom they had just written the passage (i.e., the skinhead). We reasoned that stereotypes about the group would have been rendered hyperaccessible by the monitoring aspect of the suppression task, but after the task was completed, the effortful-operating aspect of the suppression process would be relaxed. Consequently, subsequent behavior in the social interaction might be especially affected by group stereotypes among those who had previously been suppressing them. To test this possibility, we asked participants to enter the room where the interaction was to take place and choose a seat. They were told that the skinhead had stepped out for a moment, but his skinhead paraphernalia (denim jacket, etc.) were visible in one of the chairs. The question of interest was how closely the participants would choose to sit to the skinhead's seat. For the former suppressors, negative stereotypes about the group were likely to be highly accessible, leading them to prefer a greater social distance from the skinhead. They did, in fact, choose to sit farther away from the skinhead, on average, than did individuals who were not suppressing their stereotypes in the initial prose passage task. These studies show that social perceivers can successfully inhibit stereotypic responses while they are actively striving to do so, but once they stop making this effort, the stereotypes return to affect their thoughts and actions to an even greater degree.

Perhaps the clearest evidence of the hyperaccessibility that ironically results from stereotype suppression comes from Macrae, Bodenhausen, Milne, and Jetten (1994, Exp. 3). In this study, participants again completed the projective passage task that has previously been described, and again they did so either while explicitly attempting to suppress stereotypes or without any particular goal at all. As in the previous studies, suppressors produced less stereotypic passages. After completing this task, participants were asked to complete an ostensibly unrelated computerized lexical decision task. In this task, participants were presented with a series of character strings and asked to judge, as quickly as possible, whether each string was an English word or a nonword. Half of the stimuli were indeed words. Of these, half were words that had been established as being stereotypic with respect to skinheads, while the others were matched distracters which, although comparable in length and evaluative tone, were descriptively irrelevant to the skinhead stereotype. If the skinhead stereotype were made hyperaccessible because of stereotype suppression, we would expect to see faster lexical verification times from the participants who had previously been suppressing the stereotype. This was indeed the case (see Figure 7.1). Al-

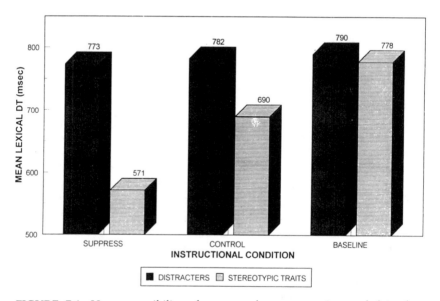

FIGURE 7.1. Hyperaccessibility of suppressed stereotypes is revealed in the faster lexical decision times for judgments of stereotypic trait terms evidenced by participants who had earlier suppressed stereotypes, compared to a control group of stereotype users and a no-stereotype-activation baseline group. Based on data from Macrae, Bodenhausen, Milne, and Jetten (1994, Exp. 3).

though decision times for the distracters was not affected by whether participants had been suppressing the stereotype or not, stereotype suppression did result in faster decision times for stereotypic words among the stereotype suppressers, relative both to participants who did not suppress stereotypes in the prose task and to a baseline condition composed of participants who completed the lexical decision task only.

So far, we have seen several examples in which the intention to suppress a stereotype can and does backfire. In each case, the effect was theoretically attributable to the unchecked operation of the monitoring process that is an integral part of mental control operations. This process ironically makes unwanted ideas particularly accessible. While the operating process is working, it can keep the unwanted thoughts successfully out of awareness, but if it is interrupted by a cognitive load, or if it simply recedes or becomes inactive because of diminishing motivation to engage in suppression, then rebound effects can begin to emerge. Unfortunately for the well-intentioned social perceiver, these hyperaccessibility-based effects are not the only source of ironic consequences of stereotype suppression. The very effortfulness of the operating process can introduce other problems for would-be stereotype suppressors.

The preferred alternative to forming stereotypic impressions of others is usually considered to be the formation of individuated impressions that incorporate the idiosyncratic personal attributes of the person into a unique mental representation (Brewer, 1988; Fiske & Neuberg, 1990). Thus, when social perceivers are trying not to stereotype others, they presumably are trying to form individuated impressions. Certainly this is the ideal that is considered appropriate in contexts such as personnel or legal decision making. But forming individuated impressions is regarded as an effortful, resource-consuming affair. If perceivers are using up a portion of their available resources in the task of trying to suppress stereotypes, this will leave fewer resources for the equally important task of forming an individuated impression of the target. Thus, although perceivers may successfully be able to inhibit stereotypes while they are actively engaged in that effort, they may be less able to process simultaneously the unique individuating information that is available as a basis for their social impressions. To borrow an analogy from the courtroom, perceivers may be so busy trying to put inadmissible (i.e., stereotypic) evidence out of mind that they fail to process adequately the admissible case evidence (i.e., individuating information).

Evidence documenting this possibility comes from studies conducted by Macrae, Bodenhausen, Milne, and Wheeler (1995). In one study, for example, participants were asked to form an impression of an elderly man while watching a videotape of him describing himself. The self-description contained material that was consisent with stereotypes about the elderly, as well as information about his personality and interests that was quite irrelevant to such stereotypes. Half of the participants were instructed to suppress their stereotypes while forming their impressions, while the remainder were given no suppression instructions. After viewing the video, participants were unexpectedly asked to recall as much of the self-description as possible. Consistent with the hypothesis that stereotype suppression efforts can reduce the amount of processing devoted to individuating information, results indicated that stereotype suppressors remembered significantly less of the stereotype-irrelevant information about the target than did the nonsuppressors. Moreover, suppressors ironically remembered more of the to-be-disregarded stereotypic material. Thus, the considerable attentional requirements of stereotype suppression appear to inhibit the processing of individuating information about stereotyped targets, at least under some circumstances.

If stereotype suppressors are not basing their impressions on their stereotypes or the individuating information, then what are they basing them on? One strong possibility is that they are simply relying on an override mechanism that directly adjusts their impressions in a nonstereotypic direction, consistent with the instruction they have been given (Baumeister & Newman, 1994; Strack, 1992). Thus, although the impression appears to be nonstereotypic, it is not necessarily really grounded in any kind of thoughtful analysis of the target's unique personal qualities. If so, then the social impression may be just as superficial as if it were based exclusively on stereotypic notions. If called on later to make judgments about the target, the person may have very little to go on other than stereotypes about the target's group, precisely because of the impoverished impression that resulted from the struggle to suppress stereotypic information. In the final section of this chapter, we explore the implications of the available research documenting these unintended aspects of stereotype suppression for genuine reductions in stereotyping, prejudice, and discrimination. In addition, we consider some alternative forms of cognitive self-regulation that may hold more promise for social perceivers who want to move beyond stereotypic impressions of others.

CAN SOCIAL PERCEIVERS DO THE RIGHT THING?

It seems that there are a substantial number of reasons to be concerned about whether stereotype suppression is a viable route to the goal of avoiding unfair bias in our assessments of others. In order to suppress stereotypes, perceivers must not only have sufficient motivation to engage in effortful inhibitory processes, they must also be aware of the possibility that stereotypes may be influencing their perceptions when they are in an intergroup situation. Unfortunately, people seem to be rather good at convincing themselves that they are not reacting to outgroup members in a prejudiced way, even when there is good evidence that they in fact are doing so. Some of the most compelling evidence of this sort comes from the work of Gaertner, Dovidio, and their colleagues on helping in interracial contexts (see Gaertner & Dovidio, 1986). This research shows that White participants encountering Blacks who are in need of assistance are significantly less helpful to these individuals than they are to Whites in identical circumstances, if there is some sort of nonracial factor that can be used to justify or rationalize the more negative response. People may be less helpful to an apparently lazy Black, convincing themselves that it is the laziness rather than the ethnicity of the person that is causing their negative reaction. However, a comparably lazy White elicits significantly more helpfulness, indicating that ethnicity is indeed a crucial factor. If social perceivers routinely engage in self-deception of this sort, they are unlikely even to be aware of the possible need to engage in stereotype suppression. On the other hand, Devine et al. (1991) have shown that people can be quite aware of the prejudice inherent in their reactions to others, and can be motivated to take corrective action, but this seems to be the case only for low-prejudice individuals, and so far it has been demonstrated primarily under circumstances in which there are no salient, nonracial justification factors available to fuel the self-deception process.

As we have seen, even when perceivers do strive to inhibit their social stereotypes, their success can be quite limited and may be accompanied by unwanted consequences. Wegner's (1994) model of the ironic processes of mental control suggests some ways of improving the success of thought suppression. The dual processes involved in thought control obviously work more effectively when the perceiver's pool of attentional resources is not drained by concomitant mental loads of one kind or another. Thus, avoiding distractions, stress, emotional reactions, and so forth while engaging in stereotype suppression should facilitate success in that endeavor. This may be easier said than done, however. Many intergroup situations are inherently stressful or anxiety-provoking (see Stephan & Stephan, 1985; Wilder, 1993), and social life in the modern world can be generally characterized as placing the perceiver under a substantial mental load much of the time.

Success in stereotype suppression also seems imperiled by anything that produces a suspension of the suppression process, because for a period of time afterward, rebound effects may emerge. How realistic is it to expect social perceivers consistently to be on guard for the unwanted emergence of stereotypes? Certainly this would require a good deal of commitment to the goal of avoiding bias. Devine's work (Devine & Monteith, 1993; Devine et al., 1991) suggests that low-prejudice people may very often have sincere commitment of this sort. Whereas low-prejudice individuals may be consistently motivated to engage in stereotype suppression in order to avoid the unpleasant compunction associated with violating their own egalitarian standards, others may be more concerned with suppressing overt stereotypic responses rather than stereotypic thoughts per se. Of course, response suppression is fraught with the same potential for counterintentional effects as is thought suppression, but those perceivers engaging merely in response suppression may be motivated to do so only when prospects for social disapproval are salient. Having publicly censored their reactions in one context, they may be particularly likely to show a rebound effect in the next context if normative pressures promoting egalitarian standards are less salient in the new context.

The distinction between response suppressors and thought suppressors calls to mind Kelman's (1958) classic distinction between compliance and internalization. As Kuran (1993) notes, public self-censorship in accordance with prevailing social norms may not necessarily produce internalization of the professed attitude or belief. However, by removing or reducing the availability of the genuine but repressed cognition from the arena of public opinion (by response suppression), thoughts that are considered "unthinkable" can die out as newer generations fail to be exposed to the repressed idea. Kuran provides examples of this phenomenon arising from the emergence of fundamentalism in Islamic cultures. In the case of social stereotypes, it does seem possible that widespread response suppression, even if based solely on normative pressure, could reduce the availability and impact of specific, erroneous stereotypic notions. Socialization is, after all, one of the primary sources through which stereotypes are acquired (Katz, 1976). But it seems highly unlikely that suppression processes, however well intentioned, could ever eliminate the tendency for people to form and use stereotypes in their perceptions of the world. As noted at the outset of this chapter, stereotypes serve too many valuable functions to be totally abandoned.

For those individuals having consistent motivation to suppress at least certain specific kinds of stereotypic thinking, it is possible that with continued practice, even the operating process involved in stereotype suppression can become relatively automatic and effortless (see Wegner,

1994). Attempting to avoid sexist language may provide an illustrative example. When first learning to be cautious in the gender assumptions inherent in pronoun usage, for instance, it may take considerable effort to construct more acceptable, neutral alternatives. With sufficient practice, avoiding sexist language can become second nature, requiring very little thought or intentional planning. Many of the ironic effects of thought suppression result from the failure of the operating process to produce an acceptable alternative to the unwanted thought or action. If the operating process associated with a given suppression activity were to become overlearned, the potential for its failure or interruption by mental loads should greatly diminish, and the unwanted side effects of mental control may become relatively rare.

Given the problematic nature of thought control, the social perceiver may be well advised to consider alternative means to the end of avoiding prejudice and bias. One possibility that may warrant investigation is the paradoxical approach of putting one's stereotypes on the table rather than trying to repress them. Perhaps by exposing and confronting these beliefs directly and consciously, rather than trying to avoid them, they will lose some of their power. Kuran (1993) similarly views thought suppression as a relatively maladaptive way of resolving social problems and controversies. Perceivers who engage in attempted thought control may often falsely convince themselves that they have successfully avoided the influence of stereotypes, making them potentially oblivious to dangers such as postsuppression rebound effects. Research on "paradoxical therapy" (Shoham-Solomon & Rosenthal, 1987; Wegner, 1994) attests to the potential benefits of reversing the usual pattern of attempted thought control.

A related strategy for cognitive self-regulation would be to abandon the intuitive-lawyer mode of thinking, in which the perceiver strives to produce a specific kind of impression or judgment (in this case, nonstereotypic), and instead to adopt the stance of the intuitive scientist (Baumeister & Newman, 1994; Fiske & Taylor, 1991). This stance involves a thorough search for evidence, full consideration of alternatives, and search and adjustment for possible biases. Obviously, it is a relatively effortful approach to social perception, but at least in important judgmental contexts, it may be a more effective recipe for producing less biased decisions than is the conscious intention to suppress one's stereotypes and prejudices. Creating the motivation necessary to support this kind of effortful analysis may be a tricky issue (see Eberhardt & Fiske, Chapter 11, this volume). For example, it has long been supposed that making people feel accountable for their decisions will motivate them to be more thoughtful and systematic in their judgment processes (Tetlock, 1983; Tetlock & Kim, 1987). However, in inter-group contexts, accountability instructions may function much like suppression instructions; that is, telling people that they must justify their judgments of an out-group member may instill a concern about being labeled "prejudiced" that results in conscious attempts to avoid stereotypes rather than conscious attempts to be as systematic and thorough as possible.

Langer, Bashner, and Chanowitz (1985) conducted research suggesting that induced mindfulness may be an effective strategy for avoiding simplistic, stereotypic generalizations. Mindfulness involves active distinction making and context-sensitive analysis rather than reliance on rigid or general patterns of thought. In their research, they showed that children who were induced to think mindfully about the physically handicapped ultimately showed more positive and less stereotypic responses to handicappers. Whereas most theories postulating more detailed and thoughtful information processing assume that it requires greater effort and cognitive resources on the part of the social perceiver (e.g., Chaiken, Liberman, & Eagly, 1989; Fiske & Neuberg, 1991; Petty & Cacioppo, 1986), Langer (1989) proposes that mindfulness is not an effortful state. Although she does assert that making the transition from mindlessness to mindfulness is effortful, once one is in a mindful mode, information processing is not taxing or onerous. The mindful person will form individuated impressions of others because he or she will move beyond rigid, general categorical knowledge to look at the unique context of a given person. Thus, cultivating a mindful orientation to the world may be a form of cognitive self-management that may be highly effective in the reduction of stereotypic biases. More research is needed to investigate the effort and attentional resource requirements associated with this form of information processing.

CONCLUSION

For a variety of reasons ranging from "political correctness" pressures to the sincere endorsement of egalitarian standards, people are often motivated to avoid the influence of many kinds of social stereotypes. One common strategy for achieving this aim is to try to banish stereotypic thoughts from consciousness. The research we have reviewed raises some serious doubts about the efficacy of this approach. The problem is not simply that the approach often fails, but rather that it often produces exactly the unintended result (i.e., greater stereotyping than might have occurred if no thought suppression had been attempted). In attempting to develop a less stereotypic worldview, social perceivers who take the path of stereotype suppression may need considerable practice before they become adept enough to avoid its pitfalls. Given the problems associated with stereotype suppression, alternative strategies for avoiding stereotypic bias may be preferable or necessary.

ACKNOWLEDGMENT

We are grateful to Marilynn Brewer, Miles Hewstone, Charles Stangor, and Dan Wegner for their helpful comments and suggestions regarding a previous version of this chapter.

REFERENCES

Allport, G. W. (1954). *The nature of prejudice.* Reading, MA: Addison-Wesley.

Bargh, J. A. (1989). Conditional automaticity: Varieties of automatic influence in social perception and cognition. In J. S. Uleman & J. A. Bargh (Eds.), *Unintended thought* (pp. 3–51). New York: Guilford Press.

Bargh, J. A. (1994). The four horsemen of automaticity: Awareness, intention, efficiency, and control in social cognition. In R. S. Wyer, Jr., & T. K. Srull (Eds.), *Handbook of social cognition* (2nd ed., Vol. 1, pp. 1–40). Hillsdale, NJ: Erlbaum.

Baumeister, R. F., & Newman, L. S. (1994). Self-regulation of cognitive inference and decision processes. *Personality and Social Psychology Bulletin, 20,* 3–19.

Biernat, M., & Vescio, T. K. (1993). Categorization and stereotyping: Effects of group context on memory and social judgment. *Journal of Experimental Social Psychology, 29,* 166–202.

Bodenhausen, G. V. (1988). Stereotypic biases in social decision making and memory: Testing process models of stereotype use. *Journal of Personality and Social Psychology, 55,* 726–737.

Bodenhausen, G. V. (1990). Stereotypes as judgmental heuristics: Evidence of circadian variations in discrimination. *Psychological Science, 1,* 319–322.

Bodenhausen, G. V. (1993). Emotion, arousal, and stereotypic judgments: A heuristic model of affect and stereotyping. In D. M. Mackie & D. L. Hamilton (Eds.), *Affect, cognition, and stereotyping: Interactive processes in group perception* (pp. 13–37). San Diego: Academic Press.

Bodenhausen, G. V., & Macrae, C. N. (1994). Coherence versus ambivalence in cognitive representations of persons. In R. S. Wyer, Jr., & T. K. Srull (Eds.), *Advances in social cognition* (Vol. 7, pp. 149–156). Hillsdale, NJ: Erlbaum.

Brewer, M. B. (1988). A dual process model of impression formation. In R. S. Wyer, Jr., & T. K. Srull (Eds.), *Advances in social cognition* (Vol. 1, pp. 1–36). Hillsdale, NJ: Erlbaum.

Carver, C. S., & Scheier, M. F. (1981). *Attention and self-regulation: A control-theory approach to human behavior.* New York: Springer-Verlag.

Chaiken, S., Liberman, A., & Eagly, A. H. (1989). Heuristic and systematic information processing within and beyond the persuasion context. In J. S. Uleman & J. A. Bargh (Eds.), *Unintended thought* (pp. 212–252). New York: Guilford Press.

Darley, J. M., & Fazio, R. H. (1980). Expectancy-confirmation processes arising in the social interaction sequence. *American Psychologist, 35,* 867–881.

Deaux, K., & Emswiller, T. (1974). Explanations of successful performance on sex-linked tasks: What is skill for the male is luck for the female. *Journal of Personality and Social Psychology, 29,* 80–85.

Dennett, D. C. (1984). *Elbow room: The varieties of free will worth having.* Cambridge, MA: MIT Press.

Devine, P. G. (1989). Stereotypes and prejudice: Their automatic and controlled components. *Journal of Personality and Social Psychology, 56,* 5–18.

Devine, P. G., & Monteith, M. J. (1992). The role of discrepancy-associated affect in prejudice reduction. In D. M. Mackie & D. L. Hamilton (Eds.), *Affect, cognition, and stereotyping: Interactive processes in group perception* (pp. 317–344). San Diego, CA: Academic Press.

Devine, P. G., Monteith, M. J., Zuwerink, J. R., & Elliot, A. J. (1991). Prejudice with and without compunction. *Journal of Personality and Social Psychology, 60,* 817–830.

Ditto, P. H., & Lopez, D. F. (1992). Motivated skepticism: Use of differential decision criteria for preferred and nonpreferred conclusions. *Journal of Personality and Social Psychology, 63,* 568–584.

Dovidio, J. F., Evans, N., & Tyler, R. B. (1986). Racial stereotypes: The contents of their cognitive representations. *Journal of Experimental Social Psychology, 22,* 22–37.

Duncan, B. L. (1976). Differential social perception and attribution of intergroup violence: Testing the lower limits of stereotyping of blacks. *Journal of Personality and Social Psychology, 34,* 590–598.

Fiedler, K., Eckert, C., & Poysiak, C. (1989). Asymmetry in human discrimination learning: Feature positive effect or focus of hypothesis effect? *Acta Psychologica, 70,* 109–127.

Fincham, F. D., & Jaspars, J. M. (1980). Attribution of responsibility: From man as scientist to man as lawyer. In L. Berkowitz (Ed.), *Advances in experimental social psychology* (Vol. 13, pp. 81–138). New York: Academic Press.

Fiske, S. T. (1989). Examining the role of intent: Toward understanding its role in stereotyping and prejudice. In J. S. Uleman & J. A. Bargh (Eds.), *Unintended thought* (pp. 253–286). New York: Guilford Press.

Fiske, S. T., & Neuberg, S. L. (1990). A continuum model of impression formation from category-based to individuating processes: Influences of information and motivation on attention and interpretation. In M. P. Zanna (Ed.), *Advances in experimental social psychology* (Vol. 3, pp. 1–74). San Diego, CA: Academic Press.

Fiske, S. T., & Taylor, S. E. (1991). *Social cognition* (2nd ed.). New York: Mc-Graw-Hill.

Frey, D. (1986). Recent research on selective exposure to information. In L. Berkowitz (Ed.), *Advances in experimental social psychology* (Vol. 19, pp. 41–80). New York: Academic Press.

Fyock, J., & Stangor, C. (1994). The role of memory biases in stereotype maintenance. *British Journal of Social Psychology, 33,* 331–343.

Gaertner, S. L., & Dovidio, J. F. (1986). The aversive form of racism. In J. F. Dovidio & S. L. Gaertner (Eds.), *Prejudice, discrimination, and racism* (pp. 61–89). Orlando, FL: Academic Press.

Gilbert, D. T. (1991). How mental systems believe. *American Psychologist, 46,* 107–119.

Gilbert, D. T., & Hixon, J. G. (1991). The trouble of thinking: Activation and application of stereotypic beliefs. *Journal of Personality and Social Psychology, 60,* 509–517.

Greenberg, B. S., & Brand, J. E. (1994). Minorities and the mass media: 1970s to 1990s. In J. Bryant & D. Zillmann (Eds.), *Media effects: Advances in theory and research* (pp. 273–314). Hillsdale, NJ: Erlbaum.

Hamilton, D. L., & Rose, T. L. (1980). Illusory correlation and the maintenance of stereotypic beliefs. *Journal of Personality and Social Psychology, 39,* 832–845.

Hamilton, D. L., & Sherman, J. W. (1994). Stereotypes. In R. S. Wyer, Jr., & T. K. Srull (Eds.), *Handbook of social cognition* (2nd ed., Vol. 2, pp. 1–68). Hillsdale, NJ: Erlbaum.

Harris, R. J. (1994). *A cognitive psychology of mass communication* (2nd ed.). Hillsdale, NJ: Erlbaum.

Hasher, L., & Zacks, R. T. (1979). Automatic and effortful processes in memory. *Journal of Experimental Psychology: General, 108,* 356–388.

Hatvany, N., & Strack, F. (1980). The impact of a discredited key witness. *Journal of Applied Social Psychology, 10,* 490–509.

Hewstone, M. (1990). The 'ultimate attribution error'? A review of the literature on intergroup causal attribution. *European Journal of Social Psychology, 20,* 311–335.

Hewstone, M. (1994). Revision and change of stereotypic beliefs: In search of the elusive subtyping model. In W. Stroebe & M. Hewstone (Eds.), *European review of social psychology* (Vol. 5, pp. 69–109). Chichester, UK: Wiley.

Jost, J. T., & Banaji, M. R. (1994). The role of stereotyping in system-justification and the production of false consciousness. *British Journal of Social Psychology, 33,* 1–27.

Judd, C. M., & Park, B. (1993). Definition and assessment of accuracy in social stereotypes. *Psychological Review, 100,* 109–128.

Jussim, L. (1991). Social perception and social reality: A reflection-construction model. *Psychological Review, 98,* 54–73.

Katz, I., Hass, R. G., & Wackenhut, J. (1986). Racial ambivalence, value duality, and behavior. In J. F. Dovidio & S. L. Gaertner (Eds.), *Prejudice, discrimination, and racism* (pp. 35–59). Orlando, FL: Academic Press.

Katz, P. A. (1976). The acquisition of racial attitudes in children. In P. A. Katz (Ed.), *Toward the elimination of racism* (pp. 125–154). New York: Pergamon Press.

Kelman, H. C. (1958). Compliance, identification, and internalization: Three processes of attitude change. *Journal of Conflict Resolution, 2,* 51–60.

Kruglanski, A. W. (1989). *Lay epistemics and human knowledge: Cognitive and motivational bases.* New York: Plenum Press.

Kunda, Z. (1990). The case for motivated reasoning. *Psychological Bulletin, 108,* 480–498.

Kuran, T. (1993). The unthinkable and the unthought. *Rationality and Society, 5,* 473–505.

Langer, E. (1989). *Mindfulness.* Reading, MA: Addison-Wesley.

Langer, E., Bashner, R., & Chanowitz, B. (1985). Decreasing prejudice by increasing discrimination. *Journal of Personality and Social Psychology, 49,* 113–120.

Macrae, C. N., Bodenhausen, G. V., Milne, A. B., & Jetten, J. (1994). Out of mind but back in sight: Stereotypes on the rebound. *Journal of Personality and Social Psychology, 67,* 808–817.

Macrae, C. N., Bodenhausen, G. V., Milne, A. B., & Wheeler, V. (1995). *On resisting the temptation for simplification: Counterintentional effects of stereotype suppression on social memory.* Manuscript submitted for publication.

Macrae, C. N., Hewstone, M., & Griffiths, R. J. (1993). Processing load and memory for stereotype-based information. *European Journal of Social Psychology, 23,* 77–87.

Macrae, C. N., Milne, A. B., & Bodenhausen, G. V. (1994). Stereotypes as energy-saving devices: A peek inside the cognitive toolbox. *Journal of Personality and Social Psychology, 66,* 37–47.

Miller, G. A., Galanter, E., & Pribram, K. H. (1960). *Plans and the structure of action.* New York: Holt, Rinehart & Winston.

Mischel, W., & Patterson, C. J. (1976). Substantive and structural elements of effective plans for self-control. *Journal of Personality and Social Psychology, 34,* 942–950.

Mischel, W., Shoda, Y., & Rodriguez, M. L. (1989). Delay of gratification in children. *Science, 244,* 933–938.

Monteith, M. J. (1993). Self-regulation of prejudiced responses: Implications for progress in prejudice-reduction efforts. *Journal of Personality and Social Psychology, 65,* 469–485.

Monteith, M. J., Devine, P. G., & Zuwerink, J. R. (1993). Self-directed versus other-directed affect as a consequence of prejudice-related discrepancies. *Journal of Personality and Social Psychology, 64,* 198–210.

Myrdal, G. (1944). *An American dilemma: The Negro problem and modern democracy.* New York: Random House.

Newman, J. P., Wolff, W. T., & Hearst, S. E. (1980). The feature-positive effect in adult human subjects. *Journal of Experimental Psychology: Human Learning and Memory, 6,* 630–650.

Pendry, L. F., & Macrae, C. N. (1994). Stereotypes and mental life: The case of the motivated but thwarted tactician. *Journal of Experimental Social Psychology, 30,* 303–325.

Pettigrew, T. F. (1979). The ultimate attribution error: Extending Allport's cognitive analysis of prejudice. *Personality and Social Psychology Bulletin, 5,* 461–476.

Petty, R. E., & Cacioppo, J. T. (1986). The elaboration likelihood model of persuasion. In L. Berkowitz (Ed.), *Advances in experimental social psychology* (Vol. 19, pp. 124–203). New York: Academic Press.

Pratto, F., & Bargh, J. A. (1991). Stereotyping based upon apparently individuating information: Trait and global components of sex stereotypes under attention overload. *Journal of Experimental Social Psychology, 27,* 26–47.

Richardson, W. K., & Massel, H. K. (1982). The feature-positive effect in adult humans: Within-group design. *American Journal of Psychology, 95,* 125–138.

Ross, L., & Nisbett, R. E. (1991). *The person and the situation: Perspectives of social psychology.* New York: McGraw-Hill.

Sagar, H. A., & Schofield, J. W. (1980). Racial and behavioral cues in black and white children's perceptions of ambiguously aggressive acts. *Journal of Personality and Social Psychology, 39,* 590–598.

Schuman, H., Steeh, C., & Bobo, L. (1985). *Racial attitudes in America: Trends and interpretations.* Cambridge, MA: Harvard University Press.

Shoham-Solomon, V., & Rosenthal, R. (1987). Paradoxical interventions: A meta-analysis. *Journal of Consulting and Clinical Psychology, 55,* 22–28.

Sidanius, J., & Pratto, F. (1993). The inevitability of oppression and the dynamics of social dominance. In P. M. Sniderman, P. E. Tetlock, & E. G. Carmines (Eds.), *Prejudice, politics, and the American dilemma* (pp. 173–211). Palo Alto, CA: Stanford University Press.

Simon, H. (1957). *Models of man.* New York: Wiley.

Slusher, M. P., & Anderson, C. A. (1987). When reality monitoring fails: The role of imagination in stereotype maintenance. *Journal of Personality and Social Psychology, 52,* 653–662.

Snyder, M. (1984). When belief creates reality. In L. Berkowitz (Ed.), *Advances in experimental social psychology* (Vol. 18, pp. 247–305). New York: Academic Press.

Spence, J. T., & Helmreich, R. (1972). Who likes competent women? Competence, sex-role congruence of interests, and subjects' attitude toward women as determinants of interpersonal attraction. *Psychology of Women Quarterly, 5,* 147–163.

Stangor, C., & Duan, C. (1991). Effects of multiple task demands upon memory for information about social groups. *Journal of Experimental Social Psychology, 27,* 357–378.

Stangor, C., Lynch, L., Duan, C., & Glass, B. (1992). Categorization of individuals on the basis of multiple social features. *Journal of Personality and Social Psychology, 62,* 207–218.

Steele, C. M., & Josephs, R. A. (1990). Alcohol myopia: Its prized and dangerous effects. *American Psychologist, 45,* 921–933.

Stephan, W. C., & Stephan, C. W. (1985). Intergroup anxiety. *Journal of Social Issues, 41*(3), 157–175.

Strack, F. (1992). The different routes to social judgments: Experiential versus informational strategies. In L. L. Martin & A. Tesser (Eds.), *Construction of social judgment* (pp. 249–275). Hillsdale, NJ: Erlbaum.

Tajfel, H. (1969). Cognitive aspects of prejudice. *Journal of Social Issues, 25,* 79–97.

Tajfel, H., & Turner, J. C. (1986). The social identity theory of intergroup behavior. In S. Worchel & W. G. Austin (Eds.), *Psychology of intergroup relations* (pp. 7–24). Chicago: Nelson-Hall.

Taylor, S. E., Fiske, S. T., Etcoff, N. L., & Ruderman, A. (1978). Categorical bases of person memory and stereotyping. *Journal of Personality and Social Psychology, 36,* 778–793.

Tetlock, P. E. (1983). Accountability and complexity of thought. *Journal of Personality and Social Psychology, 45,* 74–83.

Tetlock, P. E., & Kim, J. I. (1987). Accountability and judgment processes in a personality prediction task. *Journal of Personality and Social Psychology, 52,* 700–709.

Weber, R., & Crocker, J. (1983). Cognitive processes in the revision of stereotypic beliefs. *Journal of Personality and Social Psychology, 45,* 961–977.

Wegner, D. M. (1994). Ironic processes of mental control. *Psychological Review, 101,* 34–52.

Wegner, D. M., & Erber, R. (1992). The hyperaccessibility of suppressed thoughts. *Journal of Personality and Social Psychology, 63,* 903–912.

Wegner, D. M., & Erber, R. (1993). Social foundations of mental control. In D. M. Wegner & J. W. Pennebaker (Eds.), *Handbook of mental control* (pp. 36–56). Englewood Cliffs, NJ: Prentice Hall.

Wegner, D. M., Erber, R., & Zanakos, S. (1993). Ironic processes in the mental control of mood and mood-related thought. *Journal of Personality and Social Psychology, 65,* 1093–1104.

Wegner, D. M., & Pennebaker, J. W. (Eds.). (1993). *Handbook of mental control.* Englewood Cliffs, NJ: Prentice Hall.

Wilder, D. (1993). The role of anxiety in facilitating stereotypic judgments of out-group behavior. In D. M. Mackie & D. L. Hamilton (Eds.), *Affect, cognition, and stereotyping: Interactive processes in group perception* (pp. 87–109). San Diego, CA: Academic Press.

Wilson, T. D., & Brekke, N. (1994). Mental contamination and mental correction: Unwanted influences on judgments and evaluations. *Psychological Bulletin, 116,* 117–142.

Word, C. O., Zanna, M. P., & Cooper, J. (1974). The nonverbal mediation of self-fulfilling prophecies in interracial interaction. *Journal of Experimental Social Psychology, 10*, 109–120.

Wyer, R. S., Jr., & Srull, T. K. (1989). *Memory and cognition in its social context.* Hillsdale, NJ: Erlbaum.

Zárate, M. A., & Smith, E. R. (1990). Person categorization and stereotyping. *Social Cognition, 8*, 161–185.

8

When Stereotypes Lead to Stereotyping: The Use of Stereotypes in Person Perception

MARILYNN B. BREWER

The structure of the present volume, as represented in the introductory chapter, makes an important distinction between *stereotypes* as beliefs about social groups and the role that such beliefs play in guiding perception, thinking, remembering, learning, and behavior. For purposes of this chapter, the concept of *stereotyping* will be used specifically to refer to the role of group stereotypes in the perception of individual persons who are categorized as members of the stereotyped group. In other words, stereotyping is the *use* of stereotypic knowledge in forming an impression of an individual.

At least two conditions, then, are prerequisite to stereotyping: (1) the existence of a set of beliefs or mental representation of a social category, and (2) the classification or categorization (whether conscious or unconscious) of an individual as a member (exemplar) of that category. Within the social cognition literature, there is an interesting debate about whether categorization automatically activates associated category stereotypes (e.g., Gilbert & Hixon, 1991; Stangor & Lange, 1994; von Hippel, Sekaquaptewa, & Vargas, 1995), but neither availability *nor* activation of stereotypes is a sufficient condition for the actual use of category-based knowledge in judgments of particular individuals

(Darley & Gross, 1983; Devine, 1989). Impressions of individual category members are rarely equivalent to category stereotypes and, conversely, impressions based on experience with category exemplars do not always generalize to the category as a whole (Brewer & Miller, 1988; Cook, 1984). Thus, the interrelationship between stereotypes and stereotyping is neither simple nor straightforward.

Even when the preconditions of stereotyping are met, multiple processing mechanisms—both automatic and controlled—intervene between the activation of category-based knowledge and judgments of individual category members. At least three different information-processing pathways may attenuate the relationship between categorization and stereotyping:

1. Categorization may occur without activation of the associated stereotype because the categorization is irrelevant to current processing goals. This is the basis of Brewer's (1988; 1994) distinction between category-based and *personalized* modes of information processing in person perception. The dual-process model assumes that stereotypes will not be accessed when a strong interpersonal orientation characterizes the relationship between perceiver and target. Instead, relevant trait dimensions, such as kindness, intelligence, or power, will provide the schematic framework for impression formation (Bodenhausen & Lichtenstein, 1987).

2. Category stereotypes may be activated but not used as the basis of impression formation or judgments. One such route involves active, conscious *suppression* of the stereotyping process (Devine, 1989; Stangor & Lange, 1994; see Bodenhausen & Macrae, Chapter 7, this volume). A second route does not require effortful attention on the part of the perceiver but instead involves various aspects of the information processing context that *compete* with specific category knowledge as a basis for perception and judgment of a target individual. These include salient target-specific information, contextual cues, and alternative processing goals that make competing category stereotypes available and relevant. For instance, I may be aware that Mr. Jones is both African American and a lawyer, but the occupational stereotype may be more salient and relevant to my judgment and impressions than his ethnic identity.

3. The stereotype may be activated and used in the initial stages of impression formation, but gradually modified as individuating information about the target person becomes available and attended to. This is the basic premise of a number of different models that have been proposed to describe the interplay of category knowledge and individuating

information in the impression formation process (e.g., Brewer, 1988; Fiske & Neuberg, 1990; Kruglanski, 1990). Despite their differences, these models share a generic conceptualization of the information processing sequence involved in achieving a fit between individuating information and expectancies based on available category stereotypes (Leyens, Yzerbyt, & Schadron, 1992). The multistep process starts with category-based impressions that are successively strengthened or modified as a function of the perceived fit between information about the target and the prior expectancies.

The extent of modification of the category stereotype achieved in the final impression depends on perceiver motivation and available cognitive resources (Pendry & Macrae, 1994). Given sufficient individuating information, motivation, and cognitive capacity, the final impression formed of the individual person may deviate substantially from the original category stereotype. Such individuated impressions are nonetheless the product of category-based processing (Brewer, 1988) in that category stereotypes (1) constitute the "default" option for limited information processing (Pendry & Macrae, 1994) and (2) provide a framework for selecting, interpreting, and organizing individuating information (Bodenhausen, 1988; Macrae, Milne, & Bodenhausen, 1994; von Hippel et al., 1995). In effect, the category-based model of impression formation is one of feature matching and differentiation. Starting with category beliefs, the perceiver incorporates individuating information about the target to the extent that he or she is able and motivated to differentiate that individual from the category as a whole.

The purpose of the present chapter is to review those aspects of the information processing environment that influence the degree of correspondence between activated category stereotypes and impressions of individuals who are acknowledged category members. The question to be addressed is when does categorization result in stereotyped judgments of individuals, and when do individual impressions deviate from stereotypes *even when the perceiver is not actively suppressing* the use of category stereotypes in forming an impression?

INDIVIDUATING INFORMATION

There are many aspects of the information available about an individual target that could influence the degree of fit between the impression of that person and category stereotypes. The sheer *amount* of individuating information available, as well as the extent to which that information is *vivid* and *salient* as opposed to bland or abstract; the extent to which it is *relevant* rather than irrelevant to the judgment task at hand; or the extent to which it is *unambiguously inconsistent* rather than ambiguous or consistent with prior expectations can all determine whether behavioral information will successfully compete with category stereotypes as the basis of impression formation. The impact of each of these dimensions of stimulus information has been studied in its own right (for review see Higgins & Bargh, 1987), but for purposes of the present discussion, I will collapse these into the single dimension of *strength* of individuating information.

A Little Information Goes a Long Way

The traditional view, implicit if not explicit, in stereotyping research has assumed an inverse relationship between the amount and strength of information available about a specific person and reliance on a category stereotype in forming an impression of that individual. If individuating information is weak or absent, category stereotypes provide the default option for impression formation. As more individuating information is available and attended to, reliance on category stereotypes is reduced— at least up to the point at which information is so complex (or mixed) that perceivers fall back on stereotypes to handle the information overload, and stereotype-consistent information is attended to and remembered better than stereotype-inconsistent information (Bodenhausen & Lichtenstein, 1987; Macrae et al., 1994). This view suggests either an inverse linear relationship between amount and strength of individuating information and stereotyping (see Figure 8.1a), or perhaps a U-shaped curvilinear relationship in which stereotyping is least evident when there is a moderate (manageable) amount of relevant and salient individuating information available (Figure 8.1b).

Recent research casts doubt on this view of when perceivers rely on category stereotypes to form a judgment or impression of an individual (Leyens et al., 1992). It appears that category information alone is not considered an acceptable basis for making judgments about an individual category member, except possibly for highly prejudiced perceivers (Darley & Gross, 1983; Devine, 1989). Thus, when perceivers have only category labels and no judgment-relevant individuating information to go on, they are reluctant to make strong judgments, and stereotyping is diluted (Denhaerinck, Leyens, & Yzerbyt, 1989; Hilton & Fein, 1989; Locksley, Hepburn, & Ortiz, 1982).

Leyens et al. (1992) account for this reluctance to stereotype on the

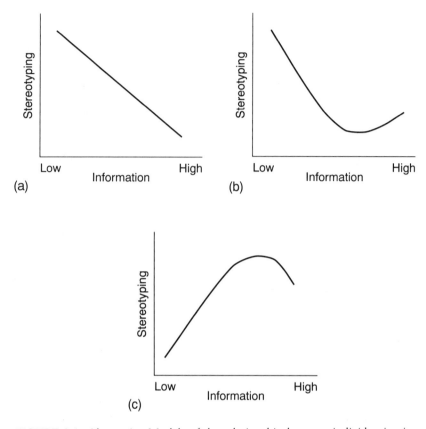

FIGURE 8.1. Alternative Models of the relationship between individuating information and stereotyping.

basis of category membership alone in terms of the concept of "social judgeability." Before making a judgment or trait attribution about an individual with any confidence, the perceiver must first feel that the amount of information provided is sufficient to warrant making any judgment. Ironically, although for most perceivers category classification alone does not meet the criterion for social judgeability, a combination of category information and individuating information does exceed threshold, and frees the perceiver to use category knowledge or stereotypes in forming an impression (Yzerbyt, Schadron, Leyens, & Rocher, 1994). As a consequence, evidence for category-based impressions should be highest when a moderate amount of individuating information is available to bolster judgments (Figure 8.1c).

Evidence regarding the impact of individuating information on stereotyping indicates that the *perception* of having suitable information about the target is sufficient to generate confident, category-based judgments, even when the information is ambiguous (Darley & Gross, 1983) or "pseudorelevant" to the judgment task (Hilton & Fein, 1989). Of particular interest is recent research indicating that fictitious individuating information can increase stereotyping, even when it is totally illusory (Yzerbyt et al., 1994). In a series of experiments, Yzerbyt and his colleagues devised a method for presenting subjects with "placebo information" about a target individual. Students in these experiments listened to the introductory portion of an interview in which the interviewee introduced himself by giving his last name, address, age, and occupation (either library archivist or comedian). The tape recording contained no further individuating information about the target person. The occupational categories had been selected to be associated with stereotypes of introverted versus extraverted, respectively, and subjects were later asked to make ratings of the interviewee on this dimension.

Subsequent to the interview, subjects engaged in a supposed vigilance task in which they listened to a cassette tape through headphones in which a male voice was heard on one channel and a female voice on the other. Subjects were instructed to follow one text in this dichotic listening task and to ignore information in the unattended channel. Later, subjects in the "illusory-information" condition were told that the distractor channel had contained further information from the earlier interview, and that they would have received this information unconsciously, even though they could not be expected to be aware of the material they had heard. Subjects in the no-information condition were not told anything about the content of the unattended channel. (In reality, the distractor channel had not contained any relevant information, and no subjects were able to correctly recount what had been presented in this channel.)

In the final phase of the experiment, subjects were asked to make a series of ratings about the person heard in the earlier interview. Subjects in the illusory-information condition were significantly less likely to give "Don't know" judgments than were subjects in the category-information-only condition, and rated the target more extremely on the introversion–extraversion scale in accord with category stereotypes. The results of these experiments provide dramatic evidence that a little individuating information (whether real or imagined) can actually increase reliance on category stereotypes in making judgments of target persons.

Too Much Information?

Figure 8.1c implies that category-based impressions will be maximized in the presence of an intermediate amount of individuating information, but reduced when the amount or strength of such information is increased. At first glance, this prediction appears to be inconsistent with recent research indicating that perceivers rely more heavily on category stereotypes under conditions of information overload or reduced cognitive capacity (Bodenhausen, 1990; Bodenhausen & Lichtenstein, 1987; Macrae et al., 1994; Pendry & Macrae, 1994). However, for the most part these studies have looked at the effects of cognitive overload created by factors extraneous to the information itself, such as arousal (Bodenhausen, 1993), task complexity (Bodenhausen & Lichtenstein, 1987), time pressure (Pratto & Bargh, 1991), or competing cognitive activities (Gilbert & Hixon, 1991; Pendry & Macrae, 1994; Stangor & Duan, 1991). These are factors that are independent of the information available about the target individual but affect the ability of the perceiver to attend to and integrate a large amount of information, or information that is complex or inconsistent. In effect, the results of this research indicate that when the amount of available information is high *and* the cognitive resources of the perceiver are taxed, impressions will be consistent with category stereotypes (Macrae, Hewstone, & Griffiths, 1993).

When cognitive capacity is not an issue, however, the presence of rich individuating information can be expected to reduce category-based impression formation for a number of reasons. First, the more information that is available, the more likely it is that stereotype-inconsistent features of the individual will be evident that reduce the fit between category-based expectancies and available data. In fact, under low processing load, perceivers display preferential recall for stereotype-inconsistent information (Macrae et al., 1993). According to the continuum model of category-based processing, this is the basis of individuated impressions (Fiske & Neuberg, 1990). Stereotypic impressions are modified to the extent that stereotype-incongruent information is available, attended to, and integrated into the final impression formed (Fiske, Neuberg, Beattie, & Milberg, 1987).

Second, the more information presented, the more likely it is that alternative categorizations of the individual will be activated simultaneously, generating competing stereotypic representations (Rothbart & John, 1985). The availability of alternative categorization cues is particularly likely when visual and behavioral information about the stimulus person is presented, rather than just linguistic labels. As Zárate and

Smith (1990) point out, much of our research on category-based processing comes from studies in which category information is presented in the form of linguistic descriptions (e.g., "a Black male") that make a single categorization particularly salient. This stands in contrast to the stimulus environment presented by interaction with a real person, in which cues to socioeconomic, age and personality-category information are equally available.

Research by Gilbert and Hixon (1991) suggests that the amount of individuating information and other cognitive demands interact to determine the activation and application of stereotypes in impression formation. When rich stimulus information is available, competing cognitive tasks reduce the likelihood that a particular category stereotype will be activated in the presence of a specific individual. However, given that a single stereotype has been activated, that stereotype is more likely to be utilized in forming an impression when cognitive resources are being used up in competing tasks than when cognitive capacity is devoted solely to the impression-formation task.

SOCIAL CONTEXT

Another characteristic of laboratory research on impression formation that stands in contrast to most real-world stimulus environments is the focus on one individual target person at a time. Typically, verbal descriptors or other cues to categorization are provided in connection with individuating information about a single category member. Without competing information about other individuals or social groups, the perceiver is able to focus on information that differentiates this particular individual from the category as a whole. In fact, the demands implicit in the stiuation are to do just that.

Information processing may change considerably when information about a specific individual is embedded in a social context in which information about many other individuals is presented simultaneously. A multiperson social context has several aspects that may influence stereotyping, either directly or indirectly.

First, the need to form impressions of several individuals simultaneously increases cognitive load and demands on cognitive resources. It is just this combination of rich stimulus information and competing cognitive demands that increases reliance on activated category stereotypes in forming impressions of individual category members (Gilbert & Hixon, 1991; Pendry & Macrae, 1994; Stangor & Duan, 1991).

Second, the order in which information about different individuals is received may affect how incoming information is organized in memory. If impressions are formed successively, with all information about a specific individual presented at once, this would facilitate organizing information at the person-level and encourage formation of differentiated, individuated impressions. In most naturalistic social settings, however, information about multiple individuals is all jumbled up, with the stream of information about Person A interrupted by information about Person B and so forth. In this stimulus environment, processing of information may not be organized around individual persons at all. Instead, information may be stored in memory in terms of other organizing frameworks, such as specific conversations, or content categories (Ostrom, Pryor, & Simpson, 1981; Sedikides & Ostrom, 1988).

Finally, and perhaps most important, social context determines which person categories are activated and the way in which category-based knowledge is used in the impression-formation process. The relative importance of category-based stereotypes versus individuating information depends, in part, on whether the social situation induces an *intragroup* or an *intergroup* judgment context.

If all individuals in a multiperson context share a common category identity, then the category stereotype provides a frame of reference for forming impressions of individual group members. With category knowledge held constant as a standard of comparison, within-category variability provides the basis for judgments of individuals (Biernat & Manis, 1994). Under these circumstances, individual impressions are more likely to be influenced by features that differentiate one individual from another than by features that category members have in common. Interestingly, the same individuating information has been found to lead to more extreme or confident judgments when the person has been categorized as a group member than when the same person is judged outside of a group context (Leyens et al., 1992; Wilder, 1981).

On the other hand, when a multiperson group can be segregated into two or more salient subcategories, differences *between* subgroups become more important than differences among individuals *within* categories as the basis of impression formation. Under these circumstances, impressions will be dominated by stereotype-consistent information, and individuating information will be ignored or assimilated (Doise & Sinclair, 1973; Tajfel, 1969).

Stereotyping in Intergroup Contexts

The impact of subcategorization on memory for individuating information has been demonstrated in a number of experiments (Arcuri, 1982;

Taylor & Falcone, 1982; Taylor, Fiske, Etcoff, & Ruderman, 1978). Typically in these experiments, participants are presented with audiovisual recordings of six to eight individuals engaged in a group discussion, with the composition of the group consisting of members of two different social categories (e.g., three males, three females; three black males, three white males, etc.). During the course of the group discussion, individuating information is provided about each group member in the form of statements attributed to that individual. Following presentation of the stimulus tape, subjects are given a recognition test in which they receive a list of statements made during the discussion and are asked to identify the photo of the specific person who made that statement. Correct identifications provide an index of individuation, whereas recognition errors provide information on confusions in memory between one group member and another.

Consistently, when a group of individuals can be divided into meaningful subsets based on shared category membership, confusions between individuals within the same category exceed confusions between categories. Furthermore, stereotyping of individual category members is enhanced when judgments of the individual are made in the context of a group divided into two approximately equal subcategories, compared to judgments of the same individual made in a more individuating context (Oakes & Turner, 1986).

Physical features provide a basis for category-based processing to the extent that they represent social categories that are meaningful or important to the perceiver. Physical cues such as clothing or hairstyle do not produce subtyping, whereas socially meaningful cues such as sex and race do affect the rate of intracategory confusions to intercategory errors (Stangor, Lynch, Duan, & Glass, 1992). In a recent series of experiments using the recognition paradigm, Brewer, Weber, and Carini (1995) demonstrated that recognition errors based on visual similarity are influenced by whether the visual cue was associated with a meaningful category distinction.

A videotaped group discussion was produced in which six same-sex college students participated, with three of the group members wearing red sweatshirts, and three wearing blue sweatshirts. The topic of the discussion was relations between the United States and Russia, and during the course of the discussion, each participant presented distinctive suggestions about how relations could best be improved. Sweatshirt color and type of suggestion were correlated such that the students in red sweatshirts all made suggestions involving institutional arrangements, whereas all the blue-sweatshirt students provided suggestions that were more people-oriented.

Some of the subjects watched the videotape without being given any prior information about the significance of the red and blue sweatshirts and were told only that they would be viewing a discussion among a group of six individuals. The remaining subjects were told that the six individuals had been divided according to their performance on a perceptual estimation task, and that the color of sweatshirt signified whether they had been classified as "overestimators" or "underestimators." These instructions were intended to convey that the categorization was a meaningful one, without providing any explicit information about the nature of the differences between the groups.

In the recognition test that followed presentation of the videotape, subjects were given photographs of the six participants (including sweatshirt color), and a list of 12 statements that had been made during the course of discussion (2 statements per group member). The subjects' task was to identify which participant had made each statement. Recognition errors were scored as *intracategory* confusions when a statement was misattributed to another person of the same subcategory (red or blue) as the correct individual, and as *intercategory* confusions when the misattribution was to a member of the other category.

Figure 8.2 presents the results for mean intracategory and intercategory confusions for both experimental conditions. Although the stimulus information was the same in all cases, subjects in the meaningful categorization condition made more errors overall, and more intracategory errors in particular. In the context of meaningful intergroup distinctions, subjects showed more interest in understanding differences at the category level than at the individual level. Thus, memory for specific information was both more selective (limited to category-relevant material) and less individuated than for subjects in the control condition.

In-Group/Out-Group Differentiation

In the domain of social categorization (as opposed to object categories), perceivers themselves can be classified as members of some categories and not others. Thus, any categorization of another person is implicitly also a classification of that individual into an in-group (a category in which the perceiver is also a member) or an out-group (Dovidio & Gaertner, 1993).

Apart from the substantive content associated with specific social categories, there are some "generic" stereotypes associated with the in-group/out-group distinction itself. Research on in-group bias and ethnocentrism indicates that in-groups are generally evaluated more positively than out-groups, but more specifically that in-groups are stereotyped as

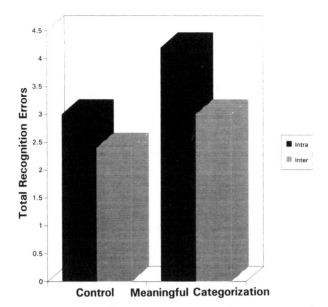

FIGURE 8.2. Intracategory and intercategory recognition errors as a function of category meaning. Data from Brewer, Weber, and Carini (1995, p. 31).

trustworthy, honest, friendly, and peaceful, whereas out-groups are more likely to be perceived as untrustworthy, deceitful, and competitive (Brewer, 1986; Brewer & Campbell, 1976; Schopler & Insko, 1992). These stereotypes are applied even when an in-group/out-group distinction is created arbitrarily, with no prior group stereotypes (Brewer, 1979; Brewer & Silver, 1978). What is of particular interest here, however, is how stereotypes derived from in-group/out-group distinctions interact with other preexisting category stereotypes to influence the impressions formed of specific individuals.

Although in-group/out-group differentiation is implicit in all social categorization, stereotypes associated with this distinction are not necessarily activated in all impression formation situations. When a single individual is categorized on the basis of age, academic major, or occupation, for instance, the fact that the individual is thereby an out-group member may not be particularly salient. The salience of in-group/out-group categorization, and its impact on impression formation, depends on the social context. In general, groups of individuals are more likely to be perceived in in-group/out-group terms than are single individuals (Doise & Sinclair, 1973; Hogg & Turner, 1987; Insko & Schopler,

1987). When the persons to be judged are all members of a single social category, the perceiver may become aware of his or her own status as an outsider or insider with respect to that social group.

When a group of individuals is classified either as an in-group or as an out-group, impressions of in-group members are more likely to be individuated than impressions of out-group members. This expectation is derived from research on the "out-group homogeneity effect"—the finding that out-groups as a whole are judged to be less variable or heterogeneous than are in-groups (Ostrom & Sedikides, 1992). On dimensions related to group stereotypes, more members of out-groups are estimated to have stereotype-consistent traits than are members of in-groups (Park & Judd, 1990; Park & Rothbart, 1992). Thus, out-group classification interacts with specific category stereotypes to enhance the utilization of category-based knowledge in impression formation. In-group classification, on the other hand, appears to reduce the perceived relevance of category stereotypes and increases the weight given to individuating information in judgments of individual group members.

The out-group homogeneity effect may be limited to social contexts in which only one social category is represented. When that category is an in-group, more attention is paid to intragroup differentiation than when the category is an out-group (Brewer, 1993). However, when members of an in-group category and members of an out-group category are both present in the social setting, the intergroup context may eliminate the out-group homogeneity effect. In this situation, in-group/out-group categorization is superimposed on another category distinction. For instance, for a male observing a group of male and female individuals, the in-group/out-group distinction converges with categorization based on gender. When the perceiver is a White college student and the targets are Black students and White students, in-group/out-group categorization converges with racial categories, and so forth.

Research on cross-categorization effects indicates that superimposed (convergent) categories enhance intercategory differentiation at the expense of intracategory differences (Arcuri, 1982; Deschamps & Doise, 1978). In the recognition experiments conducted by Brewer et al. (1995), intracategory confusions were increased when a meaningful in-group/out-group distinction was superimposed onto the initial subcategorization. In intergroup contexts, reliance on category stereotypes may be increased, and individuation of category members decreased, for *both* in-group and out-group categories.

In some social contexts, salient in-group/out-group distinctions may crosscut other category distinctions. For instance, in organizational settings, departments or work teams may consist of both male and female employees. In that case, differentiation based on work roles crosscuts categorization based on gender, and the in-group/out-group stereotype competes with gender stereotypes as a basis for forming impressions of individual group members. In general, just as convergent categorizations enhance category-based processing, crosscutting categorizations are expected to reduce reliance on category stereotypes in favor of individuating information. There is even some evidence that when in-group classification conflicts with negative category stereotypes, the in-group positivity bias overrides alternative category-based processing (Maass & Schaller, 1991).

SOCIAL RELATIONSHIPS

In most experimental research on impression formation, the role of the perceiver is that of an objective observer, with no interpersonal connections to the target individual. When social relationships between the perceiver and target are introduced, the motivation to attend to individuating information, and the organization of information in the impression formed are significantly altered. Even anticipated interaction makes a difference (Darley & Berscheid, 1967).

The Importance of Interdependence

Fiske and Neuberg (1990) have proposed that any form of *outcome dependency* between perceiver and target alters the perceiver's motivation to attend to individuating information and reduces category-based processing. Thus, when subjects are expecting to participate in a cooperative task with a member of a stereotyped group, their impression of that individual is more individuated and less category-based than when no cooperative interdependence is anticipated (Erber & Fiske, 1984; Neuberg & Fiske, 1987). Individuation is also evident when perceivers expect to be in a competitive relationship with the target person (Ruscher & Fiske, 1990). However, competitors are individuated only in the case of *interpersonal* competition. When competition is at the group level (e.g., between pairs or teams), interdependence may enhance individuation within the in-group, but impressions of out-group opponents are more likely to be category-based (Miller, Brewer, & Edwards, 1985; Ruscher, Fiske, Miki, & van Manen, 1991).

Fiske and Neuberg (1990) argue that outcome dependency alters the processing goal that guides impression formation because of the perceiver's need to be able to predict the behavior of the target person in order to achieve desired outcomes. Accordingly, *accuracy* becomes a more important goal than in noninterdependent impression-formation contexts. When Neuberg and Fiske (1987, Exp. 3) explicitly introduced an accuracy motivation to the impression-formation task, they obtained evidence of individuation that paralleled the results obtained under conditions of outcome dependency. Apparently, both self-conscious accuracy motivation and interdependence reduce reliance on category stereotypes and/or increase attention to specific individuating information.

Another way to interpret the effects of interdependence on stereotyping is in terms of information relevance. Social relationships between perceiver and target may alter the relevance of specific category stereotypes to the judgment task at hand. The perceiver may adopt an alternative schema that replaces the social category stereotype as a basis for selecting and organizing incoming information. The resulting impression may not necessarily be more complete or accurate than one based on other categorizations, but it will incorporate different individuating features that do not correspond to the category stereotype.

From this perspective, stereotyping under conditions of social interdependence between perceiver and target will depend on the fit or relevance of category knowledge to the nature of the social relationship. For instance, when interdependence is role-based (e.g., doctor–patient, storekeeper–customer), stereotypes of that role category are likely to be highly relevant to forming an impression of a specific category member (more so, for instance, than when I am asked to form an impression of someone who happens to be a doctor but outside of the doctor–patient relationship). Similarly, if the perceiver's stereotype of African Americans includes athletic prowess, then that category knowledge is going to be more relevant when interdependence involves participation on a sports team than for a relationship such as college roommate.

When category stereotypes are relevant to social role relationships, the social relationship may function as a superimposed category that strengthens, rather than reduces, reliance on category-based impression formation. On the other hand, when category knowledge does not correspond to role relationships, social interdependence may serve as a crosscutting categorization that weakens the influence of category stereotypes and promotes more individuated impression formation (Marcus-Newhall, Miller, Holtz, & Brewer, 1993).

Types of Social Relationships

In an ambitious and elegant analysis of the structure of human social relations, Alan Fiske (1991) provided a basic taxonomy of forms of social interdendence that may be relevant to understanding the interaction between social-categorization processes and processes of interpersonal relationships. The taxonomy is based on distinctions among four elementary relational models that Fiske labels as *communal sharing, authority ranking, equality matching*, and *market pricing*.

The extent to which a particular interpersonal relationship embodies one or another of these relational models may determine the influence of category stereotypes on the impressions participants in the relationship have of each other. Communal sharing relationships, for instance, stem from common in-group membership, so in-group/out-group distinctions may be the only relevant social categorization utilized in such relationships. Relations based on authority ranking may produce asymmetric impressions in which high ranking individuals make stereotype-based judgments of subordinates, but lower ranking individuals develop highly individuated impressions of authority figures (Fiske, 1993). Finally, market pricing (exchange) relationships are generally depersonalized and promote impressions based on relevant category stereotypes, whereas equality matching represents the kind of reciprocal interpersonal relationship that should promote personalized rather than category-based impression formation (Brewer, 1988).

CATEGORY-BASED JUDGMENTS AND SOCIAL POLICIES

At the outset of this chapter, *stereotyping* was defined as the utilization of category stereotypes in the impression formed of an individual category member. Category stereotypes themselves are generally assessed by presenting respondents with a group label and asking them to indicate what features are characteristic of the group as a whole, or of a "typical" group member. As Stangor and Lange (1994) point out, the group representations obtained by this method are not likely to be the same as those that would be derived if respondents were asked to make judgments about a set of individual category members and then these judgments were averaged to generate a group stereotype.

When the respondent's task is to report impressions associated with a group as a whole, the only mental representation likely to be activated is the one directly associated with that category label. When respondents make judgments of individual category members, any number of features are made available that may activate competing representations and associations, as has been discussed throughout this chapter. To the extent that multiple representations are activated simultaneously, the influence of any one category stereotype can be expected to be limited (Stangor & Lange, 1994).

Lord, Lepper, and Mackie (1984) have suggested that this difference in judgment task may account for apparent inconsistencies between social attitudes assessed at the general level, and behavior as assessed in specific situations. In the abstract, evaluations of social objects or social groups are determined by reactions to an imagined group representative or an "attitude prototype." When the perceiver encounters an individual instance or member of the social category that matches the attitude prototype, behavior toward that individual case will be consistent with the generic attitude. However, if the instance is atypical, attitude–behavior consistency will be low.

In a recent extension of this analysis of attitude–behavior consistency, Lord and his colleagues (Lord, Deforges, Fein, Pugh, & Lepper, 1994) have applied this reasoning to attitudes toward social policy issues. Positions taken on many social policies may be shaped by the respondent's mental representation of the prototypical member of a social category associated with that policy. For instance, attitudes toward social welfare may be a reflection of whether the respondent holds derogatory stereotypes of the typical welfare recipient. Attitudes toward capital punishment may reflect the perceiver's mental representation of violent criminals, and so forth. Although individuals may have strong attitudes on the issues themselves, these judgments may not be applied to particular welfare clients or criminal cases, depending on whether the specific instances match the generic prototype.

CONCLUDING THOUGHTS

Much of the content of this chapter has cast doubt on the link between stereotypes as mental representations of social categories and stereotyping in the impressions and judgments formed of specific individuals. If category stereotypes are not consistently utilized in individual instances, does this mean that category representations are ultimately relatively unimportant in real world social contexts?

The same factors that sometimes reduce stereotyping in person perception are also those that account for reliance on category stereotypes in many, if not most, social settings. Stereotyping is most likely when task demands are high, information is complex, and subcategorization of individuals based on socially meaningful distinctions is available—all characteristics of information processing in most multiperson social environments. Under these circumstances, the processing of stereotype-consistent information is facilitated at the expense of incongruent or stereotype-irrelevant individuating information. Such stereotyping is likely to be the rule rather than the exception in real world social settings. Furthermore, category stereotypes are often utilized in contexts in which no individuating information is available, as previously described research on the relationship between category stereotypes and social policy illustrates. Many important social decisions—particularly those involving social policies—are made on behalf of groups or social categories rather than specific individuals. Stereotyping functions at the group level as well as at the level of perception of individuals, and in the former case it is much less likely to be modified by competing representations or information processing goals. In many cases, category stereotypes guide behavior directly—not just indirectly through their influence on person perception. After all, we go to war against groups, not against individuals.

REFERENCES

Arcuri, L. (1982). Three patterns of social categorization in attribution memory. *European Journal of Social Psychology, 12,* 271–282.

Biernat, M., & Manis, M. (1994). Shifting standards and stereotype-based judgments. *Journal of Personality and Social Psychology, 66,* 5–20.

Bodenhausen, G. V. (1988). Stereotypic biases in social decision making and memory: Testing process models of stereotype use. *Journal of Personality and Social Psychology, 55,* 726–737.

Bodenhausen, G. V. (1990). Stereotypes as judgmental heuristics: Evidence of circadian variations in discrimination. *Psychological Science, 1,* 319–322.

Bodenhausen, G. V. (1993). Emotion, arousal, and stereotypic judgments: A heuristic model of affect and stereotyping. In D. Mackie & D. Hamilton (Eds.), *Affect, cognition, and stereotyping: Interactive processes in group perception* (pp. 13–37). New York: Academic Press.

Bodenhausen, G. V., & Lichtenstein, M. (1987). Social stereotypes and information processing strategies: The impact of task complexity. *Journal of Personality and Social Psychology, 52,* 871–880.

Brewer, M. B. (1979). In-group bias in the minimal intergroup situation: A cognitive–motivational analysis. *Psychological Bulletin, 86,* 307–324.

Brewer, M. B. (1986). The role of ethnocentrism in intergroup conflict. In S. Worchel & W. Austin (Eds.), *Psychology of intergroup relations* (pp. 88–102). Chicago: Nelson-Hall.

Brewer, M. B. (1988). A dual process model of impression formation. In T. Srull & R. Wyer (Eds.), *Advances in social cognition* (Vol. 1, pp. 1–36). Hillsdale, NJ: Erlbaum.

Brewer, M. B. (1993). Social identity, distinctiveness, and in-group homogeneity. *Social Cognition*, *11*, 150–164.

Brewer, M. B. (1994). Associated Systems Theory: If you buy two representational systems, why not many? In R. Wyer & T. Srull (Eds.), *Advances in social cognition* (Vol. 7, pp. 141–147). Hillsdale, NJ: Erlbaum

Brewer, M. B., & Campbell, D. T. (1976). *Ethnocentrism and intergroup attitudes: East African evidence*. New York: Sage.

Brewer, M.B., & Miller, N. (1988). Contact and cooperation: When do they work? In P. Katz & D. Taylor (Eds.), *Eliminating racism: Profiles in controversy* (pp. 315–326). New York: Plenum Press.

Brewer, M. B., & Silver, M. (1978). In-group bias as a function of task characteristics. *European Journal of Social Psychology*, *8*, 393–400.

Brewer, M. B., Weber, J. G., & Carini, B. (1995). Person memory in intergroup contexts: Categorization versus individuation. *Journal of Personality and Social Psychology*, *69*, 29–40.

Cook, S.W. (1984). Cooperative interaction in multiethnic contexts. In N. Miller & M. Brewer (Eds.), *Groups in contact: The psychology of desegregation* (pp. 155–185). San Diego: Academic Press.

Darley, J. M., & Berscheid, E. (1967). Increased liking as a result of the anticipation of personal contact. *Human Relations*, *20*, 29–39.

Darley, J. M., & Gross, P. H. (1983). A hypothesis-confirming bias in labeling effects. *Journal of Personality and Social Psychology*, *44*, 20–33.

Denhaerinck, P., Leyens, J-P., & Yzerbyt, V. Y. (1989). The dilution effect and group membership: An instance of the pervasive impact of out-group homogeneity. *European Journal of Social Psychology*, *19*, 243–250.

Deschamps, J.C., & Doise, W. (1978). Crossed category memberships in intergroup relations. In H. Tajfel (Ed.), *Differentiation between social groups* (pp. 141–158). London: Academic Press.

Devine, P. G. (1989). Stereotypes and prejudice: Their automatic and controlled components. *Journal of Personality and Social Psychology*, *56*, 5–18.

Doise, W., & Sinclair, A. (1973). The categorization process in intergroup relations. *European Journal of Social Psychology*, *3*, 145–157.

Dovidio, J. F., & Gaertner, S. L. (1993). Stereotypes and evaluative intergroup bias. In D. Mackie & D. Hamilton (Eds.), *Affect, cognition, and stereotyping: Interactive processes in group perception* (pp. 167–193). New York: Academic Press.

Erber, R., & Fiske, S. T. (1984). Outcome dependency and attention to inconsistent information. *Journal of Personality and Social Psychology*, *47*, 709–726.

Fiske, A. P. (1991). *Structures of social life: The four elementary forms of human relations*. New York: Free Press.

Fiske, S. T. (1993). Controlling other people: The impact of power on stereotyping. *American Psychologist*, *48*, 621–628.

Fiske, S. T., & Neuberg, S. L. (1990). A continuum of impression formation, from category-based to individuating processes: Influences of information and motivation on attention and interpretation. In M. Zanna (Ed.), *Ad-*

vances in experimental social psychology (Vol. 23, pp. 1–74). New York: Academic Press.

Fiske, S. T., Neuberg, S. L., Beattie, A., & Milberg, S. (1987). Category-based and attribute-based reactions to others: Some informational conditions of stereotyping and individuating processes. *Journal of Experimental Social Psychology, 23*, 399–427.

Gilbert, D. T., & Hixon, J. G. (1991). The trouble of thinking: Activation and application of stereotypic beliefs. *Journal of Personality and Social Psychology, 60*, 509–517.

Higgins, E. T., & Bargh, J. A. (1987). Social cognition and social perception. *Annual Review of Psychology, 38*, 369–425.

Hilton, J. L., & Fein, S. (1989). The role of typical diagnosticity in stereotype-based judgments. *Journal of Personality and Social Psychology, 57*, 201–211.

Hogg, M. A., & Turner, J. C. (1987). Intergroup behaviour, self-stereotyping and the salience of social categories. *British Journal of Social Psychology, 26*, 324–340.

Insko, C. A., & Schopler, J. (1987). Categorization, competition and collectivity. In C. Hendrick (Ed.), *Review of personality and social psychology* (Vol. 8, pp. 213–251). Beverly Hills, CA: Sage.

Kruglanski, A. W. (1990). Motivations for judging and knowing: Implications for causal attribution. In E. T. Higgins & R. M. Sorrentino (Eds.), *Handbook of motivation and cognition: Foundations of social behavior* (Vol. 2, pp. 333–368). New York: Guilford Press.

Leyens, J-P., Yzerbyt, V. Y., & Schadron, G. (1992). The social judgeability approach to stereotypes. In W. Stroebe & M. Hewstone (Eds.), *European review of social psychology* (Vol. 3, pp. 91–120). Chichester, UK: Wiley.

Locksley, A., Hepburn, C., & Ortiz, V. (1982). Social stereotypes and judgments of individuals: An instance of the base rate fallacy. *Journal of Experimental Social Psychology, 18*, 23–42.

Lord, C. G., Desforges, D., Fein, S., Pugh, M., & Lepper, M. (1994). Typicality effects in attitudes toward social policies: A concept mapping approach. *Journal of Personality and Social Psychology, 66*, 658–673.

Lord, C. G., Lepper, M., & Mackie, D. (1984). Attitude prototypes as determinants of attitude-behavior consistency. *Journal of Personality and Social Psychology, 46*, 1254–1266.

Maass, A., & Schaller, M. (1991). Intergroup biases and the cognitive dynamics of stereotype formation. In W. Stroebe & M. Hewstone (Eds.), *European review of social psychology* (Vol. 2, pp. 189–209). Chichester, UK: Wiley.

Macrae, C. N., Hewstone, M., & Griffiths, R. (1993). Processing load and memory for stereotype-based information. *European Journal of Social Psychology, 23*, 77–87.

Macrae, C. N., Milne, A. B., & Bodenhausen, G. V. (1994). Stereotypes as energy-saving devices: A peek inside the cognitive toolbox. *Journal of Personality and Social Psychology, 66*, 37–47.

Marcus-Newhall, A., Miller, N., Holtz, R., & Brewer, M. B. (1993). Cross-cutting category membership with role assignment: A means of reducing inter-group bias. *British Journal of Social Psychology, 32*, 125–146.

Miller, N., Brewer, M. B., & Edwards, K. (1985). Cooperative interaction in de-segregated settings: A laboratory analogue. *Journal of Social Issues, 41*(3), 65–79.

Neuberg, S. L., & Fiske, S. T. (1987). Motivational influences on impression formation: Outcome dependency, accuracy-driven attention, and individu-ating processes. *Journal of Personality and Social Psychology, 53*, 431–444.

Oakes, P., & Turner, J. C. (1986). Distinctiveness and the salience of social cate-gory memberships: Is there an automatic perceptual bias towards novelty? *European Journal of Social Psychology, 16*, 325–344.

Ostrom, T. M., Pryor, J., & Simpson, D. (1981). The organization of social in-formation. In E. T. Higgins, C. P. Herman, & M. Zanna (Eds.), *Social cog-nition: The Ontario symposium* (Vol. 1, pp. 3–38). Hillsdale, NJ: Erlbaum.

Ostrom, T. M., & Sedikides, C. (1992). Out-group homogeneity effects in nat-ural and minimal groups. *Psychological Bulletin, 112*, 536–552.

Park, B., & Judd, C. M. (1990). Measures and models of perceived group vari-ability. *Journal of Personality and Social Psychology, 59*, 173–191.

Park, B., & Rothbart, M. (1982). Perception of out-group homogeneity and lev-els of social categorization: Memory for the subordinate attributes of in-group and out-group members. *Journal of Personality and Social Psycholo-gy, 42*, 1051–1068.

Pendry, L. F., & Macrae, C. N. (1994). Stereotypes and mental life: The case of the motivated but thwarted tactician. *Journal of Experimental Social Psy-chology, 30*, 303–325.

Pratto, F., & Bargh, J. A. (1991). Stereotyping based on apparently individuat-ing information: Trait and global components of sex stereotypes under at-tention overload. *Journal of Experimental Social Psychology, 27*, 26–47.

Rothbart, M., & John, O. (1985). Social categorization and behavioral episodes: A cognitive analysis of the effects of intergroup contact. *Journal of Social Issues, 41*(3), 81–104.

Ruscher, J., & Fiske, S. T. (1990). Interpersonal competition can cause individu-ating processes. *Journal of Personality and Social Psychology, 58*, 832–843.

Ruscher, J., Fiske, S. T., Miki, H., & van Manen, S. (1991). Individuating processes in competition: Interpersonal versus intergroup. *Personality and Social Psychology Bulletin, 17*, 595–605.

Schopler, J., & Insko, C. A. (1992). The discontinuity effect in interpersonal and intergroup relations: Generality and mediation. In W. Stroebe & M. Hew-stone (Eds.), *European review of social psychology* (Vol. 3, pp. 121–151). Chichester, UK: Wiley.

Sedikides, C., & Ostrom, T. M. (1988). Are person categories used when orga-nizing information about unfamiliar persons? *Social Cognition, 6*, 252–267.

Stangor, C., & Duan, C. (1991). Effects of multiple task demands upon memory for information about social groups. *Journal of Experimental Social Psychology*, 27, 357–378.

Stangor, C., & Lange, J. E. (1994). Mental representations of social groups: Advances in understanding stereotypes and stereotyping. In M. Zanna (Ed.), *Advances in experimental social psychology* (Vol. 26, pp. 357–416). New York: Academic Press.

Stangor, C., Lynch, L., Duan, C., & Glass, B. (1992). Categorization of individuals on the basis of multiple social features. *Journal of Personality and Social Psychology*, 62, 207–218.

Tajfel, H. (1969). Cognitive aspects of prejudice. *Journal of Social Issues*, 25(4), 79–97.

Taylor, S. E., & Falcone, H. (1982). Cognitive bases of stereotyping: The relationship between categorization and prejudice. *Personality and Social Psychology Bulletin*, 8, 426–432.

Taylor, S. E., Fiske, S. T., Etcoff, N. L., & Ruderman, A. (1978). Categorical and contextual bases of person memory and stereotyping. *Journal of Personality and Social Psychology*, 36, 778–793.

von Hippel, W., Sekaquaptewa, D., & Vargas, P. (1995). On the role of encoding processes in stereotype maintenance. In M. Zanna (Ed.), *Advances in experimental social psychology* (Vol. 27, pp. 177–254). New York: Academic Press.

Wilder, D. A. (1981). Perceiving persons as a group. In D. Hamilton (Ed.), *Cognitive processes in stereotyping and intergroup behavior* (pp. 213–257). Hillsdale, NJ: Erlbaum.

Yzerbyt, V. Y., Schadron, G., Leyens, J-P., & Rocher, S. (1994). Social judgeability: The impact of meta-informational cues on the use of stereotypes. *Journal of Personality and Social Psychology*, 66, 48–55.

Zárate, M. A., & Smith, E. R. (1990). Person categorization and stereotyping. *Social Cognition*, 8, 161–185.

9

Stereotyping, Prejudice, and Discrimination: Another Look

JOHN F. DOVIDIO
JOHN C. BRIGHAM
BLAIR T. JOHNSON
SAMUEL L. GAERTNER

By most historical accounts, Lippmann introduced the term "stereotype" to behavioral scientists in 1922. Lippmann used this term to represent the typical picture that comes to mind when thinking about a particular social group. Despite some noteworthy early interest in the *content* of stereotypes (e.g., Katz & Braly, 1933), research on stereotyping (the *process*) did not achieve mainstream status in psychology until the 1970s. Stimulated by more general interest in cognitive social psychology, more studies of stereotyping (668) were published from 1973 to 1977 than in the previous 50 years combined (Ashmore & Del Boca, 1981). Empirical interest remains unabated. Our literature search for this chapter revealed that over 1,500 articles on stereotyping appeared in print from 1983 to 1992.

   This level of empirical interest would seem to suggest that stereotyping has important consequences for attitudes and behaviors toward social groups. But not everyone agrees. Allport (1954), for instance, proposed that stereotyping was not a determining factor in prejudice or discrimination. He wrote that stereotypes are "primarily rationalizers. . . . While it does no harm (and may do some good) to combat them in schools and colleges, and to reduce them in mass media of communication, it must not be thought that this attack alone will eradicate the roots of prejudice" (Allport, 1954, p. 204). More recently, Jost and Banaji (1994) concluded similarly that "individuals generate beliefs about themselves and stereotypes about social groups in such a way that existing situations are justified" (p. 3). For example, people may make dispositional attributions, such as "lazy," to members of a group to provide a causal explanation for the group's disadvantaged economic status. Thus, stereotypes may be a consequence, rather than a cause, of discrimination. Additionally, a relationship between stereotyping and discrimination appears difficult to demonstrate empirically. In a review of the pre-1970 literature on ethnic stereotypes, Brigham (1971a) found that "there is not a simple relationship between the expression of ethnic stereotypes and their 'use' in behavior toward specific ethnic group members" (p. 28). The present chapter conceptually and empirically reexamines the interrelationships among racial stereotypes, prejudice, and discrimination in view of progress in understanding the dynamics of prejudice and stereotyping, methodological advancements in measuring these concepts, and the accumulated research on these topics since Brigham's review.

We have focused this chapter around Whites' attitudes, stereotypes, and behavior toward Blacks.[1] We recognize potential limitations in the generalizability of our conclusions to other types of intergroup relations, but we have done so for several reasons. First, the relationship between Blacks and Whites has been an enduring issue throughout much of the history of the United States. Although other significant types of intergroup conflict have occurred in this country, and the population of other "minority" groups (i.e., Latinos) is approaching that of Blacks (Gonzales, 1990), racial conflict has historically occupied center stage. The American public's attention to domestic issues of inequality and disparity has been focused on the plight of Black Americans (Hacker, 1992; Jaynes & Williams, 1989). Public concern and public opinion about Black–White relations have, in turn, contributed to the enactment of formal antidiscrimination policies that benefit a range of other groups, as well. Second, perhaps because of the historical prominence of race relations in the United States, racial attitudes appear to be particularly strong and self-relevant, and racial stereotypes are common and consensual (Dovidio & Gaertner, 1986; Karlins, Coffman, & Walters, 1969). Third, this magnitude of public concern for race relations is reflected in the focus of studies in the psychological literature. Studies of Whites' racial attitudes provided the largest database for our empirical and conceptual analyses. In contrast, studies of prejudice toward other groups

(Ramirez, 1988) and about Blacks' attitudes toward Whites (Brigham, 1993) are still relatively rare.

DEFINITIONS OF PREJUDICE, DISCRIMINATION, AND STEREOTYPE

There are a number of common themes among the definitions of prejudice, discrimination, and stereotype that have been proposed. "Prejudice" is generally considered an attitude; "discrimination," a type of behavior; and "stereotype," a set of beliefs. Nevertheless, despite this general agreement, there are a number of different distinctions made in defining each of these concepts. Because of the emphasis of the present volume on stereotyping, we review the definitions of "prejudice" and "discrimination" relatively briefly. However, we later return to issues relating to prejudice and discrimination and consider their relationship to stereotyping.

Prejudice

"Prejudice" is widely defined as a negative attitude, but theorists disagree about whether a negative attitude must have other characteristics to be classified as a prejudice. Some researchers have asserted that *any* negative attitude represents prejudice. Ashmore (1970, p. 253), for example, defined prejudice as "a negative attitude toward a socially defined group and any person perceived to be a member of that group." Other researchers have argued that a prejudicial attitude has, by definition, something wrong with it. Thus, Allport (1954) defined "prejudice" as "an antipathy based on faulty and inflexible generalization. It may be felt or expressed. It may be directed toward a group as a whole, or toward an individual because he [*sic*] is a member of that group" (p. 9). Brigham (1971a) defined "prejudice" as a negative attitude that (by whatever criterion) is seen as unjustified by an observer, while Jones (1986, p. 288) used the term "prejudice" to refer to "a faulty generalization from a group characterization (stereotype) to an individual member of that group irrespective of either (1) the accuracy of the group stereotype, or (2) the applicability of the group characterization to the individual in question." Prejudice is also generally conceptualized, like other attitudes, as having a cognitive component (e.g., irrationally based beliefs about a target group), an affective component (e.g., dislike), and a conative component (e.g., a behavioral predisposition to avoid the target group; Harding, Proshansky, Kutner, & Chein, 1969). Prejudice is typically measured using standardized scales reflecting people's degree of endorsement of a range of statements about attributes of the group, feelings about the group, and support for policies that affect the group (Brigham, 1993; Dovidio & Fazio, 1991).

Discrimination

In the context of intergroup relations, "discrimination" has a pejorative meaning. It implies more than simply distinguishing among social objects; it also implies inappropriate treatment to individuals due to their group membership—a selectively *unjustified* negative behavior toward members of the target group. According to Allport (1954), discrimination involves denying "individuals or groups of people equality of treatment which they may wish" (p. 51). Jones (1972) defined "discrimination" as "those actions designed to maintain own-group characteristics and favored position at the expense of the comparison group" (p. 4). Racial discrimination has been measured in psychological studies in terms of direct harm, failure to help, nonverbal behaviors, and explicit evaluations of out-group members.

Stereotype

A "stereotype" was originally described by Lippmann (1922) as a "picture inside [one's] head" that helped to manage the complexity of one's environment by simplifying the social world. Despite this initial functional view of stereotyping, early conceptions of stereotypes emphasized their flawed nature. Lippmann himself asserted that stereotypes were products of faulty thought processes that led to largely incorrect beliefs. Many other theorists endorsed this approach, conceptualizing stereotypes as overgeneralizations resulting from irrational processes (e.g., Allport, 1954; Bogardus, 1959; Fishman, 1956; Katz & Braly, 1935; Sanford, 1956), and as beliefs characterized by inordinate rigidity and resistance to change (e.g., Adorno, Frenkel-Brunswik, Levinson, & Sanford, 1950; Bogardus, 1959; Fishman, 1956; Rokeach, 1960). Other theorists pointed to more specific issues. Campbell (1967) emphasized the role of erroneous causal perceptions, such as when stereotypes reflect attributions to racial rather than to environmental causes, or when stereotypes are used to rationalize one's hostility toward the group. Brown (1965) summarized the objectionable aspects of stereotypes as their ethnocentrism and their implication that groups have inborn and unalterable psychological characteristics.

Brigham (1971a) attempted to identify the common thread in these approaches by proposing that a "stereotype" is a generalization about a group or its members that is considered *unjustified* by observers. A stereotype may be recognized as unjustified if it reflects faulty thought processes or overgeneralization, factual incorrectness, inordinate rigidity, an inappropriate pattern of attribution, or a rationalization for a prejudiced attitude or discriminatory behavior. This definition sought to capture the pejorative sense in which the term is usually used in everyday discourse. More recently, Judd and Park (1993; also see Ryan, Park, & Judd, Chapter 4, this volume) have identified another dimension of possible stereotype inaccuracy, "dispersion inaccuracy." Specifically, a trait attribution could be accurate in its estimate of central tendency (i.e., the average level of a characteristic within a group), but it may still be an inaccurate overgeneralization in that it underestimates the variability of that trait within the group.

In line with the cognitive orientation that has characterized research on stereotyping during the past two decades, however, more recent theorists have stressed the information-processing and schematic characteristics of stereotypes, while deemphasizing any necessary objectionable aspects. For example, Hamilton and Trolier (1986) defined "stereotypes" simply as "cognitive categories that are used by the social perceiver in processing information about people" (p. 128). From this perspective, although stereotypes may be limited in their characterizations of individuals and groups, they are not necessarily as distorted, insidious, and rigid as Lippmann initially hypothesized (McCauley, Stitt, & Segal, 1980). Many other theorists have adopted similar cognitive, affectively neutral definitions (e.g., Ashmore & Del Boca, 1981; Dovidio, Evans, & Tyler, 1986; Sherman, Judd, & Park, 1989), describing stereotypes as necessary and normal schemas used to process social information about categories of people. However, Fiske (1987, pp. 114–115), a leading cognitive theorist, also has cautioned,

> Cognitive approaches to stereotyping do not adequately account for interracial encounters. . . . In particular, they fail to address critical issues regarding intention, motivation, and behavior. . . . Cognitive approaches to stereotyping have until recently neglected such motivational factors in their rush to show how normal stereotyping is.

Adding to the complexity of this concept is the fact that there are two quite different senses of stereotype. Ashmore and Del Boca (1979) have argued for a distinction between cultural and individual stereotypes. "Cultural stereotypes" represent a communitywide, consensual set of beliefs. "Individual stereotypes" are a set of associations held by an individual about a social group. Measures of cultural stereotypes are typically adjective checklist or rating scale techniques that represent stereotypes as consensual characterizations of the group. For example, Katz and Braly (1935) assessed stereotypes by determining the number of traits required to account for 50% of subjects' responses on their checklist. Measures of individual stereotypes may also involve rating scales, but their primary emphasis is on individual differences in the endorsement of cultural stereotypes. Alternatively, these measures may involve free-response formats to assess unique, individual beliefs about characteristics of social groups (see Stangor & Lange, 1994). The focus of the present chapter is on how *individual stereotypes* are related to individual differences in prejudice and discrimination.

Cognitive and Affective Characteristics of Stereotypes

Despite considerable debate about the specific structure and organization of stereotypic representations (see Stangor & Schaller, Chapter 1, this volume), there is widespread consensus that stereotypes are cognitive schemas (Hamilton & Sherman, 1994). People within a culture consensually ascribe certain traits to social groups (e.g., Karlins et al., 1969) and perceive that these groups possess distinctive characteristics (McCauley & Stitt, 1978). These group schemas, which may be spontaneously accessible, significantly influence how information is encoded, stored, and retrieved: "Once cued, schemas affect how quickly we perceive, what we notice, how we interpret what we notice, and what we perceive as similar and different" (Fiske & Taylor, 1991, p. 122). In general, the activation of stereotypes produces an information processing advantage for stereotypical traits (Macrae, Stangor, & Milne, 1994). Thus, stereotypes may represent the cognitive component within the tripartite view of intergroup attitudes (Harding et al., 1969). If stereotypes are conceptualized as only one of the three components of intergroup attitudes, and intergroup attitudes—like many other global measures of attitudes—are only modestly associated (i.e., $r \cong .30$) with behavior (McGuire, 1985), then Brigham's (1971a) conclusion about the limited relationship between stereotyping and discrimination seems quite logical and reasonable.

Stereotypes, however, may involve affective reactions as well as cognitive representations; that is, when stereotypes are activated, both cognitive and affective information becomes accessible (Fiske, 1982; Fiske, Neuberg, Beattie, & Milberg, 1987; Fiske & Pavelchak, 1986). Affective responses involve a "range of preferences, evaluations, moods, and emotions" (Fiske & Taylor, 1991, p. 410). In this chapter, as in much of the previous literature on stereotyping (e.g., Clark & Fiske,

1982), these affective aspects of stereotypes are represented primarily by overall *evaluative* responses. We recognize that cognitive information (e.g., perceived characteristics) may also be valenced, but we use the term "cognitive" to represent primarily *semantic* information (i.e., trait associations). Although cognitive and affective responses may have been originally linked in the formation of the stereotype, the cognitive and affective consequences of stereotype activation may be independent. Information about groups, like information about persons (Wyer & Gordon, 1984), may be represented twice in memory, independently in a trait-behavior cluster (based on its descriptive implications) and in an evaluation-based representation (based on its affective implications; Dovidio & Gaertner, 1993; Stephan & Stephan, 1993). For example, Dovidio et al. (1986) found that priming racial categories not only made specific trait information about groups (e.g., materialistic for Whites, musical for Blacks) more accessible for White subjects, it also facilitated more global evaluative reactions (more positive for Whites than for Blacks), over and above the association with specific traits. This view of stereotypes as involving both cognitive and affective associations raises questions about the traditional distinction between stereotypes and prejudice. Specifically, the distinction becomes less clear if stereotypes involve two of the three components of intergroup attitudes.

Some recent conceptualizations place primary emphasis on the evaluative nature of stereotypes (Eagly & Mladinic, 1989; Esses, Haddock, & Zanna, 1993; Stangor, Sullivan, & Ford, 1991). These measures examine the evaluative associations with individual stereotypes (see Stangor & Lange, 1994). In the Esses et al. measure, for example, subjects are first asked to describe specific groups with words or phrases. Respondents are then instructed to assign a valence to each characteristic (+ + to − −). Finally, they are asked to estimate the percentage of the group members that possess each of the characteristics identified (see also Brigham, 1971b, 1972). The measure of stereotypes is the average valence, weighted by the probability of occurrence of all of the characteristics ascribed to the group by an individual: Σ(probability of a group member possessing a particular characteristic × valence of that characteristic, from +2 to −2)/(number of characteristics attributed to the group). Note that evaluation and specific semantic associations may be independent. Equally negative but semantically distinct characteristics, such as dishonest and cowardly, could contribute similarly to the Esses et al. stereotype measure.

This view of stereotypes as an overall evaluation of groups has two implications. First, evaluative measures of individual stereotypes may address a different aspect of stereotyping than do cognitive measures (such as the extent to which an individual's trait attributions to a group match the cultural stereotype). As a consequence, evaluative and cognitive measures of stereotyping may not be strongly related. Consistent with this proposition, Stangor et al. (1991) found across two studies that correlations between cognitive and evaluative measures of Whites' stereotypes of Blacks ranged from .13 to .26. Similarly, Dovidio et al. (1986) found that the extent to which people associated traditionally stereotypic traits with Blacks and Whites (a cognitive measure of stereotyping) was only modestly (and nonsignificantly) related ($r = .25$) to the degree to which they had more positive evaluative associations with Whites than with Blacks (an evaluative measure of stereotyping). Second, focusing on the evaluative aspect tends to align stereotypes closely with some definitions of attitudes. For example, Fishbein (1963; see also Ajzen, 1985; Smith & Clark, 1973) proposed that an attitude is a function of the strength of the belief that an object has certain characteristics and the evaluations of those characteristics: Attitude = Σ(strength of characteristic association × evaluation of the characteristic). Although not identical, there are thus important similarities between some operational and conceptual definitions of stereotypes and of attitudes.

In summary, the traditional distinctions of stereotypes as a set of cognitive associations, prejudice as an attitude, and discrimination as behavior have been replaced by more complex views. The more elaborate, multidimensional view of stereotypes, in particular, raises important conceptual and empirical questions about the relationships among stereotypes, prejudice, and discrimination. In the next section, we examine these potential relations.

RELATIONSHIPS AMONG STEREOTYPES, PREJUDICE, AND DISCRIMINATION

The traditional view of stereotypes, prejudice, and discrimination suggested a relatively straightforward relationship among these phenomena. As illustrated in Figure 9.1, to the extent that stereotypes represent the cognitive component of prejudice, a greater degree of stereotyping would be expected to be positively related to prejudice. This analysis assumes that stereotypes represent *negative* trait attributions (e.g., Allport, 1954; Brigham, 1971a), because prejudice is defined as a negative attitude. Prejudice, as a negative attitude, would then directly predict (negative) discrimination.

It is also possible that stereotyping could relate to discrimination in ways independent of attitudes. This could occur for conceptual or

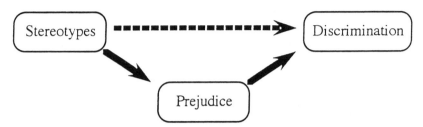

FIGURE 9.1. Potential relationship among stereotypes, prejudice, and discrimination.

methodological reasons. Conceptually, stereotypes and prejudice would have different effects if (1) the beliefs associated with the attitude of an individual are not entirely the same as those represented by cultural stereotypes, or (2) the affective and conative components of attitudes moderate the impact of cognitive beliefs. Methodologically, measures of stereotypic beliefs may be more restricted in their range of cognitive assessments than typical measures of attitudes. Whereas stereotypes may involve the association of characteristics and roles with specific groups, the cognitive component of racial attitudes may involve a multidimensional set of perceptions. For example, using a factor analytic approach, Cook and his colleagues identified 9 to 15 content dimensions that characterized Whites' racial attitudes (Ard & Cook, 1977; Brigham, Woodmansee, & Cook, 1976; Woodmansee & Cook, 1967; see also Brigham, 1977, 1993).

However, Brigham's (1971a) review of the literature over two decades ago challenged a straightforward view of the relation of stereotyping to prejudice and discrimination. Our objective in the present chapter is to extend this analysis of the relationships among racial stereotyping, prejudice, and discrimination both empirically and conceptually. Empirically, Brigham's conclusions were based on a narrative review of pre-1970 studies. We apply meta-analytic techniques to a literature enriched by over 20 additional years of research. Conceptually, we propose further distinctions involving stereotyping, prejudice, and discrimination.

We suggest that a conceptually productive approach is to consider how different aspects of stereotyping and prejudice relate to one another and predict discrimination. For example, as we noted earlier, stereotypes, like attitudes, can involve both cognitive and affective components. Thus, cognitive and affective measures of stereotyping may relate differently to measures of prejudice. Behavior is also a multidimensional concept. With respect to discrimination, Crosby, Bromley, and Saxe (1980) suggested that evaluation concerns are critical. Their literature review revealed that Whites were more likely to discriminate against Blacks when their actions were anonymous. Concerns about one's self-image, rather than one's public image, are also important. Whites are more likely to exhibit bias against Blacks when this action can be justified on the basis of some factor other than race, and thereby does not challenge one's nonprejudiced self-image (Gaertner & Dovidio, 1986). Thus, the general approach that guides the remainder of this chapter concerns how different aspects of stereotypes and prejudice relate to different types of interracial behaviors.

In the following section we examine the overall relationship between racial attitudes and discrimination. We explore the role of prejudice at this time for two reasons: First, in most conventional views, prejudice is considered to be a primary determinant of discriminatory behavior; second, our discussion of prejudice raises important measurement issues that apply to stereotypes as well.

RACIAL PREJUDICE AND DISCRIMINATION

Because of their deep-seated nature in American culture (Feagin & Feagin, 1978; Jones, 1986, 1993), negative racial attitudes persist in contemporary society. In a recent nationwide poll, White Americans still described Blacks as significantly less intelligent, less hard-working, and more violent than Whites (Davis & Smith, 1991). Substantial proportions of Whites also continued to feel that it was their right to keep Blacks out of their neighborhoods (18%) and that there should be laws against interracial marriage (18%). Perhaps because of their apparent link to social problems, the study of racial attitudes has had an enduring place in social psychology.

As illustrated in Figure 9.1, the traditional assumption has been that racial attitudes are strong predictors of discrimination. Concerns about the failure of racial stereotypes to predict discrimination often imply that they are inferior to attitudes in this regard. Nevertheless, the issue of how well racial attitudes generally predict interracial behavior is a largely unanswered question. Whereas one might assume that racial attitudes, like other types of strong attitudes, are effective predictors of behavior, this may not be the case. In fact, the issue of attitude–behavior inconsistency is a recurring theme in the area of racial and ethnic attitudes.

Crosby et al. (1980), for example, argued that the increase in positive racial attitudes in the 1960s and 1970s, reflected in surveys and polls, involved primarily Whites' compliance with egalitarian norms rather than fully internalized, nonprejudiced beliefs. Thus, they reasoned, Whites' interracial behavior may be more negative than these attitudes suggest. Consistent with this interpretation, Crosby et al. concluded in their review of unobtrusive studies of discrimination that anti-Black attitudes among Whites were strong and were manifested in discriminatory behavior. In contrast, there is also evidence that Whites' interracial responses may be more positive than measures of attitudes imply. Dovidio and Mullen (1992) conducted a recent review of 23 studies and 64 tests of Whites' evaluations and impressions of particular Black and White persons. Despite prevailing negative attitudes toward Blacks, across these studies White subjects responded consistently more favorably to Blacks than to Whites. Thus, the answer to a seemingly straightforward question about whether racial attitudes predict interracial behaviors may not be straightforward at all.

In our initial attempt to answer the question of whether Whites' attitudes predict discrimination against Blacks, we performed a meta-analysis of 35 different tests from 23 relevant studies that assessed individual differences in racial attitudes and behaviors.[2] There was a significant relationship between negative racial attitudes and discrimination ($r = .32$). Moreover, this relationship was similar whether the group was the target of discrimination ($r = .33$) or an individual member of the group was the target ($r = .32$). Although the magnitude of these effects is modest, similar to the effect size that some years ago led attitude researchers (e.g., Wicker, 1969) to question attitude–behavior consistency, the relationships are respectable given the range of situations and other potential determinants of behavior involved. Nevertheless, we observed that the magnitude of the attitude–behavior relationship did vary considerably across studies, which suggests the complexities of this relationship. In the following sections we consider two dimensions that could potentially moderate the relationship between prejudice and discrimination.

Prejudice and Behavioral Reactions

Earlier in this chapter we made a distinction between affect and cognition for both stereotypes and prejudice. This distinction, which Zajonc (1980) argued is fundamental in human functioning, also applies to behavior. With respect to interracial behavior, Whites' affective reactions toward Blacks may be manifested in voice tone (Weitz, 1972), facial expressions (Butler & Geis, 1990), or other nonverbal cues (Word, Zanna, & Cooper, 1974). Cognitive reactions may be reflected in a White person's decision to help a Black person (Crosby et al., 1980) or to support or oppose a government policy (McConahay, 1986). On the basis of this conceptual analysis, we examined the relationship between Whites' prejudice and their primarily affective or cognitive reactions to Blacks. Twenty-three studies were reliably coded as involving predominantly affective responses (e.g., general evaluations, emotional expressions), whereas 10 involved predominantly cognitive measures (e.g., specific attributional judgments).

Because measures of prejudice, like measures of other attitudes, generally assume a three-component model (McConahay, 1986), they typically do not distinguish between "affective" and "cognitive" attitudes. Methodologically, this aspect of attitude measures prevented us from being able to code reliably the attitude measures as affective or cognitive. Conceptually, because attitude measures presumably involve the *combination* of affective and cognitive components, there is little *a priori* reason to expect attitudes to be a better predictor of affectively- or cognitively-oriented behavior; our analysis is primarily exploratory. Empirically, there was no significant difference in the strength of the relationship between attitude measures and affective or cognitive interracial responses by Whites: The magnitudes of the attitude-affective behavior relationship ($r = .32$) and the attitude-cognitive behavior relationship ($r = .35$) were comparable. Whereas this investigation of the affective-cognitive distinction as a moderator of the racial attitude-behavior relationship was exploratory, the next dimension that we considered was more conceptually based. This dimension concerns *how* racial attitudes are expressed.

Racial attitudes are more socially sensitive than most other attitudes (Dovidio & Fazio, 1991). As a consequence, a person's "true" attitude may be difficult to assess accurately. Individuals may express public attitudes that reflect more their impressions of socially desirable responses than their private opinions (Roese & Jamieson, 1993). It is well-documented in laboratory research that subjects are concerned about the evaluations of others and are motivated to behave in positive and appropriate ways (e.g., Weber & Cook, 1972). As a consequence of social desirability influences, traditional measures of racial attitudes that are based on self-reports may produce more egalitarian and nonprejudiced responses among Whites toward Blacks than do behavioral measures that are less reactive or more spontaneous (Crosby et al., 1980). Indeed, there is experimental evidence that respondents systematically alter their expressed racial attitudes and behaviors to appear in a more socially desirable—unprejudiced and egalitarian—light (e.g., McConahay, Hardee, & Batts, 1981).

The systematic consideration of social values in the expression of an attitude may occur at another level besides public concern. Specifically, at a private level, individuals may distort their expressed racial attitudes in ways that reinforce a positive self-image and reflect an ideal self-concept; that is, respondents may be unwilling to admit to themselves that they are prejudiced. The importance of maintaining a non-prejudiced self-image is a central aspect of many current conceptualizations of racial attitudes, such as the aversive racism framework (Gaertner & Dovidio, 1986; Kovel, 1970).

The Nature of Contemporary Racial Attitudes of Whites

Contemporary forms of racism are more subtle and indirect than the old-fashioned form (see Dovidio & Gaertner, 1986, 1991; Pettigrew, 1988). Aversive racism, for example, represents a modern, subtle form of bias that characterizes many White Americans who possess strong egalitarian values. Many of these people also possess negative racial feelings and beliefs of which they either are unaware or try to dissociate from their nonprejudiced self-images. Gaertner and Dovidio (1986) proposed that aversive racism is an adaptation resulting from an assimilation of an egalitarian value system with (1) impressions derived from human cognitive mechanisms that contribute to the development of stereotypes and prejudice, and (2) feelings and beliefs derived from historical and contemporary cultural racist contexts. The aversive racism perspective assumes that cognitive and motivational biases, and socialization into the historically racist culture of the United States, with its contemporary legacy, lead most White Americans to develop negative feelings and beliefs about Blacks (and other minorities). Because of current cultural values, however, most Whites also have convictions concerning fairness, justice, and racial equality. Both the existence of almost unavoidable racial biases and the desire to be egalitarian form the basis of an ambivalence that aversive racists experience.

The concepts of ambivalence and subtlety of expression also apply to other perspectives on contemporary racism, such as symbolic racism (Sears, 1988) and modern racism (McConahay, 1986). According to symbolic (and modern) racism theory, Whites acquire negative feelings toward Blacks early in life. These feelings persist into adulthood but are expressed indirectly and symbolically, in terms of opposition to busing or resistance to preferential treatment, rather than directly or overtly, as in support for segregation. McConahay adds that because modern racism involves the rejection of traditional racist beliefs and the displacement of anti-Black feelings onto more rationalizable abstract social and political issues, modern racists, like aversive racists, are relatively unaware of their racist feelings.

In general, these recent conceptions of racial attitudes suggest that contemporary forms of racial prejudice among Whites are complex and subtly expressed. These considerations are obviously relevant to how racial attitudes are measured. Understanding the nature of contemporary racial attitudes of Whites as complex and conflicted, involving nonconscious negative feelings and the conscious desire to be nonprejudiced, also has relevance to understanding issues relating to racial attitude–interracial behavior consistency. Unfortunately, there has been relatively little theoretical or empirical work on Blacks' racial attitudes (Brigham, 1993; C. Thompson, Neville, Weathers, Poston, & Atkinson, 1990; V. Thompson, 1991), and it is thus unclear whether parallel conflicts and complexities characterize Blacks' racial attitudes.

Understanding the Relation between Interracial Attitudes and Behavior

One way of exploring the implications of the aversive racism framework is within the context of the MODE Model (Dovidio & Fazio, 1991; Fazio, 1990). The acronym MODE refers to *m*otivation and *o*pportunity as *de*terminants of the processing mode by which behavioral decisions are made. The MODE Model suggests that attitude–behavior processes are of essentially two types. The basic difference centers on the extent to which a behavioral decision involves conscious deliberation versus a spontaneous, unconscious reaction to an attitude object or issue:

> An individual may analyze the costs and benefits of a particular behavior, and, in doing so, deliberately reflect upon the attitudes relevant to a behavioral decision. These attitudes may serve as one of the possibly many dimensions that are considered in arriving at a behavior plan, which may then be enacted. Alternatively, attitudes may guide an individual's behavior in a more spontaneous manner, without the individual's having actively considered the relevant attitudes and without the individual's necessary awareness of the influence of the attitude. Instead, the attitude may influence how the person interprets the event that is occurring and, in that way, affect the person's behavior. (Fazio, 1990, p. 78)

The theoretical distinction between spontaneous and deliberative processing has implications for attitude measurement and behavioral prediction in general, and specifically with respect to contemporary racial attitudes. The MODE Model suggests that to optimize the accuracy of predictions, one should consider the type of decision process that is expected to operate in the behavioral context. With respect to racial attitudes in particular, a critical factor involves whether the attitude measure and the behavior both tap the conscious egalitarian component, both reflect the unconscious negative component of the racial attitude, or involve different processes. Thus, the central issue is how different aspects of attitudes relate to actions under different circumstances.

Given the ambivalence of Whites' racial attitudes, it is not surprising that our meta-analysis indicated that the attitude–behavior relationship in this arena is highly variable. The MODE Model, however, is useful in understanding the complexities of this relationship. Specifically, it suggests that attitude–behavior consistency will vary with the correspondence of the processes involved in the assessment of attitudes and the measurement of behavior. Because both traditional attitudinal self-report measures and conscious, public behaviors reflect individuals' deliberations that involve responsiveness to egalitarian social norms and personal standards, there should be correspondence between assessed attitudes and this type of behavior. In contrast, the relationship between self-report measures of prejudice and spontaneous behaviors, which are less likely to be shaped by social norms or conscious ideals, should be weaker, as Crosby et al.'s (1980) analysis suggested. Spontaneous behaviors, however, should be better predicted by measures of *implicit attitudes*, which reflect unconscious feelings and beliefs (Greenwald & Banaji, 1995), than by traditional measures of prejudice. Implicit attitudes can be assessed using a variety of response latency (priming, lexical decision) and incidental memory paradigms, and indirect measures of bias (see Dovidio & Fazio, 1991; Greenwald & Banaji, 1995).

Although there has been little direct work contrasting these factors with respect to racial attitudes, evidence across studies is generally consistent with the notion that deliberative self-reported racial attitudes are better predictors of deliberative than of spontaneous behaviors. For example, traditional measures of assessing prejudice, such as the Woodmansee and Cook (1967) Multifactor Racial Attitude Inventory (MRAI), are generally reactive and obtrusive, and raise social desirability concerns. Consistent with our hypothesis, shortened versions of the MRAI correlate significantly with highly deliberated actions, such as self-reports of racially oriented voting behavior (Weigel & Howes, 1985), but not with spontaneous reactions, such as incidental helping (Dovidio & Gaertner, 1981).

Another meta-analytic examination of the relationship between interracial attitudes and Whites' discrimination in spontaneous and deliberative situations also demonstrates the importance of correspondence between attitudinal and behavioral processes. As expected, the attitude–behavior relation was significantly stronger in studies in which attitude and behavior measures both involved deliberative processes ($r = .35$) than in studies in which attitude measures involved deliberative processes, but in which behavior was spontaneous ($r = .16$). Because of the relatively recent development of the implicit attitude measurement techniques (see Dovidio & Fazio, 1991), the prediction that spontaneous discriminatory behaviors should be better predicted by measures of automatic activation remains largely untested. We will, however, return to this issue when we consider measures of stereotyping.

Dimensions of the Attitude–Behavior Relationship

In summary, the relationship between Whites' racial attitudes and discrimination is statistically significant but modest. Nevertheless, the effect size, $r = .32$, is remarkably close to the typical magnitude of the attitude–behavior relationship ($r \cong .30$) described by McGuire (1985) across a range of areas. We propose, however, that the nature of this relationship could be better understood by examining how different aspects of racial attitudes relate to different types of behaviors. Although many types of moderators are possible, we suggest that two important dimensions are affective–cognitive and spontaneous–deliberative. Zajonc (1980) argued that the first distinction is a fundamental one; affect and cognition may involve separate systems of psychological functioning that can operate independently. However, perhaps because attitudes are a function of both affect and cognition, attitudes related equivalently to affective and cognitive measures of Whites' responses to Blacks. The second distinction, spontaneous–deliberative, is based on Fazio's (1990) integration and analysis of attitude–behavior relations across a range of social and nonsocial issues. As we proposed, traditional self-report measures of prejudice, which involve conscious deliberation, self-reflection, and social desirability concerns, are significantly better predictors of deliberative forms of interracial behavior than of spontaneous forms.

We recognize that because these distinctions are relatively recent, particularly in the area of racial attitudes, our analysis is limited and incomplete. For example, whereas we could demonstrate that correspondence in deliberative processing significantly enhances the attitude–behavior relationship, we could not test the effects of correspondence in spontaneous reactions. Empirical interest in this topic and the technologies for assessing spontaneous attitudes are not yet widespread. Greenwald and Banaji (1995), for instance, conducted a census of attitude studies published in 1989 and found that 100% used at least one direct measure of attitude, but only 13% included some form of indirect measure. Similarly, the affective–cognitive distinction is not one traditionally made in measures of racial attitudes. We also note that the affective–cognitive and spontaneous–deliberative distinctions may not be independent. Zajonc (1980) proposed that affect may "precede in time . . . the sorts of perceptual and cognitive operations commonly assumed to be the basis for these affective judgments. Affective reactions to stimuli are often the first reactions" (p. 151). From this perspective, affective and spontaneous reactions are likely to be highly correlated. Nevertheless, we believe that these two distinctions are conceptually useful devices and are important to understanding the relationships among stereotypes, prejudice, and discrimination. In the next section we explore the relationship between stereotypes and prejudice.

RACIAL STEREOTYPES AND PREJUDICE

Both traditional and contemporary views of stereotyping suggest a positive relationship between stereotypes and prejudice. First, as noted earlier, researchers have commonly considered stereotypes as the cognitive component of racial attitudes (e.g., Harding et al., 1969; Jones, 1986). Brigham (1971a) reasoned that "in order to feel negatively toward a group, one must be able to perceive the different individuals of the given ethnic group as having certain constant characteristics, as being similar to other individuals in the same group, and as being different from individuals not of that ethnic group" (p. 26). Thus, stereotypes may form the cognitive basis for racial prejudice. Second, several researchers have proposed that stereotypes perform a function for prejudiced people by allowing them to rationalize their hostility and negative feelings toward that particular group (e.g., Simpson & Yinger, 1965). Third, stereotypes and prejudice could be related more indirectly. Individual differences on dimensions such as authoritarianism that are relevant to intergroup relations may relate to both stereotyping and prejudice (Saenger & Flowerman, 1954). This common influence could thus produce a positive relationship.

In addition to these traditional perspectives, the affective–cognitive and spontaneous–deliberative distinctions that we have made in this chapter suggest that, at least under some conditions, stereotyping and racial prejudice should be positively correlated. As we noted earlier, racial attitudes, like other attitudes, are assumed to involve both cognitive and affective components. Consequently, both cognitive and affective measures of stereotypes would be likely to be positively related to racial prejudice. Zanna and Rempel (1988) have argued that the relative impact of affect and cognitions varies for different issues and groups. With respect to racial attitudes, the question remains as to which is the better predictor, cognitive or affective measures of stereotypes. Stangor et al.'s (1991) analysis suggests that affect may be the more potent determinant of prejudice. Affective responses are more likely to be based on direct and highly self-relevant experiences than are cognitive responses. Methodologically, affective measures may be more self-relevant also because they typically reflect individual, rather than consensual, stereotypes. Cognitive responses, in contrast, may largely be learned from secondary sources, or may subsequently develop as rationalizers for negative attitudes and behaviors (Harding et al., 1969; Jost & Banaji, 1994). In general, more direct and self-relevant experiences produce stronger attitudinal responses (e.g., Fazio, Powell, & Herr, 1983). Consistent with this hypothesis, Stangor et al. (1991) found that Whites' self-reported feelings (e.g., ratings of being afraid, angry, respectful, and sympathetic) toward nine different social groups (including Blacks) were a better predictor of intergroup attitudes than were cognitive measures of individual stereotypes (endorsement of traditional stereotypic characteristics of Blacks, such as athletic or lazy). We examine whether this reasoning applies to the comparison between affective (operationalized in terms of primarily evaluative measures) and cognitive measures of stereotyping. Specifically, to the extent that measures of both stereotypes and prejudice have strong affective components, measures of stereotypes that focus on overall evaluations should be substantially associated with prejudice—and more so than cognitive measures of stereotyping, which reflect the correspondence of an individual's particular trait attributions to a group with the cultural stereotype.

With respect to the spontaneous–deliberative dimension, deliberative measures of stereotyping and prejudice—the traditional measurement techniques—should both be influenced by changing public norms and personal standards; that is, common forces should produce more egalitarian responses among Whites in terms of both stereotyping and prejudice. At an aggregate level, this seems to be the case. Table 9.1 summarizes the racial stereotypes of demographically similar samples of White college students across the 60-year period from 1933 to 1993, using an adjective checklist technique. Over time, there has been a convergence between the expressed stereotypes of Whites and of Blacks in terms of both the specific characteristics expressed and the overall evaluation of these groups. Two traditional measures of attitudes reveal

TABLE 9.1. Percentage of White Subjects Selecting a Trait to Describe White and Black Americans: 1933–1993

	1933	1951	1967	1982	1988	1990	1993
			White Americans				
Industrious	48	30	23	21	13	10	11
Intelligent	47	32	20	10	6	15	10
Materialistic	33	37	67	65	41	46	48
Ambitious	33	21	42	35	35	33	48
Progressive	26	27	28	45	32	23	24
Pleasure loving	26	27	28	45	32	23	24
Alert	23	7	7	2	1	4	2
Efficient	21	9	15	8	5	3	5
Aggressive	20	8	15	11	27	23	16
Straightforward	19	—	9	7	8	4	5
Practical	19	—	12	14	10	14	14
Sportsmanlike	19	—	9	6	4	3	10
Individualistic	—	26	15	14	24	19	29
Conventional	—	—	18	20	8	11	16
Scientific	—	—	15	4	3	3	1
Ostentatious	—	—	15	6	6	5	2
Conservative	—	—	—	15	22	26	30
Stubborn	—	—	—	20	8	10	11
Tradition loving	—	—	—	19	22	13	16
Loyal to family	—	—	—	—	20	19	18
Nationalistic	—	—	—	—	24	6	12
Boastful	—	—	—	—	13	10	3
Ignorant	—	—	—	—	10	12	15
Arrogant	—	—	—	—	—	26	13
Aggressive	—	—	—	—	—	—	16
Naive	—	—	—	—	—	—	10
			Black Americans (formerly "Negroes")				
Superstitious	84	41	13	6	2	3	1
Lazy	75	31	26	13	6	4	5
Happy-go-lucky	38	17	27	15	4	1	2
Ignorant	38	24	11	10	6	5	5
Musical	26	33	47	29	13	27	12
Ostentatious	26	11	25	5	0	1	1

(continued)

TABLE 9.1. *cont.*

	1933	1951	1967	1982	1988	1990	1993
			Black Americans (*cont.*)				
Very religious	24	17	8	23	20	19	17
Stupid	22	10	4	1	1	3	0
Physically dirty	17	—	3	0	1	0	1
Naive	14	—	4	4	2	3	1
Slovenly	13	—	5	2	1	1	0
Unreliable	12	—	6	2	1	4	1
Pleasure loving	—	19	26	20	14	14	14
Sensitive	—	—	17	13	15	9	4
Gregarious	—	—	17	4	6	2	4
Talkative	—	—	14	5	5	8	13
Imitative	—	—	13	9	4	3	0
Aggressive	—	—	—	19	16	17	24
Materialistic	—	—	—	16	10	3	13
Loyal to family	—	—	—	39	49	41	39
Arrogant	—	—	—	14	7	7	5
Ambitious	—	—	—	13	16	24	
Tradition loving	—	—	—	13	22	16	16
Individualistic	—	—	—	—	24	17	19
Passionate	—	—	—	—	14	17	19
Nationalistic	—	—	—	—	13	13	19
Straightforward	—	—	—	—	12	15	24
Intelligent	—	—	—	—	—	14	5
Sportsmanlike	—	—	—	—	—	13	8
Quick-tempered	—	—	—	—	—	12	13
Artistic	—	—	—	—	—	12	6
Argumentative	—	—	—	—	—	—	14
Loud	—	—	—	—	—	—	11
Passionate	—	—	—	—	—	—	19
Progressive	—	—	—	—	—	—	11
Radical	—	—	—	—	—	—	10
Revengeful	—	—	—	—	—	—	11
Suspicious	—	—	—	—	—	—	10
Talkative	—	—	—	—	—	—	13

comparable trends. Table 9.2 presents the responses of White subjects from demographically similar populations on Bogardus's (1925) social distance scales from 1949 to 1992. Figure 9.2 presents the results of nationwide surveys of Whites' willingness to vote for a well-qualified Black presidential candidate. As with the stereotyping data, prejudice in Whites appears to have dramatically declined.

It should be noted, however, that similar patterns at an aggregate level do not necessarily mean that stereotyping and prejudice are related at an individual level. In fact, Stangor et al. (1991) observed: that "despite the voluminous research concerning patterns of social stereotype ascription, there has surprisingly been very little empirical research concerning the relationship between stereotyping and prejudice. . . . Moreover, the findings of this research are not clear cut" (p. 360). For example, Brigham's (1971a) analysis indicated that stereotyping and prejudice were only weakly and inconsistently related. Moreover, research involving social groups other than Blacks (which may involve less negative attitudes and stereotypes) has revealed that the degree of consensual stereotyping of these groups is largely unrelated to attitudes toward these groups (Gardner, 1973, 1993; Gardner, Lalonde, Nero, & Young, 1988; Gardner, Wonnacott, & Taylor, 1968; Lalonde & Gardner, 1989). This section further explores this relationship. Following the format of our examination of the link between racial prejudice and discrimination, we first summarize the overall relationship between measures of racial stereotyping of Whites and measures of Whites' racial prejudice. Then we consider, conceptually and empirically, the moderating roles of the affective–cognitive and spontaneous–deliberative dimensions.

TABLE 9.2. Social Distance Ratings in Three Generations of College Students: 1949–1992

Willing to admit Blacks (Negroes) to:	1949	1968	1992
Employment in my occupation	78%	98%	99%
My club as personal friends	51%	97%	96%
My street as neighbors	41%	95%	95%
Close kinship by marriage	0%	66%	74%

Note. Data from Bogardus (1925).

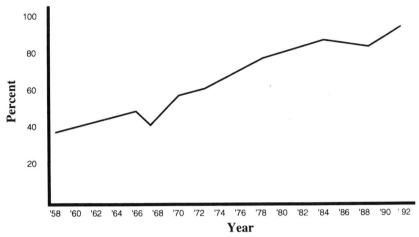

FIGURE 9.2. Percent of Whites willing to vote for a "well-qualified" Black presidential candidate. Data from Davis and Smith (1991).

What Is the Relationship between Racial Stereotypes and Prejudice?

Both racial prejudice and stereotyping in Whites have been measured in a variety of ways. Traditional measures of the "old-fashioned" form of racism reflect social distance, hostility, and derogatory beliefs. As noted earlier, more contemporary forms of racial prejudice are assessed using more indirect self-report measures, such as the Symbolic Racism Scale (Kinder & Sears, 1981) or Modern Racism Scale (McConahay, 1986). McConahay proposed that these indirect self-report measures are more likely to permit negative responses, because a prejudiced answer to an item in each case can be rationalized by a non-race-related attribution or ideology. Recent evidence suggests that scores on traditional and contemporary measures are moderately related, as Brigham (1993) found a mean correlation of .56 between Whites' scores on two largely traditional measures and two contemporary measures (Modern Racism and Symbolic Racism).

As discussed earlier in this chapter and in the other chapters of this volume, stereotypes are assessed in a wide variety of ways. Cognitive measures of individual stereotypes focus on the specific traits that are perceived to characterize a social group. They generally involve the degree to which an individual's attributions of specific traits to a group, or estimates of the proportion of group members that possess a characteristic, correspond to cultural stereotypes (Brigham, 1972; McCauley et al., 1980). Affective measures of individual stereotypes emphasize the general evaluation of the group as a function of the characteristics that are viewed as typical. As we noted earlier, in these measures, attributions of specific traits and estimated proportions are typically summarized into an overall evaluation score (Eagly & Mladinic, 1989; Esses et al., 1993; Stangor et al., 1991). Esses et al. (1993) propose that these types of affective measures are generally better predictors of attitudes than are cognitive measures. They reason that "consensual stereotypes of an out-group may vary in valence, including both positive and negative characteristics. This would explain why a measure that takes into account only the extent to which consensual stereotypes of an out-group are endorsed, irrespective of the proportion of these that are positive or negative, is a poor predictor of attitudes toward the group" (p. 142).

As an alternative to self-report measures, a variety of priming, memory, and response latency techniques have recently been developed to assess stereotyping (see Greenwald & Banaji, 1995). Devine (1989), for example, assessed Whites' racial stereotypes by subliminally priming White subjects with Black stereotypic characteristics (as part of a "vigilance" task) and then measuring their attributions of hostility to another person's ambiguous social behaviors, which were described in a brief scenario. Banaji and Greenwald (1995) used a variation of Jacoby, Kelley, Brown, and Jasechko's (1989) "false-fame" paradigm to examine gender stereotyping. Jacoby et al. found that previous exposure to nonfamous names increased the likelihood that people would subsequently incorrectly identify these people as being famous; Banaji and Greenwald demonstrated that this effect occurred more strongly for male than female names—indicating the operation of implicit gender stereotypes. Alternatively, Dovidio, Gaertner, and their colleagues have used response latency techniques to assess racial stereotypes (see Dovidio & Gaertner, 1993; also, Dovidio & Fazio, 1991). In some studies, subjects are presented with racial category primes, either supraliminally or subliminally, and are asked to make a judgment whether the word that follows could ever describe a member of that group. In other studies, a lexical decision task is used in which subjects are asked to judge whether two strings of letters (e.g., Blacks-smart) are words (Gaertner & McLaughlin, 1983). Faster response times are presumed to reflect greater stereotypic association. These associations may be assessed for either specific, traditionally stereotypic characteristics (cognitive stereotypes) or more general, nonstereotypic evaluative traits (affective stereotypes).

The advantage of such a wide variety of measures of stereotyping is that each measure may emphasize a different, and potentially important, aspect of stereotyping. For example, response latency measures have been developed, in part, to reduce the impact of social desirability and evaluation apprehension influences that may shape responses to traditional self-report measures. Consistent with this intent, as responses on these measures become more automatic and less controlled, Whites' negative associations with Blacks are more likely to be manifested (Dovidio & Gaertner, 1993). The disadvantages of the varied techniques are both methodological and conceptual. Methodologically, there is substantial variance among the different measurement techniques that is not yet well understood. Conceptually, different types of measures, even using similar techniques, may be only modestly related. As we noted earlier, cognitive and affective measures of individual racial stereotypes are only modestly correlated (rs between .13 and .26; Dovidio et al., 1986; Stangor et al., 1991). Nevertheless, following the analysis of Brigham (1971a) but recognizing the wide methodological variance in the literature, we performed an updated, meta-analytic test of the overall relationship between racial prejudice and stereotyping.

Our meta-analysis of 30 hypothesis tests from 12 research reports of Whites' views of Blacks challenges the assumption of many contemporary researchers that stereotypes are unrelated to attitudes. Across these tests, individual differences in racial stereotyping were significantly related to racial prejudice. The effect size, $r = .25$, was modest, although not much smaller than the racial prejudice–discrimination effect (.32) reported earlier, or the general attitude–behavior relationship (.30). It is also consistent with the relationship that Stephan, Ageyev, Coates-Shrider, Stephan, and Abalakina (1994) found between three measures of Americans' individual stereotypes (level of endorsement of consensual stereotypes, evaluations of consensual stereotypic group traits, and a multiplicative combination of these measures) and global attitudes toward Russians and Iraqis (average multiple $r = .31$). Because effects of this magnitude might not attain traditional levels of statistical significance in any one study, particularly if the sample size is relatively small, it is not surprising the researchers who base their conclusions on their own individual works could conclude that stereotypes and prejudice are unrelated. Collectively, however, a consistent and statistically significant pattern emerges: Racial stereotypes and racial prejudice are positively associated. In the following sections we consider whether this relationship is moderated, as we hypothesize, by the cognitive–affective and spontaneous–deliberative dimensions.

Moderators of the Stereotype–Prejudice Relationship

As we noted earlier, there are arguments suggesting why cognitive measures of stereotypes or affective measures would be particularly likely to relate to prejudice under some conditions. The arguments for cognitive measures suggest that stereotypes comprise the cognitive component of attitudes (e.g., Jones, 1986), or that negative stereotypes serve as rationalizers for negative attitudes and feelings. If the cultural stereotype is largely negative (as with Whites' stereotype of Blacks), then the degree to which an individual endorses this stereotype and prejudice should be closely related. Alternatively, other researchers have suggested that evaluative, primarily affective, measures of individual stereotypes should be more strongly related to attitudes. As Esses et al. (1993) observed, "merely looking at the degree to which an individual expresses stereotypes of a group that are in accord with stereotypes expressed by others often tells us very little about the individual's overall evaluation of the groups" (pp. 141–142). Because both individual evaluative stereotypes and attitudes involve favorable or unfavorable responses to a particular group, these measures should be more highly correlated—particularly if, as Stangor et al. (1991) suggest, racial attitudes have a substantial affective basis.

Which measure of Whites' racial stereotypes is the better predictor of prejudice? Our analysis of the literature indicates not only that both cognitive and evaluative measures of individual stereotypes are significantly related to racial prejudice, but also they are virtually equally related. The effect size for the cognitive measures of stereotypes was .26; the effect size for evaluative measures of stereotypes was .24. Thus, at least with respect to Whites' stereotypes of and attitudes toward Blacks, neither measure has a distinct empirical advantage over the other in terms of relating to prejudice.

One explanation for these equivalent relationships may be that, because the traditional stereotype of Blacks by Whites has involved predominantly negative characteristics, cognitive and evaluative individual stereotypes are highly associated, and therefore they are equally related to racial prejudice. Inconsistent with this explanation, however, we observed earlier in this chapter that evaluative and cognitive measures of stereotypes are only moderately related ($rs \leq .26$). Alternatively, cognitive and evaluative stereotypes may *independently* but modestly relate to racial prejudice. Direct empirical evidence favors this latter interpretation.

Across two studies, Stangor et al. (1991) attempted to examine methodologically and statistically the independent relationships of cognitive and affective measures of stereotypes with attitudes toward Blacks. Methodologically, these researchers attempted to unconfound measures of cognitive and evaluative individual stereotypes. They assessed cognitive stereotypes by asking subjects to indicate the percentage of Blacks who possessed six stereotypic characteristics that were evaluatively balanced: three positive (athletic, rhythmic, sociable) and three negative (aggressive, lazy, inferior). Evaluative stereotypes were assessed by asking subjects to list thoughts about Blacks. These open-ended responses were then scored by independent coders for favorability. Statistically, Stangor et al. examined the independent relationships by computing the partial correlation between racial attitude and each measure of stereotypes (cognitive and evaluative), controlling for the other stereotype measure. Across these two studies, racial stereotypes were weakly related to racial attitudes. Furthermore, as we found in our meta-analysis, there was no significant difference in the magnitude of the relationship between cognitive and evaluative measures—although evaluative stereotypes were a better predictor of attitudes toward Blacks (mean partial $r = .19$) than were cognitive stereotypes (mean partial $r = .06$). Thus, neither evaluative nor cognitive measures of stereotypes has a clear-cut or consistent advantage over the other for predicting racial attitudes. For both, the magnitude of the relationship is generally modest.

We note, however, that conclusions about both the magnitude and directions of these relationships may not necessarily generalize to other target groups. Stronger endorsement of consensual stereotypes of Blacks may relate to negative racial attitudes, because these stereotypes have traditionally been negative. In contrast, greater degrees of endorsement by Whites of the consensual stereotype of Whites, because the stereotype has traditionally been positive, would likely be associated with more *positive* attitudes toward that group. Consistent with this reasoning, Lalonde and Gardner (1989) found that there was a significant positive correlation between consensual stereotypes of the in-group and favorable in-group attitudes. Thus, how cognitive and evaluative stereotypes relate to intergroup attitudes is likely moderated by the specific groups in question.

Another dimension we proposed that could moderate the relationship between racial stereotypes and prejudice is the spontaneous–deliberative distinction. Following the reasoning that we presented for understanding the relationship between prejudice and discrimination, we hypothesized that deliberative measures of Whites' racial stereotypes would show a stronger relationship to prejudice than would more spontaneous measures. Measures of both stereotypes and prejudice would involve reflection on and consideration of social and personal egalitarian values. The effect sizes for deliberative and spontaneous measures were both individually significant, but as expected, the effect size for the relationship between deliberative measures of stereotyping and prejudice ($r = .26$) was significantly larger than the effect size for spontaneous measures of stereotypes and prejudice ($r = .19$). This difference supports our thesis that it is important to move beyond the question of *whether* there is a relationship between stereotypes and prejudice to issues of *how*, theoretically and empirically, these two phenomena are related.

STEREOTYPES AND DISCRIMINATION

There are a number of theoretical reasons to expect a positive relationship between stereotypes and discrimination in situations in which the stereotype is largely negative. First, stereotypes may directly influence behavior. The cognitive approach to stereotyping asserts that stereotypes are cognitive structures that, like other schemas, influence the way people perceive, process, store, and retrieve information (see Hamilton & Sherman, 1994; also see Mackie, Hamilton, Susskind, & Rosselli, Chapter 2, this volume). Thus, stereotypes are likely to affect behaviors that are based on these biased processes. For example, stereotypes represent a set of social expectations that can guide interpersonal behaviors to produce a self-fulfilling prophecy (Jussim, 1991; Snyder, 1981; Tajfel, 1981). Second, discrimination can affect stereotyping. At a personal or societal level, stereotypes may serve to justify discrimination (Jost & Banaji, 1994). At the personal level, negative stereotypes can have an "ego-justification" function. Lippmann (1922) and Allport (1954) both posited that people may stereotype others to justify their treatment of them. In addition, stereotypes may be the product of "system-justification." Jost and Banaji (1994) argue that stereotypes arise from "the psychological process whereby an individual perceives, understands, and explains an existing situation or arrangement with the result that the situation or arrangement is maintained" (p. 16); that is, people may make dispositional attributions (e.g., lazy) to explain Blacks' disadvantaged economic status in society. These attributions represent stereotypes that contribute to perpetuation of the economic status quo. Third, stereotypes and discrimination may be related because they share a common underlying source, such as an authoritarian personality or salient anti-Black norms within a person's reference group. Thus, there are a variety of theoretical approaches that suggest a positive relationship between stereotypes and discrimination.

Given this rich and convergent theoretical context, two aspects of our literature review were surprising. First, studies that examine the relationship between racial stereotypes and discrimination are rare. We found only three published reports of individual differences in racial stereotypes and discrimination, and these studies (to be discussed) generally investigated behavioral intentions rather than actual interpersonal behaviors. Perhaps one reason for the paucity of work connecting stereotypes to discrimination is that research on social cognition, which has dominated recent work on stereotyping, has mainly focused on *intra*personal processes (e.g., memory, perceptions, and attributions) rather than on actual interpersonal interactions. It is also possible that earlier conclusions about the lack of relationship between stereotypes and discrimination have discouraged researchers from pursuing this topic.

Second, despite the conceptual arguments that racial stereotypes and discrimination should be positively related, the findings of the three studies are inconsistent and, at best, moderate in strength. Feldman and Hilterman (1977) found no correlation between Whites' stereotypes of Blacks and performance evaluations of specific Blacks in a simulated work situation. Brigham (1971b) examined the relationships of an attitude measure (a version of the MRAI) and a cognitive measure of Whites' stereotypes of Blacks with evaluations of individual Black defendants and behavioral intentions toward Black offenders (i.e., severity of recommended sentences) in hypothetical juvenile court cases. Cognitive stereotypes did predict general evaluations of Black defendants; subjects who endorsed traditional stereotypes evaluated Black defendants less positively ($r = .34$, compared to an $r = .38$ for the relationship between the measure of racial attitudes and evaluations). On the average, though, the degree to which subjects endorsed specific stereotypic characteristics of Blacks as a group only weakly related to how they evaluated particular Black juvenile offenders on these same dimensions. Furthermore, there was little relationship ($r = .04$) between the cognitive stereotype measure and behavioral intentions, represented by the severity of recommended punishments. If Bogardus's social distance measures are considered as indices of behavioral intentions, the findings of Stangor et al. (1991, Exp. 2) are also relevant. Although neither relationship was statistically significant by itself, an evaluative measure of Whites' stereotypes tended to relate more strongly ($r = .24$) to social distance toward Blacks than did a cognitive measure of stereotypes ($r = .10$). Across these three studies, the average effect size was significant, but weak ($r = .16$) and inconsistent.

Given the theoretical reasons to expect a relationship between negative stereotypes and discrimination, the weakness of this relationship is surprising. But, given that social expectations are just one of many elements influencing behavior in a specific situation, these results may not be so surprising. Features of the situation may make norms or other types of information salient, which may override or moderate the influence of stereotypes. As Stangor and Lange (1994, p. 379) observed, "It is known that social expectations have small overall effects upon responses to others (Jussim, 1991), and their use is highly determined by context (Deaux & Major, 1987; Smith & Zárate, 1992). Thus predicting when stereotypes will or will not be used as a basis for judgment is not a trivial matter."

Moderators of the Stereotype–Discrimination Relationship

With the developing technology for assessing implicit as well as explicit stereotypes and attitudes (see Dovidio & Fazio, 1991; Greenwald & Banaji, 1995), it is becoming increasingly possible to empirically address the complexity of the relations among racial stereotyping, prejudice, and discrimination. For example, Dovidio and colleagues conducted two preliminary studies that investigated some of the hypothesized relations (Dovidio et al., 1994). These studies examined the independent contributions of implicit evaluative stereotypes and explicit racial attitudes to the prediction of different types of behavior. Implicit evaluative stereotypes were assessed using a response latency technique (Dovidio et al., 1986); they represented a stereotype measure that, in terms of our previous spontaneous–deliberative and cognitive–affective distinctions, was spontaneous and affectively oriented. Expressed racial attitudes were measured by McConahay's (1986) Old-Fashioned and Modern Racism Scales. Across the two studies, the behaviors that were examined represented the four possible combinations of the spontaneous–deliberative and cognitive–affective dimensions. The general position, as described in this chapter, was that implicit evaluative stereotypes (as measured by response latencies) would best predict spontaneous behaviors (particularly affective ones), and that self-reported attitudes would best predict deliberative or public behaviors.

The procedures for both studies were similar. Each study involved two parts, conducted in separate rooms and ostensibly unrelated. One part involved the assessment of self-reported racial attitudes and implicit stereotypes; the other part included measures of race-related behaviors. With respect to assessing racial attitudes, subjects performed a response latency task and completed two self-report measures of racial attitudes. One self-report measure was McConahay's (1986) Old-Fashioned Racism Scale, which involves the endorsement of traditional stereotypes (e.g., "Black people are generally not as smart as Whites") and support of segregation. The other self-report measure was McConahay's (1986) Modern Racism Scale. This scale measures "the expression [of racial prejudice] in terms of abstract ideological symbols and symbolic behaviors of the feelings that Blacks are violating cherished values and making illegitimate demands for changes in the racial status quo" (McConahay & Hough, 1976, p. 38). The measure of implicit evaluative stereotypes was a latency measure based on a modified version of the priming procedure used by Perdue, Dovidio, Gurtman, and Tyler (1990; see also Dovidio & Gaertner, 1993). Specifically, the latency measure was the sum (in milliseconds) of the extent to which subjects were faster to respond to positive words and slower to respond to negative words following a White rather than a Black subliminal prime.

The second part of the two studies involved different measures of behaviors that varied along the deliberative–spontaneous and affective–cognitive dimensions. The first study examined deliberative and spontaneous cognitive responses. Deliberative responses involved judgments of the guilt or innocence of Black defendants in a simulated trial. Spontaneous responses were measured in a variation of Gilbert and Hixon's (1991) word-completion task. Subjects were presented with two decision-making tasks, supposedly unrelated, on alternate trials. On half of the trials, subjects were asked to classify faces presented on a computer screen as Black or White, by pressing a key. These faces served as primes for the alternate task. On alternate trials, subjects were instructed to complete words "as quickly as possible" by pressing a key corresponding to an appropriate letter (e.g., an "a," "i," or "u" to complete "B_D"). The measure of racial bias was the extent to which subjects created more negative words following Black than White faces. The second study examined deliberative and spontaneous affective and evaluative responses related to subjects' interactions with Black and White interviewers. Deliberative responses were represented by subjects' relative evaluations of the interviewers and their description of their own behaviors with the interviewers. Spontaneous responses involved subjects' nonverbal behaviors (e.g., eye blinking, gaze aversion) that normally reflect discomfort or other negative feelings.

The results were generally supportive of our predictions. Measures of stereotypes and attitudes that were more consistent on the cognitive–affective and particularly the spontaneous–deliberative dimension with the behavior being examined were better predictors. As illustrated in Table 9.3, expressed racial attitudes, which represented deliberative measures of both affective and cognitive orientations toward Blacks, best predicted cognitive, deliberative behaviors, such as ratings of guilt. Our measure of implicit (spontaneous) evaluative stereotypes (i.e., the response latency measure) tended to be negatively related to judgments of guilt. Also, self-reported attitudes predicted less favorable deliberative evaluations of Black relative to White interviewers; implicit stereo-

TABLE 9.3. The Relationships between Old-Fashioned Racism, Modern Racism, and Implicit Evaluative Stereotypes (Latency Measure) on Deliberative and Spontaneous Responses

	Old fashioned racism r(beta)[a]	Modern racism r(beta)	Implicit evaluative stereotypes r(beta)
Deliberative responses			
Judgments of guilt	.40* (.56*)	.30 (.19)	−.04 (−.50*)
Interviewer evaluations	−.07 (−.35)	.22 (.44*)	.02 (.01)
Spontaneous responses			
Negative word completions	.08 (−.16)	.15 (−.10)	.39* (.56*)
Rate of blinking	.07 (.02)	.12 (.18)	.45* (.48*)
Eye contact	.13 (.11)	.22 (.25)	−.39* (−.37*)

[a]Beta values for predicting the dependent measure from old-fashioned racism, modern racism, and implicit evaluative stereotypes simultaneously.
*p < .05.

types did not. Thus, explicit attitudes toward Blacks were most highly related to explicit cognitive and evaluative responses to Blacks.

In contrast, our response latency measure of stereotypes best predicted subjects' spontaneous interracial reactions. Specifically, as indicated in Table 9.3, spontaneous evaluative stereotypes significantly predicted spontaneous, negative, racially-biased word completions, whereas expressed racial attitudes did not. Similar effects were obtained for spontaneous interpersonal behaviors. Subjects with more negative implicit stereotypes blinked more frequently and maintained less eye contact with the Black relative to the White interviewer. Although these findings are preliminary, they do demonstrate the conceptual and empirical value of attempting to understand how different types of stereotypes, prejudice, and discrimination interrelate. As with our analyses of stereotypes and prejudice, correspondence along the spontaneous–deliberative dimension appears to be a particularly important factor.

SUMMARY AND IMPLICATIONS

Our review of the literature raises several issues relevant to research on stereotyping in general and racial stereotypes in particular. In some ways, our results challenge many of the assumptions of researchers in these areas. In particular, racial stereotypes, prejudice, and discrimination have traditionally been considered closely related phenomena. Whites' negative racial attitudes and stereotypes are commonly assumed to be substantial causes of bias and discrimination (see Dovidio & Gaertner, 1986). Nevertheless, the overall empirical relationships among these phenomena are generally moderate. Individual racial stereotyping is only modestly related to prejudice ($r = .25$) and to discrimination ($r = .16$) across studies. Racial attitudes are moderately related to discrimination ($r = .32$). The finding that personal attitudes contribute only moderately to discrimination supports arguments that attempts to eliminate racial discrimination need also to consider the nature of inter*group* relations (e.g., Gaertner et al., 1993; see also Chapter 10 by Hewstone in this volume) and structural solutions (Feagin & Feagin, 1978; Jones, 1986; Pettigrew & Martin, 1987) as well as interpersonal processes.

Our research also raises questions about assumptions concerning a stereotype–behavior link. Researchers of race relations have typically assumed a relationship between racial stereotyping and bias in Whites. This assumption is frequently supported by data, at least at the aggregate level. For example, presumably because Blacks are stereotyped as being aggressive and violent, Whites perceive ambiguous behaviors as more violent when the actor is Black than when the actor is White (Sagar & Schofield, 1980). Nevertheless, our review of the literature raises questions about the usefulness of *individual differences* in stereotyping as a predictor of interracial behaviors. Despite the apparent relationship between stereotypes and discrimination at a global level, the extent to which individuals express racial stereotypes is only modestly related to their interracial responses. Cross-cultural evidence with other social groups shows a similar pattern. Lynskey, Ward, and Fletcher (1991) found that Pakeha (Anglo-origin) subjects in New Zealand reported more positive stereotypes of their own group than of the Pacific Island-origin Maoris and, to a lesser extent, made more favorable attributions for the behavior of in-group than out-group members. Nevertheless, at an individual level, there was no correlation between bias in stereotypes and favorableness of attributions.

In other ways, however, our results extend previous research. Specifically, our analyses of the relationships among stereotypes, prejudice, and discrimination demonstrated the importance of understanding the fundamental processes that relate these phenomena. Research on attitudes in general has moved from the issue of whether there is a relationship to behavior, to what the nature of that relationship is (Fazio,

1990). As recent attempts have illustrated (e.g., Esses et al., 1993; Stangor et al., 1991), this appears to be a productive avenue for research on intergroup stereotypes, as well. Although other moderators are possible (see, e.g., Stangor & Lange, 1994), we investigated the moderating roles of affective–cognitive and spontaneous–deliberative dimensions on the interrelationships among stereotypes, attitudes, and behaviors. Consistent with our expectations, our meta-analysis revealed that greater correspondence of stereotypes, prejudice, and discrimination measures on the spontaneous–deliberative dimension produced stronger relationships among these phenomena. The affective–cognitive dimension was generally much less critical. One potential explanation for this latter finding is that, because cognitive information is also valenced, cognitive and affective measures of stereotypes may be tapping similar underlying dimensions. The generally weak correlation between cognitive and affective stereotypes, however, makes this argument less plausible.

Because of the limited number of studies that involved different levels of these dimensions and the restricted range of experimental contexts, our research summaries should be interpreted with some caution. The relative impact of the different dimensions examined is likely moderated by contextual factors. For example, interracial behaviors were typically assessed in nonthreatening settings that did not involve intergroup conflict. Under more affectively laden circumstances, for example, our finding that attitudes predict affective and cognitive responses equivalently might not hold. Struch and Schwartz (1989), for instance, found that in-group favoritism and out-group aggression were virtually unrelated and were predicted by different variables. How racial stereotypes and attitudes relate differently to "cold" and to "hot" responses remains an open question.

Furthermore, our conclusions about the relationships among stereotypes, prejudice, and discrimination may be influenced by the domain that our analysis was restricted to—race relations. Because of their historical prominence, Whites' racial attitudes toward Blacks may represent particularly strong attitudes. Strong attitudes are better predictors of behavior than are weak attitudes (Eagly & Chaiken, 1993). Thus, the relationship between prejudice and discrimination might be even weaker for other intergroup attitudes. This aspect is also relevant to the generalizability of the moderating role of the spontaneous–deliberative dimension. According to Fazio (1990), the key to spontaneous processing is attitude accessibility. The attitude must be automatically activated from memory upon exposure to the attitude object in order to guide subsequent spontaneous behavior. The likelihood of automatic activation is a function of the strength of the association in memory between the attitude object and the cognitive representation and evaluation of the object. Thus, spontaneous processes relating stereotypes, attitudes, and behavior may operate primarily for strong attitudes—such as Whites' attitudes toward Blacks—and not for weaker, less well-formed beliefs and attitudes.

Our conclusions about the relationship between affective and cognitive dimensions of stereotypes and racial prejudice may also be qualified in their application to other groups. Racial stereotypes may be "hotter" and more affectively laden than many other types of social and nonsocial attitudes (Stangor et al., 1991). In fact, affect is central to many of the theories of contemporary racial attitudes, which emphasize the importance of unconscious negative feelings toward Blacks despite conscious, nonprejudiced thoughts and beliefs (e.g., Devine, 1989). Thus, affect may have even weaker effects in attitudes toward other groups. Nevertheless, we note that other researchers who have been concerned specifically about the contributions of affect and cognitions to intergroup attitudes have found that the pattern of responses to other social groups is similar to the reactions of Whites to Blacks. Stangor et al. (1991), for instance, found that emotional responses to nine different target groups (including Blacks) were consistently better predictors of intergroup attitudes than were measures of stereotypes. Similarly, across four different Canadian minority groups (French Canadian, Native Indian, Pakistani, and homosexual) Esses et al. (1993) found that emotions were most strongly related to attitudes, whereas stereotypes reflected significant but generally weaker effects. The generalizability of these authors' findings suggest that our conclusions may not be restricted to one particular type of intergroup relations.

Beyond examining how well our conclusions relate to different domains of intergroup relations, our analysis suggests other promising directions. For example, future research might go beyond simple correlations between these phenomena and consider the interrelationships among measures of stereotypes, prejudice, and discrimination—and when possible, their separate components; that is, the independent contributions of stereotypes and prejudice need to be examined more fully (Brigham, 1972). The relationships among the different factors within each phenomenon also could be considered further. Dovidio and Gaertner (1993) found that affective and cognitive stereotypes of Blacks may, at least under some conditions, be independent. To the extent that cognitive and affective stereotypes operate independently, traditional ways of reducing prejudice and discrimination may be limited in their effectiveness. For example, attempts at changing the cognitive component of stereotypes, even if successful, may not be sufficient to eliminate affective bias. Negative affect of Whites toward Blacks may linger and continue to influence perceptions, expectations, personal interactions, and at a larger level, public policy decisions (Feagin, 1991). In addition, because affective and spontaneous responses tend to be correlated in the existing literature, we note that the independent effects of these two dimensions require further direct study. Although in naturalistic settings affective and spontaneous reactions may also be correlated as a function of the potential primacy of the affective system relative to the cognitive system (e.g., Zajonc, 1980) and of the common use of more deliberative cognitive strategies to mask spontaneous emotional expressions (Ekman, 1985), it is still theoretically important to determine the independent contributions of these factors.

Furthermore, it would be valuable for future research on this topic to address more fully the *causal* nature of that relationships among stereotypes, prejudice, and discrimination. For example, on the one hand, stereotyping may influence behavior. Because Whites may associate certain characteristics and crimes with Blacks and other groups (Duncan, 1976; Sunnafrank & Fontes, 1981), they may process information differently about the actions of group members and respond accordingly. In fact, this is the process that is assumed to operate by many cognitive approaches to stereotyping (also see Mackie, Hamilton, Susskind, & Rosselli, Chapter 2, and Jussim & Fleming, Chapter 5, this volume). Alternatively, as suggested by Allport (1954) and more recently by Jost and Banaji (1994), discrimination may cause stereotyping. As Jost and Banaji proposed,

> System-justification is the psychological process by which existing social arrangements are legitimized, even at the expense of personal and group interest. . . . Stereotypes, which are widespread beliefs about social groups, are hypothesized to accompany any system characterized by the separation of people into roles, classes, positions, or statuses, because such arrangements tend to be explained and perceived as justifiable by those who participate in them. (pp. 2–3)

Thus, a clearer demonstration that a link between stereotypes and discrimination exists is not sufficient to demonstrate fundamental, causal relationship between the two.

Finally, our review of the literature suggests the value of methodologically and conceptually refining measures of stereotypes. Stereotypes are assessed in a wide variety of ways, with as yet an incomplete understanding of the relationships among these measures or of the relationships of these measures to intergroup attitudes or behaviors. The problems with this approach are exacerbated by the fact that different measures of stereotypes are often only weakly related. Our attempts to categorize measures as spontaneous–deliberative and cognitive–affective, although informative in many ways, suffer many of the weaknesses of any post hoc classification. The measures of attitudes, stereotypes, and discrimination that are used in the experiments that we reviewed frequently do not fit neatly into categories (such as cognitive *vs.* evaluative responses) and are not as precise as they would be if they were developed directly from this framework. We recognize that our concerns are not new; concerns such as these have been expressed by many reviewers of this literature across the past three decades (e.g., Brigham, 1971a; McCauley et al., 1980; Stangor & Lange, 1994). However, we are not proposing that there should be a uniform way of assessing stereotypes, or even that there could ever be one best way. On the contrary, the use of different methodologies may be necessary to address different critical aspects of stereotypes. Our appeal is thus for the development of more general conceptual frameworks for understanding the nature of stereotyping and its relationship to other aspects of intergroup relations. These frameworks, in turn, may suggest appropriate ways for assessing stereotypes.

CONCLUSION

A cynical view of our findings may lead one to ask, "Why study stereotyping?" Although stereotyping may be interesting in its own right, stereotypes seem to have little to do with attitudes and even less to do with discrimination. However, we believe that this view is overpessimistic and unwarranted. Despite the fact the racial attitudes are socially sensitive, readily influenced by social desirability concerns, and measured in a variety of ways, we found that Whites' prejudice systematically predicts discrimination against Blacks. Furthermore, the magnitude of the effect is comparable to the general effect size for attitude–behavior relationships. In addition, despite the conclusion of many previous researchers about the lack of relationship between stereotypes and prejudice, we demonstrated that stereotypes are significantly related to both prejudice and discrimination. Although the magnitudes of these effects are modest, our analysis suggests that understanding how stereotypes, prejudice, and discrimination relate to one another may produce even greater consistency and substantially increase our understanding of the dynamics of intergroup relations.

ACKNOWLEDGMENTS

Preparation of this chapter was facilitated by Grant No. R01 MH48721–01 from the National Institute of Mental Health. We are grateful to Stacy Taylor, Paula Guerra, Adaiah Howard, and Ana Validzic for their valuable assistance with the library reasearch and to the editors for their helpful suggestions on an earlier draft of the chapter.

NOTES

1. We recognize and acknowledge the preference of many people for the term African American instead of Blacks. However, because much of the research in this chapter specifically used the term "Blacks" as a stimulus category, we use that term as well.

2. The details of this and all subsequent meta-analyses are available from the authors. All findings that are described as significant reflect results for which $p < .05$ for the appropriate statistical test.

REFERENCES

Adorno, T., Frenkel-Brunswik, E. Levinson, D., & Sanford, R. N. (1950). *The authoritarian personality*. New York: Harper.

Ajzen, I. (1985). From intentions to actions: A theory of planned action. In J. Kuhl & J. Beckmann (Eds.), *Action-control: From cognition to behavior* (pp. 11–39). Heidelberg: Springer.

Allport, G. W. (1954). *The nature of prejudice*. Reading, MA: Addison-Wesley.

Ard, N., & Cook, S. W. (1977). A short scale for the measurement of change in verbal racial attitude. *Educational and Psychological Measurement, 37*, 741–743.

Ashmore, R. D. (1970). Prejudice: Causes and cures. In B. E. Collins (Ed.), *Social psychology: Social influence, attitude change, group processes, and prejudice* (pp. 245–339). Reading, MA: Addison-Wesley.

Ashmore, R. D., & Del Boca, F. K. (1979). Sex stereotypes and implicit personality theory: Toward a cognitive–social psychological conceptualization. *Sex Roles, 5*, 219–248.

Ashmore, R. D., & Del Boca, F. K. (1981). Conceptual approaches to stereotypes and stereotyping. In D. L. Hamilton (Ed.), *Cognitive processes in stereotyping and intergroup behavior* (pp. 1–35). Hillsdale, NJ: Erlbaum.

Banaji, M. R., & Greenwald, A. G. (1995). Implicit gender stereotyping in judgments of fame. *Journal of Personality and Social Psychology, 68*, 181–198.

Bogardus, E. S. (1925). Measuring social distance. *Journal of Applied Sociology, 9*, 299–308.

Bogardus, E. S. (1959). *Social distance*. Yellow Springs, OH: Antioch Press.

Brigham, J. C. (1971a). Ethnic stereotypes. *Psychological Bulletin, 76*, 15–38.

Brigham, J. C. (1971b). Racial stereotypes, attitudes, and evaluations of and behavioral intentions toward Negroes and Whites. *Sociometry, 34*, 360–380.

Brigham, J. C. (1972). Racial stereotypes: Measurement variables and the stereotype–attitude relationship. *Journal of Applied Social Psychology, 2*, 63–76.

Brigham, J. C. (1977). The structure of racial attitudes of blacks. *Personality and Social Psychology Bulletin, 3*, 658–661.

Brigham, J. C. (1993). College students' racial attitudes. *Journal of Applied Social Psychology, 23*, 1933–1967.

Brigham, J. C., Woodmansee, J. J., & Cook, S. W. (1976). Dimensions of verbal racial attitudes: Interracial marriage and approaches to racial equality. *Journal of Social Issues, 32*, 9–21.

Brown, R. (1965). *Social psychology.* New York: Free Press.

Butler, D., & Geis, F. L. (1990). Nonverbal affect responses to male and female leaders: Implications for leadership evaluations. *Journal of Personality and Social Psychology, 58*, 48–59.

Campbell, D. T. (1967). Stereotypes and perceptions of group differences. *American Psychologist, 22*, 817–829.

Clark, M. S., & Fiske, S. T. (Eds.). (1982). *The Seventeenth Annual Carnegie Symposium on Cognition.* Hillsdale, NJ: Erlbaum.

Crosby, F., Bromley, S., & Saxe, L. (1980). Recent unobtrusive studies of black and white discrimination and prejudice: A literature review. *Psychological Bulletin, 87*, 546–563.

Davis, J. A., & Smith, T. W. (1991). *General social surveys, 1972–1991: Cumulative codebook.* Chicago: National Opinion Research Center.

Deaux, K., & Major, B. (1987). Putting gender into context: An interactive model of gender-related behavior. *Psychological Review, 94*, 369–389.

Devine, P. G. (1989). Stereotypes and prejudice: Their automatic and controlled components. *Journal of Personality and Social Psychology, 56*, 5–18.

Dovidio, J. F., Evans, N., & Tyler, R. B. (1986). Racial stereotypes: The contents of their cognitive representations. *Journal of Experimental Social Psychology, 22*, 22–37.

Dovidio, J. F., & Fazio, R. H. (1991). New technologies for the direct and indirect assessment of attitudes. In J. Tanur (Ed.), *Questions about survey questions: Meaning, memory, attitudes, and social interaction* (pp. 204–237). New York: Russell Sage Foundation.

Dovidio, J. F., & Gaertner, S. L. (1981). The effects of race, status, and ability on helping behavior. *Social Psychology Quarterly, 44*, 192–203.

Dovidio, J. F., & Gaertner, S. L. (1986). Prejudice, discrimination, and racism: Historical trends and contemporary approaches. In J. F. Dovidio & S. L. Gaertner (Eds.), *Prejudice, discrimination, and racism* (pp. 1–34). Orlando, FL: Academic Press.

Dovidio, J. F., & Gaertner, S. L. (1991). Changes in the nature and expression of racial prejudice. In H. Knopke, J. Norrell, & R. Rogers (Eds.), *Opening doors: An appraisal of race relations in contemporary America* (pp. 201–241). Tuscaloosa: University of Alabama Press.

Dovidio, J. F., & Gaertner, S. L. (1993). Stereotypes and evaluative intergroup bias. In D. M. Mackie & D. L. Hamilton (Eds.), *Affect, cognition, and stereotyping* (pp. 167–193). San Diego: Academic Press.

Dovidio, J. F., Johnson, C., Gaertner, S. L., Validzic, A., Howard, A., & Eisinger, N. (1994, April). *Racial bias and the role of implicit and explicit attitudes.* Paper presented at the annual meeting of the Eastern Psychological Association, Providence, RI.

Dovidio, J. F., & Mullen, B. (1992). *Race, physical handicap, and response amplification.* Unpublished manuscript, Department of Psychology, Colgate University, Hamilton, NY.

Duncan, B. L. (1976). Differential social perception and attribution of intergroup violence: Testing the lower limits of stereotyping of blacks. *Journal of Personality and Social Psychology, 34,* 590–598.

Eagly, A. H., & Chaiken, S. (1993). *The psychology of attitudes.* New York: Harcourt Brace Jovanovich College Publishers.

Eagly, A. H., & Mladinic, A. (1989). Gender stereotypes and attitudes toward women and men. *Personality and Social Psychology Bulletin, 15,* 543–558.

Ekman, P. (1985). *Telling lies: Clues to deceit in the marketplace, politics, and marriage.* New York: Norton.

Esses, V. M., Haddock, G., & Zanna, M. (1993). Values, stereotypes, and emotions as determinants of intergroup attitudes. In D. M. Mackie & D. L. Hamilton (Eds.), *Affect, cognition, and stereotyping* (pp. 137–166). San Diego: Academic Press.

Fazio, R. H. (1990). Multiple processes by which attitudes guide behavior: The MODE Model as an integrative framework. In M. P. Zanna (Ed.), *Advances in experimental social psychology* (Vol. 23, pp. 75–109). Orlando, FL: Academic Press.

Fazio, R. H., Powell, M. C., & Herr, P. M. (1983). Toward a process model of attitude–behavior relation: Accessing one's attitude upon mere observation of the attitude object. *Journal of Personality and Social Psychology, 44,* 723–735.

Feagin, J. B. (1991, August). *The continuing significance of race: The Black middle-class experience.* Paper presented at the annual meeting of the American Sociological Association, Cincinnati, OH.

Feagin, J. B., & Feagin, L. B. (1978). *Discrimination American style: Institutional racism and sexism.* Englewood Cliffs, NJ: Prentice-Hall.

Feldman, J. M., & Hilterman, R. J. (1977). Sources of bias in performance evaluation: Two experiments. *International Journal of Intercultural Relations, 1,* 35–57.

Fishbein, M. (1963). An investigation of the relationship between beliefs about an object and the attitude toward the object. *Human Relations, 16,* 233–239.

Fishman, J. A. (1956). An examination of the process and function of social stereotyping. *Journal of Social Psychology, 43,* 26–64.

Fishman, J. A. (1956). An examination of the process and function of social stereotyping. *Journal of Social Psychology, 43,* 27–64.

Fiske, S. T. (1982). Schema-triggered affect: Applications to social perception. In M. S. Clark & S. T. Fiske (Eds.), *The Seventeenth Annual Carnegie Symposium on Cognition* (pp. 55–78). Hillsdale, NJ: Erlbaum.

Fiske, S. T. (1987). On the road: Comment on the cognitive stereotyping literature in Pettigrew and Martin. *Journal of Social Issues, 43,* 113–118.

Fiske, S. T., Neuberg, S. L., Beattie, A. E., & Milberg, S. J. (1987). Category-based and attribute-based reactions to others: Some informational conditions of stereotyping and individuating processes. *Journal of Experimental Social Psychology, 23,* 399–427.

Fiske, S. T., & Pavelchak, M. A. (1986). Category-based versus piecemeal-based affective responses: Developments in schema-triggered affect. In R. M. Sorrentino & E. T. Higgins (Eds.), *Handbook of motivation and cognition: Foundations of social behavior* (Vol. 1, pp. 167–203). New York: Guilford Press.

Fiske, S. T., & Taylor, S. E. (1991). *Social cognition.* New York: McGraw-Hill.

Gaertner, S. L., & Dovidio, J. F. (1986). The aversive form of racism. In J. F. Dovidio & S. L. Gaertner (Eds.), *Prejudice, discrimination, and racism* (pp. 61–89). Orlando, FL: Academic Press.

Gaertner, S. L., Dovidio, J. F., Anastasio, P. A., Bachman, B. A., & Rust, M. C. (1993). The common in-group identity model: Recategorization and the reduction of intergroup bias. In W. Stroebe & M. Hewstone (Eds.), *European review of social psychology* (Vol. 4, pp. 1–26). New York: Wiley.

Gaertner, S. L., & McLaughlin, J. P. (1983). Racial stereotypes: Associations and ascriptions of positive and negative characteristics. *Social Psychology Quarterly, 46,* 23–30.

Gardner, R. C. (1973). Ethnic stereotypes: The traditional approach, a new look. *Canadian Psychologist, 14,* 133–148.

Gardner, R. C. (1993). Stereotypes as consensual beliefs. In M. P. Zanna & J. M. Olson (Eds.), *The psychology of prejudice: The Ontario symposium* (Vol. 7, pp. 1–32). Hillsdale, NJ: Erlbaum.

Gardner, R. C., Lalonde, R. N., Nero, A. M., & Young, M. Y. (1988). Ethnic stereotypes: Implications of measurement strategy. *Social Cognition, 6,* 40–60.

Gardner, R. C., Wonnacott, E. J., & Taylor, D. M. (1968). Ethnic stereotypes: A factor analytic investigation. *Canadian Journal of Psychology, 22,* 35–44.

Gilbert, D. T., & Hixon, J. G. (1991). The trouble of thinking: Activation and application to stereotypic beliefs. *Journal of Personality and Social Psychology, 60,* 509–517.

Gonzales, J. L., Jr. (1990). *Racial and ethnic groups in America.* Dubuque, IA: Kendall/Hunt.

Greenwald, A. G., & Banaji, M. R. (1995). Implicit social cognition: Attitudes, self-esteem, and stereotypes. *Psychological Review, 102,* 4–27.

Hacker, A. (1992). *Two nations: Black, white, separate, hostile, unequal.* New York: Scribner's.

Hamilton, D. L., & Sherman, J. W. (1994). Stereotypes. In R. S. Wyer & T. K. Srull (Eds.), *Handbook of social cognition* (2nd ed., Vol. 2, pp. 1–68). Hillsdale, NJ: Erlbaum.

Hamilton, D. L., & Trolier, T. K. (1986). Stereotypes and stereotyping: An overview of the cognitive approach. In J. F. Dovidio & S. L. Gaertner (Eds.), *Prejudice, discrimination, and racism* (pp. 127–163). Orlando, FL: Academic Press.

Harding, J., Proshansky, H., Kutner, B., & Chein, I. (1969). Prejudice and ethnic relations. In G. Lindzey & E. Aronson (Eds.), *The handbook of social psychology* (2nd ed., pp. 1–76). Reading MA: Addison-Wesley.

Jacoby, L. L., Kelley, C., Brown, J., & Jasechko, J. (1989). Becoming famous overnight: Limits on the ability to avoid unconscious influences of the past. *Journal of Personality and Social Psychology, 56,* 326–338.

Jaynes, G. D., & Williams, R. M., Jr. (Eds.). (1989). *A common destiny: Blacks and American society.* Washington, DC: National Academy Press.

Jones, J. M. (1972). *Prejudice and racism.* Reading, MA: Addison-Wesley.

Jones, J. M. (1986). Racism: A cultural analysis of the problem. In J. F. Dovidio & S. L. Gaertner (Eds.), *Prejudice, discrimination, and racism* (pp. 279–314). Orlando, FL: Academic Press.

Jones, J. M. (1993, August). *Racism and civil rights: Right problem, wrong solution.* Invited address at the annual convention of the American Psychological Association, Toronto, Canada.

Jost, J. T., & Banaji, M. R. (1994). The role of stereotyping in system-justification and the production of false consciousness. *British Journal of Social Psychology, 33,* 1–27.

Judd, C. M., & Park, B. (1993). Definition and assessment of accuracy in social stereotypes. *Psychological Review, 100,* 109–128.

Jussim, L. (1991). Social perception and social reality: A reflection–construction model. *Psychological Review, 98,* 54–73.

Karlins, M., Coffman, T. L., & Walters, G. (1969). On the fading of social stereotypes: Studies in three generations of college students. *Journal of Personality and Social Psychology, 13,* 1–16.

Katz, D., & Braly, K. W. (1933). Racial stereotypes of one hundred college students. *Journal of Abnormal and Social Psychology, 28,* 280–290.

Katz, D., & Braly, K. W. (1935). Racial prejudice and racial stereotypes. *Journal of Abnormal and Social Psychology, 30,* 175–193.

Kinder, D. R., & Sears, D. O. (1981). Prejudice and politics: Symbolic racism versus threats to "the good life." *Journal of Personality and Social Psychology, 40,* 414–431.

Kovel, J. (1970). *White racism: A psychohistory.* New York: Pantheon.

Lalonde, R. N., & Gardner, R. C. (1989). An intergroup perspective on stereotype organization and processing. *British Journal of Social Psychology, 28,* 289–303.

Lippmann, W. (1922). *Public opinion.* New York: Harcourt Brace.

Lynskey, M. T., Ward, C., & Fletcher, G. J. O. (1991). Stereotypes and intergroup attributions in New Zealand. *Psychology and Developing Societies*, 3, 113–127.

Macrae, C. N., Stangor, C., & Milne, A. B. (1994). Activating social stereotypes: A functional analysis. *Journal of Experimental Social Psychology*, 30, 370–389.

McCauley, C., & Stitt, C. L. (1978). An individual and quantitative measure of stereotypes. *Journal of Personality and Social Psychology*, 36, 929–940.

McCauley, C., Stitt, C. L., & Segal, M. (1980). Stereotyping: From prejudice to prediction. *Psychological Bulletin*, 87, 195–208.

McConahay, J. B. (1986). Modern racism, ambivalence, and the modern racism scale. In J. F. Dovidio & S. L. Gaertner (Eds.), *Prejudice, discrimination, and racism* (pp. 91–125). Orlando, FL: Academic Press.

McConahay, J. B., Hardee, B. B., & Batts, V. (1981). Has racism declined in America? It depends upon who is asking and what is asked. *Journal of Conflict Resolution*, 25, 563–579.

McConahay, J. B., & Hough, J. C. (1976). Symbolic racism. *Journal of Social Issues*, 32, 23–45.

McGuire, W. J. (1985). Attitudes and attitude change. In G. Lindzey & E. Aronson (Eds.), *The handbook of social psychology* (3rd ed., pp. 233–346). New York: Random House.

Perdue, C. W., Dovidio, J. F., Gurtman, M. B., & Tyler, R. B. (1990). "Us" and "Them": Social categorization and the process of intergroup bias. *Journal of Personality and Social Psychology*, 59, 475–486.

Pettigrew, T. F. (1988, October). *The nature of modern racism.* Paper presented at the meeting of the Society for Experimental Social Psychology, Madison, WI.

Pettigrew, T. F., & Martin, J. (1987). Shaping the organizational context for Black American inclusion. *Journal of Social Issues*, 43, 41–78.

Ramirez, A. (1988). Racism toward Hispanics: A culturally monolithic society. In P. Katz & D. Taylor (Eds.), *Towards the elimination of racism: Profiles in controversy* (pp. 135–157). New York: Plenum Press.

Roese, N. J., & Jamieson, D. W. (1993). Twenty years of bogus pipeline research: A critical review and meta-analysis. *Psychological Bulletin*, 114, 363–375.

Rokeach, M. (1960). *The open and closed mind.* New York: Basic Books.

Saenger, G., & Flowerman, S. (1954). Stereotypes and prejudicial attitudes. *Human Relations*, 7, 217–238.

Sagar, H. A., & Schofield, J. W. (1980). Racial and behavioral cues in black and white children's perceptions of ambiguously aggressive acts. *Journal of Personality and Social Psychology*, 39, 590–598.

Sanford, N. (1956). The approach of the authoritarian personality. In J. L. McCary (Ed.), *Psychology of personality* (pp. 253–319). New York: Logos Press.

Sears, D. O. (1988). Symbolic racism. In P. Katz & D. Taylor (Eds.), *Towards the elimination of racism: Profiles in controversy* (pp. 53–84). New York: Plenum Press.

Sherman, S. J., Judd, C. M., & Park, B. (1989). Social cognition. *Annual Review of Psychology, 40*, 281–326.

Simpson, G. E., & Yinger, J. M. (1965). *Racial and cultural minorities*. New York: Harper & Row.

Smith, A. J., & Clark, R. D. (1973). The relationship between attitudes and beliefs. *Journal of Personality and Social Psychology, 26*, 321–326.

Smith, E. R., & Zárate, M. A. (1992). Exemplar-based model of social judgment. *Psychological Review, 99*, 3–21.

Snyder, M. (1981). On the self-perpetuating nature of social stereotypes. In D. L. Hamilton (Ed.), *Cognitive processes in stereotyping and intergroup behavior* (pp. 183–212). Hillsdale, NJ: Erlbaum.

Stangor, C., & Lange, J. (1994). Mental representations of social groups: Advances in understanding stereotypes and stereotyping. In M. Zanna (Ed.), *Advances in experimental social psychology* (Vol. 26, pp. 357–416). Orlando, FL: Academic Press.

Stangor, C., Sullivan, L. A., & Ford, T. E. (1991). Affective and cognitive determinants of prejudice. *Social Cognition, 9*, 359–380.

Stephan, W. G., Ageyev, V., Coates-Shrider, L., Stephan, C. W., & Abalakina, M. (1994). On the relationship between stereotypes and prejudice: An international study. *Personality and Social Psychology Bulletin, 20*, 277–284.

Stephan, W. G., & Stephan, C. W. (1993). Cognition and affect in stereotyping: Parallel interactive networks. In D. M. Mackie & D. L. Hamilton (Eds.), *Affect, cognition, and stereotyping* (pp. 111–136). San Diego: Academic Press.

Struch, N., & Schwartz, S. H. (1989). Intergroup aggression: Its predictors and distinctness from in-group bias. *Journal of Personality and Social Psychology, 56*, 364–373.

Sunnafrank, M., & Fontes, N. E. (1981). General and crime-related racial stereotypes and influences on juridic decisions. *Cornell Journal of Social Relations, 17*, 1–15.

Tajfel, H. (1981). Social stereotypes and social groups. In J. C. Turner & H. Giles (Eds.), *Intergroup behaviour* (pp. 144–167). Oxford: Blackwell.

Thompson, C. E., Neville, H., Weathers, P. L., Poston, W. C., & Atkinson, D. R. (1990). Cultural mistrust and racism reaction among African American students. *Journal of College Student Development, 31*, 162–168.

Thompson, V. L. S. (1991). Perceptions of race relations which affect African-American identification. *Journal of Applied Social Psychology, 21*, 1502–1516.

Weber, S. J., & Cook, T. D. (1972). Subject effects in laboratory research: An examination of subject roles, demand characteristics, and valid inferences. *Psychological Bulletin, 77*, 273–295.

Weigel, R. H., & Howes, P. W. (1985). Conceptions of racial prejudice: Symbolic racism revisited. *Journal of Social Issues, 41*, 117–138.

Weitz, S. (1972). Attitude, voice, and behavior: A repressed affect model of interracial interaction. *Journal of Personality and Social Psychology, 24,* 14–21.

Wicker, A. W. (1969). Attitudes versus actions: The relationship between verbal and overt behavioral responses to attitude objects. *Journal of Social Issues, 25,* 41–78.

Word, C. O., Zanna, M. P., & Cooper, J. (1974). The nonverbal mediation of self-fulfilling prophecies in interracial interaction. *Journal of Experimental Social Psychology, 10,* 109–120.

Woodmansee, J. J., & Cook, S. W. (1967). Dimensions of verbal racial attitudes: Their identification and measurement. *Journal of Personality and Social Psychology, 7,* 240–250.

Wyer, R. S., Jr., & Gordon, S. E. (1984). The cognitive representation of social information. In R. S. Wyer, Jr. & T. K. Srull (Eds.), *The handbook of social cognition* (Vol. 2, pp. 73–150). Hillsdale, NJ: Erlbaum.

Zanna, M. P., & Rempel, J. K. (1988). Attitudes: A new look at an old concept. In D. Bar-Tal & A. Kruglanski (Eds.), *The social psychology of knowledge* (pp. 315–334). Cambridge, UK: Cambridge University Press.

Zajonc, R. B. (1980). Feeling and thinking: Preferences need no inference. *American Psychologist, 35,* 151–175.

IV

UNDERMINING STEREOTYPES AND STEREOTYPING

10

Contact and Categorization: Social Psychological Interventions to Change Intergroup Relations

MILES HEWSTONE

> Since wars begin in the minds of men, it is in the minds of men that the defences of peace must be constructed.
>
> —UNESCO Motto

One of the most powerful journalistic images of 1994 was of the atrocities committed in the African state of Rwanda, leaving hundreds of thousands dead or brutally injured. Remarkably, the conflict between Hutu and Tutsi is some four centuries old and seemingly intractable. When members of the two groups were asked how they viewed each other, their responses were particularly pessimistic: "Asked whether the characteristics could be changed by training and upbringing, both groups answered that only very limited changes could be made; the qualities were inherent" (Tajfel, 1978, p. 85).[1]

This example gives a flavor of how difficult it may sometimes be to change strongly held stereotypes. Not least, because there is often extensive social support for stereotypes, most evident in the form of power relations, mass media representations, and social norms (Pettigrew, 1981). Yet, because stereotypical perceptions of out-groups are often negative and homogeneous, rationalizing discrimination and making cooperative intergroup interaction less likely, there is widespread agreement about the need for interventions that can bring about stereotype change. The aim of this chapter is not to review all the available evidence from an array of potential interventions (see Duckitt, 1992; Fisher, 1990; Stephan, 1985; Wilder, 1986b). Instead, I begin by highlighting some of the issues that should be raised at the outset of any review, and I then identify four main themes around which this chapter is organized.

The first point to clarify is the present focus on *social psychological* interventions and their impact on *intergroup relations.* There are, of course, alternative kinds of interventions whose impact is directed at different kinds of outcomes. For example, some more sociological interventions are aimed at structural conditions (e.g., affirmative action programs directed at differential rates of employment in ethnic groups); whereas other more educational interventions target specifically educational outcomes (e.g., academic achievement). These interventions will only be included in this chapter insofar as they influence intergroup relations, which they frequently do (see Schofield, 1989, 1991).

The second point to clarify is that the title of this chapter refers to *intergroup relations,* including behavior but especially perceptions, and not exclusively to stereotypes. This title reflects the diversity of measures found across studies—including racial attitudes, social distance scales, and sociometric measures—although studies that measure stereotypes will be highlighted. Furthermore, intergroup relations includes perceptions of in-group as well as out-group (although most work deals mainly with the latter), because theoretical analyses of intergroup discrimination have emphasized that it is often driven by a pro-in-group rather than an anti-out-group orientation (see Brewer, 1979). From the social identity theory perspective (e.g., Hogg & Abrams, 1988; Tajfel, 1978; Tajfel & Turner, 1979) that has stimulated most of the work reviewed here, the most appropriate and effective interventions may be those that affect in-group perceptions, although the consequences to out-group members may be no less pernicious when they are disadvantaged in this more subtle way (e.g., Mummendey & Schreiber, 1983) than when they are treated with open disparagement, hostility, or aggression.

In writing this chapter for this particular book, I have used four general themes to organize the large number of studies and perspectives. First, since a much-lamented failure of many interventions is that they do not "generalize," I begin by considering types of generalization that could serve as outcome measures in research and then relate the studies reviewed back to these criteria. An underlying goal of the chapter is to identify which, if any, types of generalization are achieved by which interventions. Second, I accentuate the most promising *theoretical* perspectives in this area. To take the topic of school desegregation as an example, several authors have argued that the lack of adequate theory is partly responsible for an inconclusive literature (e.g., Cohen, 1975; St. John, 1975; Schofield, 1978).

Third, I select studies that specify more exactly the *process* underlying effects. To this end, I prefer experiments to surveys, and especially studies that have successfully specified the mediational or moderational effects of key variables (see Baron & Kenny, 1986). Unfortunately, many surveys in this area suffer from various design flaws, especially when only able to evaluate ongoing programs in a relatively reactive way (see Schofield, 1991). Where the results of experiments and good surveys converge, of course, we can have more faith in the underlying theoretical model supported (Campbell & Fiske, 1959). Fourth, and finally, the title of this chapter is selected to convey two main interventions that emerge from a broad literature: those aimed at encouraging contact between members of opposed groups, and those directed at altering the structure of social categorizations underlying situations of intergroup conflict. I argue that these interventions—and the variants contained within each—are distinct but complementary, and that the next thrust of research in this area should actively seek to integrate them.

Thus this chapter begins by looking at the goal—generalized change in intergroup relations—and then considers what I view as the two most important means of achieving this.

THE NATURE OF GENERALIZED CHANGE

Before planning and evaluating any intervention, one should of course clarify the desired outcomes. In a recent theoretical analysis, Brewer and Miller (1988) argued for a distinction between three types of generalization, any of which a successful intervention might seek to achieve. They also made several useful predictions about the type of intergroup interaction likely to be associated with each type of generalization, and they pointed to some of the dangers associated with each approach to improving intergroup relations. I will refer to these predictions as I evaluate each major intervention in turn.

The first type of generalization, "change in attitudes toward the social category," is the classic outcome variable in this area—generalization from a target individual to the out-group as a whole. Evidence of this effect is quite rare (Amir, 1969, 1976). Brewer and Miller (1988) argue that this type of generalization is most likely to be effected by *category-based* interaction, in which a given in-group member responds to out-group members as interchangeable representatives of a fairly homogeneous category. Brewer and Miller see two main problems with this type of interaction. First, positive contact must be contrived, so that generalized change is in the desired direction; such change may not be easy to engender, and the contact may be constrained and superficial. Second, the distinctiveness of the out-group social category may be reinforced during the course of interaction, thus maintaining in-group/out-group distinctions in the long run.

The second type of generalization, "increased complexity of intergroup perceptions," refers to an increase in the perceived variability of the out-group. Although perceived group variability has become a central area of research on stereotyping and intergroup relations (e.g., Park, Judd, & Ryan, 1991; see Ryan, Park, & Judd, Chapter 4, this volume), we shall see that it has only very recently been incorporated as an outcome measure of stereotype change. Brewer and Miller suggest that "differentiated" interaction is most likely to accomplish increased complexity (or perceived variability) of an out-group, whereby perceivers recognize distinctions among members of a given category who are still subtyped within the larger superordinate category. The danger is that the formation of subtypes may prevent change in the perceived characteristics of the group as a whole (stereotypes).

The third type of generalization, "decategorization," refers to change in the perceived usefulness, or meaningfulness, of a social category for identifying and classifying new individuals. Brewer and Miller suggest that this form of generalization is most likely to be realized by a final type of interaction, "personalization," in which an in-group member responds to out-group individuals in terms of their relationship to self, such that self–other comparisons are made across category boundaries. Although this form of generalization may be important in some circumstances, as when group identities are quite weak and recently formed, it seems less likely to be realistic in the context of established identities, intensified by wider social and political factors.

The remainder of this chapter applies the foregoing analysis of change to an evaluation of interventions based on engineering contact between groups, and on changing the structure of social categorizations in intergroup settings. For each separate intervention, I deal with theory, research, and critique, moving toward an integration that could potentially result in all three kinds of generalization.

THE CONTACT HYPOTHESIS: GETTING
TOGETHER ... BUT HOW?

The more we get together, together, together
The more we get together, the happier we'll be
'Cause your friends are my friends
And my friends are your friends
The more we get together, the happier we'll be.
—TRADITIONAL SONG

The "contact hypothesis" refers to the simple idea that contact between members of different groups will improve relations between them. This view has been the basis of many social policy decisions advocating racial integration in North American schools, housing projects, the armed forces and so on. Allport (1954/1979) acknowledged, however, that contact could increase as well as decrease prejudice and stereotyping. He emphasized the "nature of contact" and saw that its effect would depend on the kinds of people and situations involved. I will not provide a comprehensive review of contact research here (see Amir, 1969, 1976; McClendon, 1974; Riordan, 1978). Instead, I will summarize its main points, its evaluation to date, and its main limitation, opening up the way to a more detailed analysis of recent theoretical developments and research.

Perhaps the major achievement of research on the contact hypothesis was to distill Allport's initial long list of potentially relevant factors down to the few main conditions that should be satisfied to bring about positive intergroup contact. Thus Cook (1962, 1978) predicted that less derogatory out-group attitudes would result when individuals had personal contact with members of a disliked group, but under conditions of equal status, stereotype disconfirmation, cooperation, high "acquaintance potential" and "equalitarian norms." Thus, Cook focused pragmatically on structural features of the interaction situation, that could potentially be manipulated or controlled. After contact under these conditions, people did tend to report more favorable evaluations of the individual out-group members they had come to know. But an increasing number of variables was added to this list, leading to criticisms that the contact hypothesis was now subject to so many qualifications that it had lost its initial value and appeal (Pettigrew, 1986). As Stephan (1987) pointed out, the long list of conditions considered important in creating contact situations with potential for positive outcomes made researchers realize that there are many ways in which contact can lead to negative consequences. In addition, the elaborate creation of harmonious interpersonal relations was so obviously artificial when considered against the external realities of residential segregation, widespread discrimination, and numerous intergroup inequalities (see Hewstone & Brown, 1986).

Extensive assessments of the contact hypothesis yield a complex picture, hardly surprising given the predominance of relatively uncontrolled field studies over laboratory experiments, and the wide range of applied interventions (educational settings, armed services, workplace, and housing projects). The difficulties involved in evaluating the contact hypothesis are well illustrated with the topic of racial desegregation of U.S. schools, the success or failure of which is still fiercely debated (e.g., Cook, 1979, 1985; Gerard, 1983; Schofield, 1991; Stephan, 1978). First, there have been a large number of outcome measures. Evaluations of school desegregation have ranged from short-term, individual measures (e.g., the achievement and self-esteem of minority children) to long-term, societal measures (e.g., the chances that Blacks will subsequently work in integrated settings, or will live in integrated neighborhoods; see Braddock, 1985; Greenblatt & Willie, 1980). Second, many school settings were merely "desegregated" (members of two previously segregated groups were physically copresent) rather than "integrated" (two groups mixed under conditions conducive to positive outcomes; Pettigrew, 1973; Schofield, 1991). Thus, evaluations of school desegregation tend to speak to the effects of mere contact, if even that, rather than to the effects of contact under the conditions specified by Cook and others. Third, Schofield (1991) has argued that contact *theory* did not fundamentally influence the conduct of much empirical work on school desegregation, although when it did, results were generally promising (e.g., Cook, 1978; Schofield, 1979; Schofield & Sagar, 1977).

Thus, research on the contact hypothesis has moved from the optimism based on early studies (e.g., Deutsch & Collins, 1951; Wilner, Walkley, & Cook, 1955; see Cook, 1985) to the pessimism eloquently expressed by Rothbart and John (1993): "The contact hypothesis brings to mind T. H. Huxley's remark about the tragedy that occurs when 'a lovely idea is assaulted by a gang of ugly facts'" (p. 42). A central aspect of this pessimism, to some authors *the* main shortcoming of the contact hypothesis (Hewstone & Brown, 1986), is the failure to generalize positive attitudes promoted by the contact experience ("specific attitude change") to include other members of the out-group not actually present in the contact situation ("generalized change in out-group attitudes").

The remainder of this section deals with recent theory-based approaches to contact that achieve different kinds of generalization, and shows how a cognitive approach can provide a deeper understanding of the processes underlying stereotype change in intergroup contact. These three approaches give rise to a clearer and more critical understanding of what is accomplished by interventions based on the contact hypothesis.

Contact as "Personalization"

The rationale that Cook (1978) developed for the conditions he felt would induce successful contact derived from a theory of interpersonal attraction: Contact between members of different groups allows individuals to discover that they have, after all, many similar values and attitudes (e.g., Byrne, 1969; Newcomb, 1961; Rokeach, 1960). Thus Triandis (1988, p. 47), for example, argued that the goal of intergroup contact "should be to create in the shortest possible time the largest number of . . . 'successful interpersonal relationships.'" Brewer and Miller's (1984) model of personalized contact also takes an interpersonal perspective.

Theory

To reduce the salience of category memberships, Brewer and Miller (1984, 1988) argued that contact should be "differentiated" (allowing for distinctions to be made among out-group members) but moreover "personalized" (allowing for perceptions of the uniqueness of out-group members). More recently, Miller and Harrington (1990) have suggested that changes in the perception of self and of in-group members, as well as perceptions of out-group members, are important. They view decategorized intergroup interaction (differentiation and personalization) as "mutual and reciprocal": Personalized interaction with a member of the out-group results both in personalization of self and other, and in differentiation of self from in-group, and of the out-group member from the out-group.

The goal then is a more interpersonally oriented and "non-category-based" form of responding that allows members to "attend to information that replaces category identity as the most useful basis for classifying each other" (Brewer & Miller, 1984, p. 288). With the process of personalization, members attend only to information that is relevant to the self and is not correlated with membership. In personalized contact, category identity should no longer be the sole or major determinant of how members of different groups respond to one another. It is assumed that repeated interpersonal contact of this kind disconfirms the negative stereotype of members of disliked out-groups who are seen as similar to the self. Brewer and Miller contend that the ideal approach to intergroup contact involves personalized interactions that are "more likely to generalize to new situations because extended and frequent utilization of alternative information featured in interactions undermines the availability and usefulness of category identity as a basis for future interactions, with the same or different individuals" (pp. 288–289). This kind of contact, they maintain, will bring about the third type of generalization—decategorization. Frequent individuation of out-group members will result in the category being seen as less "useful" and, thus, being used less often.

Research

Brewer, Miller, and their colleagues have investigated their model in a series of experimental studies (see Bettencourt, Brewer, Rogers-Croak, & Miller, 1992; Miller, Brewer, & Edwards, 1985). The basic paradigm in these studies follows a three-phase sequence. In the first phase, subjects are arbitrarily divided into two ad hoc groups. To bolster identification with the group, members spend time working together on a task, make evaluations of their own and the other group's product, and receive feedback indicating that the out-group was biased in its evaluations. In the second phase, previously isolated groups are brought together to form two heterogeneous teams comprised of members of each group. At this stage, the independent variables are manipulated. Brewer and Miller propose two general conditions necessary to realize positive outcomes from cooperative interventions: (1) that the nature of the cooperative interaction promotes an *interpersonal* rather than a *task* orientation toward fellow team members; and (2) that the basis for assignment to team membership (or to roles within teams) is perceived to be independent of category memberships. In a final phase, all subjects view a videotaped interaction of alleged members of both groups with whom they have not interacted. Evaluations of these groups serve as the primary measure of generalized attitude change.

The studies confirmed the hypothesized effects of personalized contact. Under conditions of both interteam cooperation and competition, groups that adopted an interpersonal focus displayed significantly less favoritism toward the videotaped groups than did subjects in either the task focus conditions, or subjects who were given no instructional manipulation. Confirming the proposed role of individuation, subjects differentiated among the out-group members more in the interpersonal conditions, and there was a strong correlation between perceived similarity of out-group members (to each other) and the degree of bias shown toward members of the videotaped teams.

One of the most important potential benefits of Brewer and Miller's model is in further improving cooperative learning techniques, which have been enthusiastically introduced into multiethnic classrooms with encouraging results. These techniques were a response to the fact that traditional classroom instruction methods permitted little contact between students (including those from different groups) that was not simply superficial (Slavin, 1985). Yet, while many of these carefully structured techniques have proved positive in improving dyadic relationships, they have not generally had an impact on perceptions of the group as a whole (for reviews see Aronson, Blaney, Stephan, Sikes, & Snapp, 1978; Aronson & Gonzalez, 1988; Johnson & Johnson, 1982, 1989, 1992; Sharan, 1990; Slavin, 1985). Miller and Harrington (1992) show how key principles from their work impact on cooperative learning; these include "minimization of the salience of social categories when forming teams and during group process" and "provision of opportunities for personalization of team members." In fact, although a number of the models of cooperative learning appear superficially similar, Miller and Harrington point to subtle differences (e.g., whether a competitive interteam reward structure is imposed on the classroom; see DeVries, Edwards, & Slavin, 1978) that do affect outcomes.

Miller and Davidson-Podgorny's (1987) thoughtful review and meta-analysis of cooperative learning studies isolates some of the key strengths and shortcomings of each technique. They point out that rules for assignment of students to subgroups are generally not explicit in the techniques, and they show that three of the variables highlighted by their theoretical model and laboratory work do moderate the impact of cooperative learning on social relations. Specifically, the effect of cooperative learning is more positive when tasks require interdependence, when pupils are randomly assigned to roles, and when there are equal proportions of minority and White students on a team.

Critique

Notwithstanding the support gleaned from several elegant studies, there are several grounds on which the personalized model of contact can be criticized. First, although decategorization does appear to have been achieved in the laboratory studies, it remains to be seen whether the "usefulness" of evaluatively laden social categories can be reduced in this way (but see Warring, Johnson, Maruyama, & Johnson, 1985).

Second, although the model seems to accomplish one form of generalization (decategorization), Brewer and Miller concede that the conditions that promote personalization will impede generalization of contact effects to the out-group as a whole (Brewer, 1988; Brewer & Miller, 1988). This is consistent with the paradox noted by Rose (1981), that intimate relationships may generalize over a wide range of situations, but not over different persons. Miller and Harrington (1992) acknowledge that the video rating used in the third phase of their paradigm is designed to test whether new out-group members are interacted with as individuals, rather than to assess generalized attitudes toward the out-group.

Third, interpretation of the results as pure effects of personalization is problematic. Because members wore large identification badges denoting initial group membership, it could be argued that categories remained salient throughout the experiment. Additionally, it is not clear whether the experimental inductions created a purely personalized form of contact, as the authors argue, since decategorization is a joint function of both differentiation, which is considered category-based, and personalization, which involves only self–other considerations and comparisons. In other words, categorizations appear to have been maintained, not erased.

Finally, the personalization strategy is based on the view that decreasing the salience of group boundaries is likely to reduce intergroup bias. Yet, as Schofield (1991) has pointed out, this conclusion is at odds with her own and others' evaluations of schools that have adopted a "color-blind" perspective. Encouraging the suppression of race or ethnicity by all those involved in a desegregated school may actually increase category salience (Saharso, 1989; Schofield, 1986). This is an interesting parallel to the cognitive experimental work showing that consciously trying *not* to think about something (including a stereotype) may increase the frequency with which one thinks about it (and make one more stereotypic in judgments and behavior; Wegner, 1989; see Bodenhausen & Macrae, Chapter 7, this volume). Thus, personalization seems to avoid the important issue highlighted by Schofield (1991), of how cultural diversity can be acknowledged, even encouraged, without worsening intergroup relations. Since membership of ethnic and other kinds of groups often provides a source of desired social identity (Tajfel, 1978), it would be impractical as well as undesirable for all parties concerned to ignore distinctive memberships (see Rist, 1979; Schofield & McGivern, 1979).

Intergroup Contact and Mutual Intergroup Differentiation

Hewstone and Brown (1986) put forward a theoretical perspective on contact, which diverges sharply from personalization, although both are derived from social identity theory. Hewstone and Brown argue, first, that contact should be "intergroup" not "interpersonal"; and second, that an appropriate model of intergroup contact should be based on "mutual intergroup differentiation."

Theory

Regarding intergroup contact, Hewstone and Brown contend (based on Brown & Turner, 1981) that the contact hypothesis is based theoretically on interpersonal relations, focuses in practice on improving interpersonal relations, and that the failure to effect a generalized change of out-group attitudes can be attributed to this interpersonal perspective. To be successful in changing out-group evaluations, they argue that

> favourable contact with an out-group member *must* be defined as an inter*group* encounter. A weak association between the contact-partner and the out-group (i.e. if the target is an *a*typical out-group member) will define the contact situation as an interpersonal, rather than an intergroup, encounter. . . . Somewhat paradoxically, this means making the group affiliations *more* salient and not less and ensuring that in some way the participants in the contact encounters see each other as representatives of their groups. (1986, p. 18)

In the light of subsequent studies (to be discussed), this position appears now to be overstated. However, I still argue that group affiliation, social categorization, should be evident in the contact situations, although not necessarily made "more salient" as originally argued. In addition, I now follow Stephenson's (1981) suggestion that Tajfel's (1978) distinction between interpersonal and intergroup forms of interaction should be restated as two orthogonal dimensions. In certain contexts it is possible to make both personal and social identity highly salient, and thus an interaction might be both highly personalized and categorized (see the preceding interpretation of Brewer and Miller's research).

In view of this clarification of our earlier position, and some misunderstandings of it, it is important to emphasize what intergroup contact should, and should not, be like. First, it is not always necessary for multiple members to be present, and two individuals acting as group representatives also constitute intergroup behavior. In fact, it has been found that having three members of each group present led to less competitive and more cooperative behavior than did a condition in which two individuals opposed each other as group representatives (Insko et al., 1987; cf. team composition in Bettencourt et al., 1992; Miller et al., 1985). Second, intergroup contact should not be confused with "category-based assignment" (Miller et al., 1985), which is a strategy more akin to tokenism. Third, Miller and Harrington (1992) argue *as if* people will behave in ways that enhance the in-group's image relative to the out-group *whenever* social categories are salient features of situational identity. In fact, although social categorization can be a sufficient condition for intergroup discrimination, this is by no means a universal response, and can be extinguished by feedback concerning how other members of the in- and out-group respond (Locksley, Ortiz, & Hepburn, 1980) or by ensuring that the in-group and out-group are rated on independent dimensions (Mummendey & Schreiber, 1983). Finally, it is worth pointing out that Hewstone and Brown are neither alone nor the first to argue for "intergroup" contact. Similar ideas were suggested many years ago by Chein, Cook, and Harding (1948) and Lewin and Grabbe (1945; see Van Oudenhoven, Groenewoud, & Hewstone, 1995).

Regarding mutual intergroup differentiation, Hewstone and Brown (1986) recommended encouraging groups to recognize mutual superiorities and inferiorities, and to accord equal values to dimensions favoring each group (for similar ideas, see Tajfel, 1981; Turner, 1981; Van Knippenberg, 1984). Mutual intergroup differentiation would be reflected in positive in-group and out-group stereotypes (see Taylor & Simard, 1979). Again, this recommendation is consistent with other prescriptions for intergroup harmony (Berry, 1984; Schofield, 1986; Stephan & Stephan, 1984).

Research

There is now considerable support for the view that out-group attitudes are generalized when memberships are clear in the contact situation. Wilder (1984, Exp. 1) systematically varied the typicality of the out-group college member in a simulated intergroup contact situation. The nature of the contact was also varied in line with traditional theorizing on contact. Thus, the contact person behaved either in a pleasant and supportive way toward the real participants, or in a less pleasant and more critical fashion. The interaction took place over a cooperative task. Wilder predicted that only in the combined conditions, in which the interaction was pleasant and the partner could be seen as typical of her college, would ratings of the out-group college become more favorable. Wilder's results were exactly in line with his prediction.

Wilder's research also highlighted a potential problem associated with the manipulation of typicality. Although his first study reported change in out-group attitudes, there was little evidence that the contact manipulation affected stereotypes of the out-group. As Wilder noted, if stereotypes are negative, then "typical" out-group members need to have some negative characteristics, but then how can we ensure positive change in out-group perception? He suggested that the key to this dilemma may lie in the specific stereotypes the out-group members exhibit in the contact setting (Wilder, 1984, 1986a). Some beliefs about the out-group directly implicate the in-group (e.g., "They think they're better than us"), whereas other beliefs do not (e.g., "they're lazy"). Wilder (1984, Exp. 2) showed that contact with a typical out-group member can improve intergroup relations when the out-group member's typicality is based on characteristics that do *not* involve negative actions directed at the in-group. Finally, Wilder (1984, Exp. 3) demonstrated that the more positive evaluation of the out-group following contact with the typical member could be interpreted in terms of ease of generalization. Subjects judged the typical out-group member's personality and behavior to be more indicative of how others in the out-group would act in the same setting.

These findings were replicated and extended in a recent study by Vivian, Brown, and Hewstone (1995). In a cooperative work situation, British subjects were led to believe that their German partner (a confederate) was either typical or atypical of his national group (Germans), which was alleged to be either more or less homogeneous than other national groups within the European Community. Presumably, contact with a typical member from a relatively homogeneous group is construed as more of an intergroup encounter than is contact with atypical members of heterogeneous groups. Although there was no difference between conditions in rating German partners (who were viewed positively as a function of cooperation), only in the typicality (and especially typicality–homogeneity) conditions was this person explicitly associated with the German out-group as a whole, leading to most positive ratings of the out-group as a whole. The effects of perceived typicality were not, however, universally positive in this study. Contact with a typical member also gave rise to some more negative evaluations of the out-group (on stereotype-confirming traits such as materialistic and boring) than did contact with atypical members. Thus, while a categorized form of contact may have some benefits, there may also be certain risks associated with this strategy (to be discussed).

In a second study, Vivian, Hewstone, and Brown (in press) found that dimensions of membership salience *moderated* the impact of traditional contact variables on European students' generalized attitudes toward a European out-group. There was evidence that different salience variables (typicality, references to nationality, perceived out-group homogeneity) each moderated the effects of at least one contact variable (amount, intimacy, and interdependence of contact). Typicality, especially, moderated the effects of contact variables in a manner consistent with the intergroup model of contact. Thus, the amount of contact and the intimacy of contact were more likely to be associated with a positive view of the out-group *if* an out-group target was perceived as typical of his or her national group.

The final study supporting intergroup contact predicted that attitudes toward out-group members who did not participate in the cooperative setting would be more favorable if social categories were made salient than if the interaction were decategorized (Van Oudenhoven et al., 1995). We found that referring explicitly to the ethnic background of a Turkish partner helped to transfer Dutch students' favorable attitude with respect to a Turkish partner to Turks in general. As in Vivian et al. (1995, Exp. 2), cooperative interaction had a positive effect on ratings of the out-group partner in all conditions, but this was only transferred to the out-group as a whole when the contact was "intergroup."

Taken together, these studies provide support for the intergroup contact model. They show that encountered members of the out-group need to be perceived as having out-group membership as an attribute, that the associative link between individual members and the out-group as a whole cannot be broken altogether, or any change of attitude will not generalize beyond those particular individuals.

There has been less empirical work on mutual intergroup differentiation. Brown and colleagues have, however, supported the idea that in work groups, group differences should be emphasized on dimensions that are accorded equal value, and that a division of labor between groups should permit mutual positive differentiation. In this way, cooperative contact need not threaten one's social identity. Again, the emphasis placed on distinctive memberships directly contradicts that of Brewer and Miller, who argue that group divisions should not be correlated with group membership. In a pair of studies, Brown and colleagues have shown that cooperative encounters involving a division of labor along group lines produce the most favorable responses to members of an out-group (Brown & Wade, 1987; Deschamps & Brown, 1983). Thus, attitudes towards the out-group were friendliest when the groups' roles were clearly defined, and least friendly when their respective roles were ambiguous.

To the extent that our model encourages the recognition of diversity rather than assimilation as a guiding social value, it can be thought of as a more pluralistic model of intergroup relations. It is therefore consistent with those scholars who contend that, in multiethnic societies, the cultural identity of each group should be maintained and positive relations between the groups valued (e.g., Berry, 1984; Berry, Kalin, & Taylor, 1977; Van Oudenhoven & Willemsen, 1989).

Critique

Although intergroup contact can boast greater success in realising generalized change in out-group attitudes, it is not without its dangers and critics (see Harrington & Miller, 1992; Miller & Harrington, 1992b). First, as noted in the case of Wilder's (1984) research, successfully manipulating typicality may involve manipulating negativity. As the research by Vivian and colleagues (1995) indicated, an intergroup form of contact may produce negative as well as positive generalized change. Thus the basic conditions for successful contact, specified by Allport (1954/1979), Cook (1978) and others, must be met when group memberships are explicit, or made salient.

Second, intergroup contact may have a negative effect on intergroup relations via its effect on intergroup anxiety (Stephan & Stephan, 1985). In principle, contact should reduce anxiety, as it has been shown to among White pupils vis-à-vis Black pupils in some desegregated schools (Collins & Noblit, 1977; Noblit & Collins, 1981; Schofield, 1981). But in cases of real intergroup conflict, an overemphasis on group memberships may increase intergroup anxiety, thereby mitigating against the desired generalization of positive out-group attitudes. Exactly this process was demonstrated by Islam and Hewstone (1993a). In a correlational study of contact between Hindu and Muslim religious groups in Bangladesh, they found that intergroup contact was positively associated with anxiety, which in turn was negatively associated with perceived out-group variability and out-group attitudes. These findings are consistent with the suggestions that anxiety narrows the focus of attention, leading to the treatment of out-group members less as individuals and more as equivalent members of a category (Stephan & Stephan, 1985). Anxiety can also weaken the impact of stereotype-disconfirming information (Wilder, 1993a, 1993b; Wilder & Shapiro, 1989). Thus, to the extent that intergroup contact brings about an increase in anxiety, it will worsen, not improve, intergroup relations.

Notwithstanding these valid criticisms of the intergroup contact model, its emphasis on typicality is also shared by cognitive analyses of stereotype change, which approach the issue of contact from a quite different theoretical background. These approaches are now considered. The studies reported in the following section can arguably also be seen as relating to the intergroup contact model (Hewstone & Brown, 1986; Vivian et al., in press).

A Cognitive Analysis of Contact: The Impact of Stereotype-Disconfirming Information

Recent approaches to the contact hypothesis have, rather than addressing Allport's and Cook's (1978) dimensions separately, proposed that they share an impact on the ways people process stereotype-relevant, and especially stereotype-disconfirming, information. This focus on information processing is the hallmark of cognitive analyses of intergroup relations.

Theory

Rothbart and John's (1985) cognitive analysis of intergroup contact is based on principles of categorization. If we accept that objects, or exemplars, differ in the degree to which they are viewed as prototypical examples of a category (what Barsalou, 1987, calls "graded structure"), then we should accept that it is the *goodness of fit* to the stereotype, and not just a few defining features, that determines whether a person becomes associated with a given category. Rothbart and Lewis (1988) showed that as prototypicality increased, the degree of inference from member to group increased. From this view, disconfirming attributes are most likely to become associated with the stereotype if they belong to an individual who is otherwise a very good fit to the category.

Rothbart and John's (1985) view implies that the more a particular episode disconfirms a stereotypic category of which it is an instance, the more likely it is to be associated with a different, possibly counterstereotypic, category. This process enhances the tendency of stereotypic beliefs to confirm themselves. Thus individuating information can "release" an exemplar from the attributes of a superordinate category, and at the same time render the stereotype immune from the attributes of the exemplar. Somewhat counterintuitively, stereotype-disconfirming information should therefore be linked to typical out-group members (see also Wilder, 1986a), a view that is consistent with Hewstone and Brown's (1986) idea that categories should be maintained in contact settings. Unless this is the case, people tend to react to stereotype-disconfirming information not with generalization, but with what Allport (1954/1979) called "re-fencing." The "special case" is excluded and the category held intact (see also Williams, 1964).

Research

Rothbart and John's (1985) prototype model has received support from experimental studies investigating three cognitive models of stereotype change: "bookkeeping," "conversion," and "subtyping" (Weber & Crocker, 1983). The bookkeeping model (Rothbart, 1981) proposes a gradual modification of stereotypes by the additive influence of each piece of disconfirming information. Any single piece of disconfirming information elicits only a minor change in the stereotype; major change occurs gradually and only after the perceiver has accumulated many disconfirming instances that deviate systematically from the stereotype. The conversion model (Rothbart, 1981) envisages a radical change in response to dramatic disconfirming information, but no change in response to minor disconfirming information. Finally, the subtyping model of stereotype change views stereotypes as hierarchical structures, in which discriminations can be created in response to disconfirming information (Ashmore, 1981; Brewer, Dull, & Lui, 1981; Taylor, 1981). This process leads to the formation of subtypes, which constitute exceptions, unrepresentative of the group as a whole. One serious consequence of subtyping is that it may insulate the superordinate stereotype from change (Weber-Kollmann, 1985).

These models were tested in a series of studies that compared stereotype change in response to disconfirming information that was either "dispersed" across several group members (each of whom slightly disconfirms the stereotype), or "concentrated" in a small number of highly disconfirming members. Weber and Crocker (1983) found that stereotypes of occupational groups (librarians and lawyers) changed more when the disconfirming information was dispersed than when it was concentrated, but only under large-sample conditions (30 vs. 6 members). They also showed that disconfirmers with high representativeness (e.g., White, middle-class, high-earning lawyers) were more successful at bringing about stereotype change than were disconfirmers with low representativeness (e.g., Black lawyers). Overall, Weber and Crocker provided strongest support for subtyping, some support for bookkeeping, and none for conversion. Generally, stereotype-disconfirming information had greater impact on perceptions of the group as a whole (generalization) when it was associated with a group member who was perceived as typical of the group.

The results from a series of studies by Hewstone and colleagues also strongly support the subtyping model (although there is some scattered support for the other models; for a review see Hewstone, 1994). These more recent studies have specified the cognitive processes underlying stereotype change. Johnston and Hewstone (1992) showed, first, that weak disconfirming members (in the dispersed condition) were rated more typical than strong disconfirming members (in the concentrated condition). Moreover, this perceived typicality was the only dependent measure that *mediated* the relatively weaker stereotyping in the dispersed condition. This mediating role of perceived typicality has also been demonstrated in three other independent studies, generalizing across manipulations, subject groups, and target groups (Hantzi, in press; Hewstone, Hassebrauck, Wirth, & Waenke, 1995; Maurer, Park, & Rothbart, 1995).

A "prototype subtyping" model seems to provide the best account of how stereotypes change in response to dispersed or concentrated patterns of disconfirming information. Stereotype change is generally effected via the perceived typicality, or goodness of fit, of mild disconfirmers in the dispersed condition; it is generally impeded by the atypicality, or badness of fit, of strong disconfirmers in the concentrated condition. Desforges et al. (1991) tested the hypothesis that contact affects attitudes, in part, by eliciting a more positive portrait of the typical group member. They found that changes in portraits of the typical mental patient were significantly correlated with changes in attitudes (see also Werth & Lord, 1992).

Some doubt remains, however, as to whether the formation of subtypes results in change, inertia, or active preservation of a stereotype (Hamilton & Sherman, 1994). Subtyping may lead to change when subtypes become sufficiently strong that they weaken and ultimately dissolve the stereotype (Pettigrew, 1981; Rothbart & John, 1985). But subtyping may simply limit generalization, resulting in inertia, if there is little overlap between a subtype, which contains some disconfirming information, and the global stereotype (e.g., Devine & Baker's [1991] example of "businessman Black" vs. "Blacks").

The third possible outcome of subtyping highlights the active, purposive nature of subtyping. According to this view, perceivers may deliberately subcategorize members who disconfirm the stereotype *for the purpose of* preserving the generic stereotype (Weber & Crocker, 1983). For example, women whose behavior disconfirms the superordinate-level gender stereotype may be subtyped as lesbians or macho women (Costrich, Feinstein, Kidder, Maracek, & Pascale, 1975; Deaux & Lewis, 1984; Jackson & Cash, 1985). This active preservation of the stereotype clearly impedes change, but may be even more pernicious. Taylor (1981) has argued that subtyping may strengthen the overall stereotype since, as the number of subtypes within it increases, *any* behavior performed by a member of the group can be fitted to at least one subtype. Hewstone, Macrae, Griffiths, Milne, and Brown (1994) reported results consistent with the view that subtyping is associated with active preservation of the stereotype. Stereotyping was stronger in two- vs. one-subtype conditions, when subtypes were based on disconfirming information. Hence, where contact allows, or worse, facilitates subtyping, generalized change in out-group attitudes will tend to be blocked.

Critique

Perhaps the most general and valid criticism of this cognitive research is that it more or less ignores affective change. Yet, Dovidio and colleagues (Chapter 9, this volume) raise an interesting issue about the relationship between cognitive and affective change. To the extent that cognitive and affective stereotypes operate independently, such ways of reducing prejudice and discrimination may be limited: Change in the cognitive component may have no impact on the affective component. Besides, some of the interventions that do work (e.g., cooperation) may actually provoke affective changes (e.g., anxiety, self-esteem) that have consequences for the processing of stereotypic information, but which are at present untapped. More speculatively, following Fiske's (1982) idea that affect is stored with a schema and is cued by categorization, research should attend to which paradigms and interventions might achieve a change in these "affective tags" and other aspects of affective responding, in addition to cognitive measures of stereotyping.

A second, general criticism concerns the paradigm used in much, but not all, of this research. The concentrated–dispersed paradigm confounds several properties (see Hewstone et al., 1994), deals with processing of presented disconfirming information that perceivers may not actively seek out (Johnston & Macrae, 1994), and should not lead us to ignore alternative manipulations of the pattern of presented information (e.g., how information is organized *within* stimulus persons; White & Zsambok, 1994). Despite these reproaches, the cognitive approach has contributed significantly to our understanding of the processes underlying stereotype change, demonstrating the mediating role of typicality.

Summary and Conclusions

The simple contact hypothesis is, in terms of attitude theory, both appealing and naive. It is appealing because, compared with attitudes based on secondhand information, attitudes based on direct experience are relatively strong, held more confidently, brought to mind more easily, and are more resistant to change. They should therefore predict subsequent behavior more accurately (Fazio, 1990). All this is desirable *if* contact is positive and leads to positive attitude change. But the contact hypothesis is naive, because it represents an inappropriate selection of target beliefs to be changed (i.e., trying to change attitudes toward groups as a whole by changing beliefs about particular members of the group; Fishbein & Ajzen, 1975).

The three approaches reviewed in this section all receive substantial empirical support. We now know which variables to manipulate in order to bring about either personalization or intergroup contact; and we know that perceived typicality plays a mediating role and intergroup contact a moderating role, in changing intergroup perceptions. There is also evidence that personalized, decategorized contact can achieve one form of generalization (decategorization), whereas intergroup contact can accomplish another form (generalized change of out-group attitudes). I will defer integration of these approaches until the end of the chapter, when I attempt to pull all three approaches together with those reviewed in the next section and ask, not "which of these approaches to use," but "when to use which of these approaches."

Cook (1985) relates how one of the factors that drew him to study the contact hypothesis was that he had "grown up in the South and had many opportunities to observe and experience *a type of interracial contact that had left prejudice untouched*" (p. 452, italics added). We have, I would argue, made progress in terms of learning what contact to provide, how to provide it, and what is likely to change. We have also learned to be careful, especially with surveys, to check that a substantial amount of contact has actually taken place (e.g., Hamilton & Bishop, 1976) and not been avoided or replaced by resegregation (e.g., Sagar & Schofield, 1984).

If anything, I am more not less sanguine when I try to answer a question we (Hewstone & Brown, 1986) raised in 1986: Is any positive contact better than none? First, prolonged isolation may reduce the likelihood of future intergroup contact, and the continued assumption of belief dissimilarity will likely reinforce the boundary between groups (Allen & Wilder, 1975). Second, Sagar and Schofield (1984) noted one rather subtle positive change in peer relations, even among students in more highly *re*segregated schools: There had been a reduction in the "almost automatic fear" with which many students, especially Whites, responded to members of the other race. According to the authors, the experience of "simple conflict-free exposure" served a fear-reducing function, even if it did not go as far as generalized change of out-group attitudes. Third, especially through cooperative learning techniques, cross-ethnic friendships do develop and access is gained to friendship networks, which can be a major source of increasing cross-friendship friendships (Miller & Harrington, 1992; Slavin, 1985). In turn, these social relations may affect minority students' academic achievement, and access to desegregated networks can help them to obtain better employment (Braddock & McPartland, 1987; Pettigrew, 1967; Schofield, 1991). Against a background of extensive racial segregation in housing, these effects are of no little significance. Indeed, consistent with the theoretical analysis of change provided by Brewer and Miller (1988), we should acknowledge the importance, and the consequences, of various forms of generalization, and not focus solely on the one type that may be hardest to realize.

CATEGORIZATION: CHANGING COGNITIVE REPRESENTATIONS OF "US" AND "THEM"

> I against my brother.
> I and my brother against my cousin.
> I, my brother and our cousin against the foreigner.
> —BEDOUIN PROVERB

The two interventions reviewed in this section start from the same premise as Brewer and Miller (1984), that since social categorization is the cause of discrimination, an improvement in intergroup relations must be brought about by reducing the salience of existing social categories. These interventions try to achieve this, however, not by eliminating categorization, but by altering which categorizations are used (see also Wilder, 1986b). Specifically, they attempt to structure a definition of group categorization in ways that reduce intergroup bias and conflict (Gaertner, Dovidio, Anastasio, Bachman, & Rust, 1993).

Like two of the recent approaches to contact, both interventions are inspired theoretically by social identity theory (Tajfel, 1978) and, more recently, self-categorization theory (e.g., Oakes, Haslam, & Turner, 1994; Turner, 1987). These perspectives emphasize that we all typically belong to several social categories and therefore may have a series of social identifications, one of which is salient at any given time. Self-categorization theory develops the earlier social identity perspective by arguing that self can be conceived on a number of levels of inclusiveness (e.g., me as an individual, me as a group member, me as a human being). The level at which the self is defined determines how one relates to others, including members of the same group. Thus self-categorization theory addresses self- as well as other stereotyping, in-group- and out-group stereotyping, and emphasizes that individuals ascribe to themselves characteristics associated with their in-group. From this perspective, attempts to change intergroup perceptions should look more closely than they have done at how interventions might change both in-group and out-group perceptions. The two interventions reviewed in this section—crossed categorization and common in-group identity—do just this.

Crosscutting Social Categorizations

Most realistic contexts involve several categorizations, some of which coincide and some of which tend to cut across each other. This means that some people who belong to an individual's membership group according to one categorization simultaneously belong to a different group according to a second categorization. A simple idea lies behind the crossed-categorization intervention. When category boundaries are crosscutting versus converging, competing bases for in-group/out-group categorization should reduce the importance of any *one* category and force the perceiver to classify other individuals on *multiple* dimensions at the same time (Miller & Brewer, 1986).

Theory

Proponents of different theories differ somewhat in their predictions concerning discrimination in favor of, or against, each of the four possible target groups created by crossing two dimensions, A/B and X/Y, and in how they see crossed categorization working (for a review see Hewstone, Islam, & Judd, 1993). There are two main theoretical positions.

According to Doise's (1978) "category differentiation model," single or simple categorization leads to two cognitive processes: an accentuation of both the differences between categories (an "interclass effect") and similarities within categories (an "intraclass effect"; see Tajfel, 1959). In contrast, the crossing of two categorizations leads to "convergence" between the categories (weakening the interclass effect) and "divergence" within each category (weakening the intraclass effect). Thus, for example, the accentuation of perceived similarities within one category (e.g., A) will be counteracted by a simultaneously aroused accentuation of perceived differences, because category A contains two different subgroups according to another (e.g., X/Y) categorization (Vanbeselaere, 1991). As a result of these processes, intergroup discrimination based on the A/B categorization can be reduced or even eliminated.

In contrast to Doise's purely cognitive model, an account of crossed-categorization phenomena based on social identity theory (e.g., Tajfel & Turner, 1979) argues that social categorization arouses self-evaluative social comparison processes whereby individuals strive to obtain a positive self-esteem. Brown and Turner (1979) hypothesized that the motivation to create positive differences between in-group and out-group(s), stemming from the need for a positive social identity, persists in a situation of crossed categorizations and leads to an additive combination of tendencies to discriminate. All out-groups will be discriminated against (relative to the double in-group), provided that both categorizations are of equal relevance to social identity, but discrimination will be strongest toward out-groups differing on two rather than on only one dimension.

A further theoretical development was necessary to take account of the fact that outside the laboratory, categorizations tend to be of unequal psychological significance, connoting differences in status, numerosity, and power. Brewer, Ho, Lee, and Miller (1987) suggested four alternative models in cases of unequal category salience:

1. *Category dominance*: A single categorization will dominate, and categorization based on the subordinate category distinction will be ignored.
2. *Additivity*: Both category distinctions are attended to, and are combined additively to form a categorization judgment.
3. *Category conjunction*: A target individual is only classified as an "in-group" member when he or she shares category membership with the subject on all available category distinctions, and all other combinations are classified as "out-group."
4. *Hierarchical ordering*: The effects of one category distinction are dependent on prior categorization on the other dimension (thus in-group/out-group differentiation on a second category distinction would be greater for a target person classified as an in-group member on the first dimension, than for a target classified as an out-group member on the first dimension).

A review of the relevant research indicates partial support for each of the models, but only a qualified success for the intervention.

Research

Deschamps and Doise (1978), in the first experimental study, showed that intergroup discrimination could be reduced by crossing gender (a strong categorization) with red/blue (a weak, experimentally created categorization). This study was criticized by Brown and Turner (1979), however, for not using categories of equal psychological significance (which could surely not "cancel each other out," the putative process according to the category differentiation model). Yet, the main finding was replicated by Vanbeselaere (1987). Using two artificial categories and improved methodology, he found bias was reduced, not eliminated, in the crossed-categorization conditions, on specific and general evaluations (see also Brown & Turner, 1979; Rehm, Lilli, & Van Eimeren, 1988; Vanbeselaere, 1991). Diehl (1989, 1990) also used two artificially created categorizations of equal psychological significance, but reported that subjects in a crossed-categorization condition discriminate against the totally different group, but not against a partly overlapping group.

Taken together, these and other studies have not yet distinguished between category-differentiation and social-identity predictions, but have fairly consistently shown the strongest discrimination against the double out-group, which is attenuated in the case of the two crossed conditions (e.g., Brown & Turner, 1979; Deschamps & Doise, 1978; Vanbeselaere, 1987). Although interpretable in terms of reduced category salience (see Messick & Mackie, 1989; Stephan, 1985; Wilder, 1986b), such studies do still constitute "intergroup" situations, because categories are not ignored when crossed (see Arcuri, 1982; Brewer, 1968; Vanbeselaere, 1987).

There has also been support for each of the four models specified by Brewer and colleagues (1987), which sometimes make similar predictions to the two earlier perspectives (see Hewstone et al., 1993). In specific circumstances, there is evidence for category dominance (e.g., Hewstone et al., 1983; Islam & Hewstone, 1993b, Exp. 2), additive (e.g., Brewer, 1968), category-conjunction (e.g., Rogers, Miller, & Hennigan, 1981) and hierarchical-ordering (e.g., Brewer et al., 1987) effects. Hewstone and colleagues (1993) therefore suggest that further research should pay closer attention to when (i.e., the situations in which) and how (i.e., the processes by which) each model might operate. In the context of a general discussion of how to improve intergroup relations, the category-dominance model seems crucial. Both category-differentiation and social-identity perspectives are severely limited by their focus on crossed categorizations of equal psychological significance. Outside the laboratory, one categorization tends to be primary whenever research relies on real social categorizations that have historical, cultural, socioeconomic and affective significance. Thus, the category dominance model appears to reflect reality in multigroup societies (e.g., race in South Africa or the United States, religion in Northern Ireland or Bangladesh, and language in Belgium or Quebec).

The idea of crossing social categories has considerable appeal and may underlie other socialpsychological interventions. As we saw in the previous section, Miller and colleagues manipulated decategorized contact by placing members of different groups on the same team. Thus, the results of their studies could be seen in terms of crossed categorization (e.g., out-group members of one's team are out-group on the original categorization but in-group on the team categorization). Indeed, Marcus-Newhall, Miller, Holtz, and Brewer (1993) made explicit the importance of crossed categorization (role assignment) in their paradigm. They reported that, compared with converging-category assignment, crosscutting categories and role assignments decrease perceptions of similarity within categories and increase perceptions of similarity across categories. This supports Doise's (1978) category-differentiation account of the underlying process. Marcus-Newhall and colleagues were even able to show that an index of perceived similarity (based on decreased similarity between individuals within the same category and increased similarity between individuals from different categories) *mediated* the effect of role assignment on bias. But there was no generalization beyond the team setting to out-group perception in general.

Crossed categorization may also be usefully incorporated into applied settings. Schofield (1991) discusses evidence that crosscutting ties can improve peer relations in desegregated schools (Schofield & McGivern, 1979) and speculates that the creation of crosscutting ties may help to account for the positive impact of cooperative-learning teams on intergroup relations (e.g., the "Jigsaw Classroom" created by Aronson et al., 1978). Finally, Duckitt (1992) refers to the understated and undeveloped role of social scientists in designing constitutions and political systems to reduce or channel interethnic conflicts (e.g., Horowitz, 1985), which may seek to reinforce crossed, rather than converging, categorizations.

Critique

A first criticism concerning this intervention concerns the lack of clarity about exactly what effect it achieves. A recent meta-analysis of crossed-categorization studies by Migdal, Hewstone, and Mullen (1995) concluded that crossed categorization does not achieve a notable reduction in the magnitude of intergroup bias observed under simple categorization conditions. Why, then, do many studies on crossed categorization appear to "work," in the sense that they yield significant results? The answer, we believe, lies both in the creation of the double out-group condition and in the frequent failure to compare bias in simple and crossed conditions within the same study (an exception is Brown & Turner, 1979, but they failed to find discrimination in the simple categorization conditions).

First, what most studies show, and most models predict, is greatest bias toward the double out-group. But from this we should not conclude that crossed categorization "reduces" intergroup bias, only that it can help to reduce bias against existing double (or multiple) out-groups. Of course, outside the laboratory, multiple categorization is the rule, rather than the exception, and the double out-group response found in crossed-categorization studies is consistent with Brewer and Campbell's (1976) discussion of increased discrimination in situations of "converging boundaries," in which multiple intergroup differences coincide. Thus, perhaps crossed categorization should be more accurately presented as a technique for reducing bias against out-groups characterized by converging boundaries (by no means a rare occurrence outside the laboratory; see Pettigrew's, 1981, discussion of "double jeopardy").

Second, the processes underlying crossed-categorization effects are far from clear, and there is evidence consistent with several explanations (including the reduction of original categorization salience, the self-esteem conferring function of social identity, and category differentiation; see Hewstone et al., 1993). Future work must be more process oriented and might include factors such as attention paid to different categorizations and perceived homogeneity of in- and out-groups (see Smith, 1992). One interesting possibility is that crossed-categorization effects may be mediated by perceptions of a common in-group identity (see the following discussion of work by Gaertner et al.).

Third, future research should be guided by a more detailed consideration of the change likely to be associated with crossed categorization. At present, there is little evidence that crossed categorization achieves any reduction in discrimination compared with simple categorization. Moreover, given that crossing categories should, at least, make perceivers aware that the out-group consists of different subgroups, this intervention should—logically—be associated with the second type of generalization, differentiation. Tajfel (1982) explicitly mentioned the hypothesis that crossed categorizations break down the perceived homogeneity of the out-group, yet there is little evidence for this effect (but see Marcus-Newhall et al., 1993).

Finally, given that category dominance is probably the norm when real, conflicting groups are studied, it may prove impossible to weaken discrimination by crossing multiple categorizations (e.g., Hewstone et al., 1993, Exp. 2). Yet, if crossed categorization can *force* continual realignments among individuals and categories via extended interactions on the basis of multiple categorizations at different points in time (Miller & Brewer, 1986), then it should be a significant component of many interventions to reduce intergroup discrimination.

Common In-Group Identity

In Sherif's (1966) famous summer camp studies, an initial attempt to reduce intergroup conflict involved bringing boys from two opposing groups into contact in pleasant surroundings. It resulted in further hostile exchanges (see also Diab, 1970; Sherif & Sherif, 1965). Sherif concluded that there needed to be some positive and functional interdependence between groups before conflict between them would abate. He created these conditions in the form of superordinate goals, goals that neither group could attain on its own and that superseded other goals each group might have had. Sherif also reported that a single superordinate goal was not sufficient to reduce intergroup conflict; a series of cumulative superordinate goals was required (see also Wilder & Thompson, 1980). A recent theoretical perspective developed by Gaertner and colleagues (1993) has built on Sherif's work emphasizing goals, to argue that it is ultimately group members' *cognitive representations* of the situation that are the critical variable mediating a reduction in intergroup bias.

Theory

The "common in-group identity" model argues that bias can be reduced by factors that transform members' perceptions of group boundaries from "us" and "them" to a more inclusive "we." Indeed, there is evidence that manipulation of the pronouns *we* and *they* can differentially influence intergroup perception and behavior (Perdue, Dovidio, Gurtman, & Tyler, 1990; see Maass & Arcuri, Chapter 6, this volume). Gaertner and colleagues argue that several features specified by the contact hypothesis are effective, in part, because they contribute to the development of a common in-group identity.

Although Gaertner et al. acknowledge that several factors influence intergroup bias and conflict, they still regard the cognitive representations of the situation as the critical mediating variable. Whereas a representation of the situation as one involving two groups is thought to maintain or enhance intergroup biases, decategorized (i.e., separate individuals) or recategorized (i.e., common in-group identity) representations are expected to reduce tension, albeit in different ways. Decategorization reduces bias through a process that moves initial in-group members away from the self and toward out-group members; thus former in-group members are seen less positively and as more evaluatively similar to out-group members. Recategorization, in contrast, should reduce bias by increasing the attractiveness of former out-group members, once they are included within the superordinate group structure.

Research

Two main experimental studies support the common in-group identity model (for a discussion of more indirect support see Gaertner et al., 1993). The first study used a two-step procedure whereby previously isolated problem-solving groups were brought together under different conditions (Gaertner, Mann, Murrell, & Dovidio, 1989). By varying the structural arrangements (i.e., integrated, segregated, or separate seating patterns), the nature of interdependence among participants, and the identifying labels given to participants (new group name, original group names, individual names), the experiment was designed to induce a "one-group," "two-groups," or "separate-individuals" representation of the intergroup situation. As predicted, subjects in one-group and separate-individuals conditions showed lower levels of intergroup bias than subjects in the two-groups condition (which maintained the salience of intergroup boundaries). Furthermore, the positive effects associated with the two former conditions were apparently controlled by different mechanisms, as specified earlier. In the one-group condition, bias was reduced primarily by increased attraction to former out-group members; in the separate-individuals condition, bias was reduced by decreased attraction to former in-group members.

The second study (Gaertner, Mann, Dovidio, Murrell, & Pomare, 1990) tested the prediction that intergroup cooperation reduces bias, at least partly, because it decreases the salience of the intergroup boundary. The results confirmed the hypothesis that a one-group representation would produce lower levels of bias than a two-groups representation. Gaertner and colleagues also provided definitive *mediational* evidence that cooperation affected bias via cognitive representations of social categorization. Consistent with the common in-group identity model, the one-group representation was the only significant predictor of out-group member evaluations; moreover, the significant effect for interdependence (cooperation vs competition) effectively disappeared once the one-group representation was controlled for.

Gaertner and colleagues also conducted a field study of factors related to the contact hypothesis in a multiethnic high school (Gaertner, Rust, Dovidio, Bachman, & Anastasio, 1994). They reported that the effect of perceptions of interdependence on out-group bias was partially mediated by perceptions that the school body was "one group" (positive

relation) and "different groups" (negative relation). The evidence of mediation was, however, much weaker, and the data could be seen to give
more support to Sherif's model, whereby goal relations have a direct effect on bias (see Vivian et al., in press). Nonetheless, like the other interventions reviewed, the common in-group identity model has considerable intuitive appeal in applied settings (e.g., Schofield & McGivern,
1979; Slavin, 1985).

Critique

The first and most obvious criticism of this approach is that it may not
be realistic. Can the recategorization process and the creation of a superordinate group identity overcome powerful ethnic and racial categorizations on more than a temporary basis? Gaertner and colleagues'
strategy is open to the same criticisms leveled at Sherif's method of inducing superordinate goals. When Sherif finally introduced superordinate goals, the conflict was to all intents and purposes over (Billig,
1976; Tajfel, 1978). Success by this method is achieved by fusing together the two groups. Thus, it can be argued that the situation is no longer
an intergroup one at all.

Second, the common in-group identity strategy is analogous to
those forms of assimilation that supposedly work by blurring and ultimately merging identities into a single, broader superordinate identity
(Duckitt, 1992), a model of intergroup relations that is now fairly uniformly rejected (e.g., Berry, 1984; van Oudenhoven & Willemsen,
1989). As Turner (1981) argued, cooperative interdependence is not,
and should not be, incompatible with psychological distinctiveness for
each separate group. Thus, a more successful strategy in practice seems
likely to involve a superordinate identity *and* distinctive subgroup identities (e.g., Brown & Wade, 1987; Deschamps & Brown, 1983).

Third, it is not clear what kind of generalization, and to what extent, is actually realized by this intervention. The reported reduction in
bias suggests a decrease in the use of the original category (i.e., decategorization), but there are no measures of generalized change in out-
group attitudes. In fact, Gaertner and colleagues propose that "*generalization* will be maximized when the salience of the intitial group
identities are [*sic*] maintained, but *within a context* of a salient superordinate common in-group identity" (1993, p. 6, italics in original). This
statement invites an integration of the common in-group identity approach and the intergroup model of contact (see next section). Of
course, whether it will be possible to make dual memberships simultane-

ously salient is an empirical question, but here integration with the crossed-categorization approach is suggested. Despite these criticisms, the common in-group identity approach is exemplary in its theoretical grounding and its methodological sophistication; it surely has a role to play in any integrated model of changing intergroup relations.

Summary and Conclusions

Interventions that manipulate social categorizations have yielded an array of supportive data. They have also reminded researchers that a change in intergroup perceptions could mean a change in perceptions of the in-group as well as the out-group. These interventions may best be viewed as "contact-enhancing" manipulations that can reduce the likelihood of applying old categorizations, can perhaps also increase the complexity of out-group perceptions, but which cannot necessarily achieve a change in generalized out-group attitudes. They may, however, when paired with cooperation that results in success, be equally important in providing undeniable evidence that members of two previously antagonistic groups can work together. Extreme care must be exercised to ensure that a realignment of categorization does not redirect conflict elsewhere. Intergroup conflict is not resolved when the presence of a new, extreme out-group leads to a previously moderate out-group being assimilated to the in-group (see Wilder & Thompson, 1988).

AN INTEGRATION

Everybody has won and all must have prizes.
—LEWIS CARROLL (*Alice in Wonderland*)

The research reviewed in this chapter indicates that different interventions bring about different kinds of changes, and never bring about all three kinds of change in one study (see Table 10.1 for an overview).

Personalized contact (Brewer & Miller, 1984) can effect both more differentiated out-group perception and a decrease in the extent to which a category is used (decategorization; e.g., Bettencourt et al., 1992). Intergroup contact (Hewstone & Brown, 1986) and contact with prototypical out-group members (Rothbart & John, 1985), can realize change in out-group attitudes (and this fact is acknowledged by other perspectives; Brewer, 1988; Gaertner et al., 1993). Yet, by encouraging group distinctiveness, we may risk increasing intergroup anxiety and tendencies to bias. This tension between the merits of emphasizing

TABLE 10.1. Changing Intergroup Perceptions: A Summary of the Impact of Different Interventions

Type of generalization	Intervention	Exemplary research	Process(es)
Change in attitudes toward the social category	Intergroup contact	Wilder (1984)	Only contact with typical members of the out-group leads to a change in perceptions of the group as a whole
		Johnston & Hewstone (1992)	Perceived typicality of disconfirming group members *mediates* stereotype change.
		Vivian et al. (in press)	Intergroup contact *moderates* intergroup bias (generalized perceptions of in-group vs. out-group).
Increased complexity of intergroup perceptions	Decategorized contact (differentiation/ personalization)	Bettencourt et al. (1992)	Personalized contact leads to greater out-group differentiation, which is (negatively) correlated with bias.
	Crossed categorization	Marcus-Newhall et al. (1993)	Perceived out-group homogeneity *mediates* bias.
Decategorization	Decategorized contact	Bettencourt et al. (1992)	Personalized contact leads to less biased perceptions of individual members of out-group versus in-group.
	Common in-group identity	Gaertner et al. (1993)	Cognitive representations of "one group" *mediate* biased perceptions of individual members of out-group versus in-group.

membership, on the one hand, and either individuality or common identity, on the other, represents what is perhaps the central issue in the field (Vivian et al., in press). Crossed categorization (Deschamps & Doise, 1978) seems best suited to achieving a change in the complexity of intergroup perception, and this can reduce bias (Marcus-Newhall et al., 1993), whereas common in-group identity (Gaertner et al., 1993) can effect decategorization (and possibly, over time, differentiation, too).

If we take the view that ultimately all three types of generalization are desirable, we should then want to plan interventions that can achieve all three outcomes. Some support for this kind of integration already exists. For example, personalized contact does seem to include some degree of category maintenance, and a revised model of intergroup contact now accepts that interpersonal and intergroup aspects of contact can and should be manipulated orthogonally. Cook's (1978, 1984) work, for example, shows how the category-based and personalization approaches can come together. He successfully brought about generalization by both making categorization salient *and* creating positive interpersonal encounters. In his 1978 study, White subjects experienced pleasant, cooperative interracial contact with Black individuals. When their well-liked Black coworker gave an account of the discrimination he experienced (*as a Black*), Cook then ensured that another White participant advocated desegregation and racial equality. This was done in such a way that the White subjects understood how the adoption of equalitarian social policies would make it less likely that their new Black friends would encounter prejudice and discrimination. Thus peer-group support served as a "cognitive booster" for generalization, from favorable interpersonal contact to positive attitudes toward the group as a whole. As Pettigrew and Martin (1987) concluded, Cook "achieves generalization to blacks as a group *by deliberately making group categorization salient*" (p. 68, italics added). The results of the study by Van Oudenhoven and colleagues (1995) can be interpreted in the same way.

The next question that arises concerns the order in which we should try to achieve the different kinds of change, because they seem to be linked to different interventions and difficult, if not impossible, to realize simultaneously. Given three types of generalization, there are at least six different orders we could investigate (in fact, there are many more possibilities, since there are at least four main types of intervention). How should we do this? The simple answer is that we do not know, but must find out. The prejudice and out-group derogation that make such interventions necessary are unlikely to be reduced by one-off interventions, and are more likely to require a graduated series of interactions involving a variety of manipulations.

It may be useful to speculate on a few possibilities that seem to merit research. First, given the acknowledged danger of fomenting intergroup conflict by maintaining or emphasizing category memberships, we should perhaps initially try to establish positive interpersonal relations (especially when intergroup relations are divisive), only later seeking to manipulate typicality. Although Van Oudenhoven and colleagues (1995) found no difference between two conditions that introduced categorization at the beginning or middle of a cooperative interaction, they suggested that gradual introduction of ethnic categorization may be more effective in generalizing out-group attitudes under more threatening circumstances (when anxiety may be high; Wilder, 1993a, 1993b).

An alternative view, of course, is that typicality should be clear from the outset, while trying to reduce category-based processing. Here research could be guided by the graded-structure approach to social categories (Barsalou, 1987) and research on the nature of stereotypic traits (Rothbart & Park, 1986). We should try to identify those stereotype-confirming traits that convey no more than the required degree of typicality to mediate stereotype change, and those disconfirming traits that are actually susceptible to change and likely to effect desired change in other traits.

A second issue concerns how to achieve both generalized change in out-group attitudes and a change in intergroup complexity. One line of reasoning suggests that we should try to change variability first, and in this way "unfreeze" cognitions (Kruglanski, 1989; Lewin, 1948). Conversely, it can be argued that a change in cognitive representation may make change more difficult to achieve. By increasing the variability of a stereotype when inconsistent group members are encountered, social perceivers can maintain the stereotype's central tendency (see Srull, 1981). Indirect support for this view comes from research showing that subtypes consisting of stereotype-disconfirming members were associated with active preservation of the stereotype (Hewstone et al., 1994).

A potential resolution to this problem is offered by new research. Maurer, Park, and Rothbart (in press) distinguished between "subtyping" (distinguishing between stereotype-confirming and disconfirming individuals) and "subgrouping" (instructions to divide group members into multiple groups). They predicted and found that the principle consequence of subtyping was preservation of the stereotype, whereas the principle consequence of subgrouping was greater perceived variability and less stereotypic perceptions of the group. Thus attempts to induce changes in perceived variability should be based on subgrouping, not subtyping.

CONCLUSIONS

> Not only are we using the tools of persuasion, but
> we've got to use tools of coercion. Not only is this
> thing a process of education, but it is also a
> process of legislation.
> —Martin Luther King, Jr.

> People of comfortable circumstance live peacefully
> together and those afflicted by poverty do not.
> —John Kenneth Galbraith

In his wide-ranging analysis of prejudice, Duckitt (1992) argues for a multilevel approach. He identifies three causal processes that establish and maintain prejudice, and proposes that change at each level would be required to effect a significant reduction in prejudice: (1) the level of social structure and intergroup relations; (2) the level of social influences to which individuals are exposed; and (3) the level of individual susceptibility. This chapter has focused on two broad interventions—contact and categorization—that address the first and second levels, but ignore the third. This can be justified on the grounds that prejudice is primarily a social, and not an individual, problem, but still it could be argued that these interventions leave untouched the problem of institutionalized discrimination, which is the core of the problem (Pettigrew, 1986).

To get at the underlying, social structural causes of prejudice, higher level interventions will surely be required, as implied by the quotations at the beginning of this section. Yet, notwithstanding the importance of legal, educational, and politicoeconomic factors, there remains a role for social psychology, because it is often individuals' subjective representations of these factors that guide perceptions and behavior. More pragmatically, since it is not in our gift, as social psychologists, to change the social structure, I argue that our time and efforts are better spent in continuing to work as we do. But in so doing, we should try to be more innovative and less reactive than we have been in the past, as in the case of evaluating school desegregation (see Cook, 1985). For example, schools in South Africa are currently being desegregated, and they surely have much to learn from the North American experience, but innovative, theory-driven programs should first be put into place there and then evaluated.

I have argued throughout for the importance of *theory*, and the value of good, testable theory is exemplified in the diverse interventions that have sprung from Tajfel's social identity theory. I have proposed that each of the main interventions reviewed can help to change intergroup relations in particular circumstances, but that an integrated approach is likely to be most effective. If we accept that there are different types of change to achieve, and that different interventions may realize different types of change, then our future interventions will need to be more complex to be more successful.

ACKNOWLEDGMENT

I gratefully acknowledge a grant from the Cardiff Research Initiative during the time at which this chapter was written.

NOTE

1. The quotation is taken by Tajfel from a book by Mason (1970), based on anthropological work in Rwanda by Maquet (1961).

REFERENCES

Allen, V. L., & Wilder, D. A., (1975). Categorization, belief similarity, and intergroup discrimination. *Journal of Personality and Social Psychology, 32,* 971–977.

Allport, G. W. (1979). *The nature of prejudice.* Cambridge/Reading, MA: Addison-Wesley. (Original work published 1954)

Amir, Y. (1969). Contact hypothesis in ethnic relations. *Psychological Bulletin, 71,* 319–42.

Amir, Y. (1976). The role of intergroup contact in change of prejudice and ethnic relations. In P. A. Katz (Ed.), *Towards the elimination of racism* (pp. 245–308). Elmsford: NY: Pergamon Press.

Arcuri, L. (1982). Three patterns of social categorization in attribution memory. *European Journal of Social Psychology, 12,* 271–282.

Aronson, E., Blaney, N., Stephan, C., Sikes, J., & Snapp, M. (1978). *The jigsaw classroom.* Newbury Park, CA: Sage.

Aronson, E., & Gonzalez, A. (1988). Desegregation, jigsaw, and the Mexican American experience. In P. A. Katz & D. A. Taylor (Eds.), *Eliminating racism: Profiles in controversy* (pp. 301–314). New York: Plenum Press.

Ashmore, R. D. (1981). Sex stereotypes and implicit personality theory. In D. L. Hamilton (Ed.), *Cognitive processes in stereotyping and intergroup relations* (pp. 37–81). Hillsdale, NJ: Erlbaum.

Baron, R. M., & Kenny, D. A. (1986). The moderator–mediator variable distinction in social psychological reasearch: Conceptual, strategic, and statistical considerations. *Journal of Personality and Social Psychology, 51,* 1173–1182.

Barsalou, L. W. (1984). Cultural relations in plural societies: Alternatives to segregation and their sociopsychological implications. In N. Miller & M. B. Brewer (Eds.), *Groups in contact: The psychology of desegregation* (pp. 11–27). San Diego: Academic Press.

Berry, J. W., Kalin, R., & Taylor, D. M. (1977). *Multiculturalism and ethnic attitudes in Canada.* Ottawa: Minstry of Supply and Services.

Bettencourt, B. A., Brewer, M. B., Rogers-Croak, M., & Miller, N. (1992). Cooperation and the reduction of intergroup bias: The role of reward structure and social orientation. *Journal of Experimental Social Psychology, 28,* 301–319.

Billig, M. (1976). *Social psychology and intergroup relations.* London: Academic Press.

Braddock, J. H., II. (1985). School desegregation and black assimilation. *Journal of Social Issues, 41,* 9–22.

Braddock, J. H., II, & McPartland, J. (1987). How minorities continue to be excluded from equal employment opportunities: Research on labor market and institutional barriers. *Journal of Social Issues, 43,* 5–39.

Brewer, M. B. (1968). Determinants of social distance among East African tribal groups. *Journal of Personality and Social Psychology, 10,* 279–289.

Brewer, M. B. (1979). In-group bias in the minimal intergroup situation: A cognitive–motivational analysis. *Psychological Bulletin, 86,* 307–334.

Brewer, M. B. (1988). A dual process model of impression formation. In T. K. Srull & R. S. Wyer (Eds.), *Advances in social cognition* (Vol. 1, pp. 1–36). Hillsdale, NJ: Erlbaum.

Brewer, M. B., & Campbell, D. T. (1976). *Ethnocentrism and intergroup attitudes: East African evidence.* New York: Halstead Press.

Brewer, M. B., Dull, V., & Lui, L. (1981). Perceptions of the elderly: Stereotypes as prototypes. *Journal of Personality and Social Psychology, 41,* 656–670.

Brewer, M. B., Ho, H. K., Lee, J. Y., & Miller, N. (1987). Social identity and social distance among Hong Kong schoolchildren. *Personality and Social Psychology Bulletin, 13,* 156–165.

Brewer, M. B., & Miller, N. (1984). Beyond the contact hypothesis: Theoretical perspectives on desegregation. In N. Miller & M. B. Brewer (Eds.), *Groups in contact: The psychology of desegregation* (pp. 281–302). Orlando, FL: Academic Press.

Brewer, M. B., & Miller, N. (1988). Contact and cooperation: When do they work? In P. Katz & D. Taylor (Eds.), *Eliminating racism: Means and controversies* (pp. 315–326). New York: Plenum Press.

Brown, R. J., & Turner, J. C. (1979). The criss-cross categorization effect in intergroup discrimination. *British Journal of Social and Clinical Psychology, 18,* 371–383.

Brown, R. J., & Turner, J. C. (1981). Interpersonal and intergroup behaviour. In

J. Turner & H. Giles (Eds.), *Intergroup behaviour* (pp. 33–65). Oxford: Blackwell.

Brown, R. J., & Wade, G. S. (1987). Superordinate goals and intergroup behavior: The effects of role ambiguity and status on intergroup attitudes and task performance. *European Journal of Social Psychology, 17,* 131–142.

Byrne, D. (1969). Attitudes and attraction. In L. Berkowitz (Ed.), *Advances in experimental social psychology* (Vol. 4, pp. 35–89). New York: Academic Press.

Campbell, D. T., & Fiske, D. W. (1959). Convergent and discriminant validation by the multitrait–multimatrix method. *Psychological Bulletin, 56,* 81–105.

Chein, I., Cook, S. W., & Harding, J. (1948). The field of action research. *American Psychologist, 3,* 43–50.

Cohen, E. (1975). The effects of desegregation on race relations. *Law and Contemporary Problems, 39,* 271–299.

Collins, T. W., & Noblit, G. W. (1977). *Crossover high.* Unpublished manuscript, Memphis State University, Memphis, TN.

Cook, S. W. (1962). The systematic analysis of socially significant events: A strategy for social research. *Journal of Social Issues, 18,* 66–84.

Cook, S. W. (1978). Interpersonal and attitudinal outcomes in cooperating interracial groups. *Journal of Research and Development in Education, 12,* 97–113.

Cook, S. W. (1979). Social science and school desegregation: Did we mislead the Supreme Court? *Personality and Social Psychology Bulletin, 5,* 420–437.

Cook, S. W. (1984). Cooperative interaction in multiethnic contexts. In N. Miller & M. B. Brewer (Eds.), *Groups in contact: The psychology of desegregation* (pp. 156–186). New York: Academic Press.

Cook, S. W. (1985). Experimenting on social issues: The case of school desegregation. *American Psychologist, 40,* 452–460.

Costrich, N., Feinstein, J., Kidder, L., Maracek, J., & Pascale, L. (1975). When stereotypes hurt: Three studies of penalties for sex-role reversals. *Journal of Experimental Social Psychology, 11,* 520–530.

Deaux, K., & Lewis, L. L. (1984). The structure of gender stereotypes: Interrelationships among components and gender label. *Journal of Personality and Social Psychology, 46,* 991–1104.

Deschamps, J.-C., & Brown, R. (1983). Superordinate goals and intergroup conflict. *British Journal of Social Psychology, 22,* 189–195.

Deschamps, J.-C., & Doise, W. (1978). Crossed category memberships in intergroup relations. In H. Tajfel (Ed.), *Differentiation between social groups* (pp. 141–158). Cambridge, UK: Cambridge University Press.

Desforges, D. M., Lord, C. G., Ramsey, S. L., Mason, J. A., Van Leeuwen, M. D., & Lepper, M. R. (1991). Effects of structured cooperative contact on changing negative attitudes toward stigmatized social groups. *Journal of Personality and Social Psychology, 60,* 531–544.

Deutsch, M., & Collins, M. E. (1951). *Interracial housing: A psychological evaluation of a social experiment.* Minneapolis: University of Minnesota Press.

Devine, P. G., & Baker, S. M. (1991). Measurement of racial stereotype subtyping. *Personality and Social Psychology Bulletin, 17,* 44–50.

DeVries, D., Edwards, K., & Slavin, R. (1978). Biracial learning teams and race relations in the classroom: Four field experiments in Teams–Games–Tournament. *Journal of Educational Psychology, 70,* 356–362.

Diab, L. N. (1970). A study of intragroup and intergroup relations among experimentally produced small groups. *Genetic Psychology Monographs, 82,* 49–82.

Diel, M. (1989). Dichotomie und Diskriminierung: Die Auswirkungen von Kreuzkategorisierungen auf die Diskriminierung im Paradigma der minimalen Gruppen [Dichotomy and discrimination: The effect of crossed categorizations on discrimination in the minimal group paradigm]. *Zeitschrift für Sozialpsychologie, 20,* 92–102.

Diehl, M. (1990). The minimal group paradigm: Theoretical explanations and empirical findings. In W. Stroebe & M. Hewstrone (Eds.), *European review of social psychology* (Vol. 1, pp. 263–292). Chichester, UK: Wiley.

Doise, W. (1978). *Groups and individuals: Explanations in social psychology.* Cambridge, UK: Cambridge University Press.

Duckitt, J. (1992). *The social psychology of prejudice.* New York: Praeger.

Fazio, R. H. (1990). Multiple processes by which attitudes guide behavior: The MODE model as an integrative framework. In M. P. Zanna (Ed.), *Advances in experimental social psychology* (Vol. 23, pp. 75–109). New York: Academic Press.

Fishbein, M., & Ajzen, I. (1975). *Belief, attitude, inention and behavior: An introduction to theory and research.* Reading, MA: Addison-Wesley.

Fisher, R. J. (1990). *The social psychology of intergroup and international conflict resolution.* New York: Springer-Verlag.

Fiske, S. T. (1982). Schema-triggered affect: Applications to social perception. In M. S. Clark & S. T. Fiske (Eds.), *Affect and cognition: The 17th Annual Carnegie Symposium* (pp. 55–77). Hillsdale, NJ: Erlbaum.

Gaertner, S. L., Dovidio, J. F., Anastasio, P. A., Bachman, B. A., & Rust, M. C. (1993). The common ingroup identity model: Recategorization and the reduction of intergroup bias. In W. Stroebe & M. Hewstone (Eds.), *European review of social psychology* (Vol. 4, pp. 1–26). Chichester, UK: Wiley.

Gaertner, S. L., Mann, J. A., Dovidio, J. F., Murrell, A. J., & Pomare, M. (1990). How does cooperation reduce intergroup bias? *Journal of Personality and Social Psychology, 59,* 692–704.

Gaertner, S. L., Mann, J., Murrell, A., & Dovidio, J. F. (1989). Reducing intergroup bias: The benefits of recategorization. *Journal of Personality and Social Psychology, 57,* 239–249.

Gaertner, S. L., Rust, M. C., Dovidio, J. F., Bachman, B. A., & Anastasio, P. A. (1994). The contact hypothesis: The role of common ingroup identity on reducing intergroup bias. *Small Group Research, 25,* 244–249.

Gerard, H. B. (1983). School desegregation: The social science role. *American Psychologist, 38,* 869–877.

Greenblatt, S. L., & Willie, C. V. (1980). The serendipitous effects of school desegregation. In W. G. Stephan & J. Feagin (Eds.), *School desegregation* (pp. 51–66). New York: Plenum Press.

Hamilton, D. L., & Bishop, G. D. (1976). Attitudinal and behavioral effects of initial integration of white suburban neighbourhoods. *Journal of Social Issues, 32,* 47–67.

Hamilton, D. L., & Sherman, J. W. (1994). Stereotypes. In R. S. Wyer & T. K. Srull (Eds.), *Handbook of social cognition* (2nd ed., Vol. 2, pp. 1–68). Hillsdale, NJ: Erlbaum.

Hantzi, A. (in press). Change in stereotypic perceptions of familiar and unfamiliar groups: The pervasiveness of the subtyping model. *British Journal of Social Psychology.*

Harrington, H. J., & Miller, N. (1992). Research and theory in intergroup relations: Issues of consensus and controversy. In J. Lynch, M. Modgil, & S. Modgil (Eds.), *Cultural diversity in the schools: Consensus and controversy* (pp. 159–178). London: Falmer Press.

Hewstone, M. (1994). Revision and change of stereotypic beliefs: In search of the elusive subtyping model. In W. Stroebe & M. Hewstone (Eds.), *European review of social psychology* (Vol. 5, pp. 69–109). Chichester, UK: Wiley.

Hewstone, M., & Brown, R. J. (1986). Contact is not enough: An intergroup perspective on the "contact hypothesis." In M. Hewstone & R. J. Brown (Eds.), *Contact and conflict in intergroup encounters* (pp. 1–44). Oxford: Blackwell.

Hewstone, M., Hassebrauck, M., Wirth, A., & Waenke, M. (1995). *Mediation of stereotype change via perceived typicality of diconfirmers.* Unpublished manuscript, University of Wales, Cardiff, and University of Mannheim.

Hewstone, M., Islam, M. R., & Judd, C. M. (1993). Models of crossed categorization and intergroup relations. *Journal of Personality and Social Psychology, 64,* 779–793.

Hewstone, M., Macrae, C. N., Griffiths, R., Milne, A., & Brown, R. (1994). Cognitive models of stereotype change: (5) Measurement, development, and consequences of subtyping. *Journal of Experimental Social Psychology, 30,* 505–526.

Hogg, M. A., & Abrams, D. (1988). *Social identifications: A social psychology of intergroup relations and group processes.* London: Routledge.

Horowitz, D. (1985). *Ethnic groups in conflict.* Berkeley: University of California Press.

Insko, C. A., Pinkley, R. L., Hoyle, R. H., Dalton, B., Hong, G., Slim, R., Landry, P., Holton, B., Ruffin, P. F., & Thibaut, J. (1987). Individual–group discontinuity: The role of intergroup contact. *Journal of Experimental Social Psychology, 23,* 250–267.

Islam, M. R., & Hewstone, M. (1993a). Dimensions of contact as predictors of intergroup anxiety, percieved out-group variability, and out-group attitude:

An integrative model. *Personality and Social Psychology Bulletin, 19,* 700–710.

Islam, M. R., & Hewstone, M. (1993b). Intergroup attributions and affective consequences in majority and minority groups. *Journal of Personality and Social Psychology, 64,* 936–950.

Jackson, L. A., & Cash, T. F. (1985). Components of gender stereotypes: Their implications for inferences on stereotypic and nonstereotypic dimensions. *Personality and Social Psychology Bulletin, 11,* 326–344.

Johnson, D. W., & Johnson, R. T. (1989). *Cooperation and competition: Theory and research.* Edina, MI: Interaction.

Johnson, D. W., & Johnson, R. T. (1992). Positive interdependence: Key to effective cooperation. In R. Hertz-Lazarowitz & N. Miller (Eds.), *Interaction in cooperative groups: The theoretical anatomy of group learning* (pp. 174–199). Cambridge, UK: Cambridge University Press.

Johnston, L., & Hewstone, M. (1992). Cognitive models of stereotype change: (3) Subtyping and the perceived typicality of disconfirming group members. *Journal of Experimental Social Psychology, 28,* 360–386.

Johnston, L., & Macrae, C. N. (1994). Changing social stereotypes: The case of the information seeker. *European Journal of Social Psychology, 24,* 581–592.

Kruglanski, A. W. (1989). *Lay epistemics and human knowledge: Cognitive and motivational bases.* New York: Plenum Press.

Lewin, K. (1948). *Resolving social conflict.* New York: Harper.

Lewin, K., & Grabbe, P. (1945). Conduct, knowledge, and acceptance of new values. *Journal of Social Issues, 2,* 53–64.

Locksley, A., Ortiz, V., & Hepburn, C. (1980). Social categorization and discriminatory behavior: Extinguishing the minimal intergroup discrimination effect. *Journal of Personality and Social Psychology, 39,* 773–783.

Maquet, J. J. (1961). *The premise of inequality in Ruanda.* Oxford: Oxford University Press.

Marcus-Newhall, A., Miller, N., Holtz, R., & Brewer, M. B. (1993). Cross-cutting category membership with role assignment: A means of reducing intergroup bias. *British Journal of Social Psychology, 32,* 125–146.

Mason, P. (1970). *Race relations.* Oxford: Oxford University Press.

Maurer, K. L., Park, B., & Rothbart, M. (in press). Subtyping versus subgrouping processes in stereotype representation. *Journal of Personality and Social Psychology.*

McClendon, M. J. (1974). Interracial contact and the reduction of prejudice. *Sociological Focus, 7,* 47–65.

Messick, D. M., & Mackie, D. M. (1989). Intergroup relations. *Annual Review of Psychology, 33,* 45–81.

Migdal, M., Hewstone, M., & Mullen, B. (1995). *The impact of crossed categorization on intergroup discrimination: A meta-analysis.* Unpublished manuscript, University of Syracuse and University of Wales, Cardiff.

Miller, N., & Brewer, M. B. (1986). Social categorization theory and team learning procedures. In R. S. Feldman (Ed.), *The social psychology of education* (pp. 172–198). Cambridge, UK: Cambridge University Press.

Miller, N., Brewer, M. B., & Edwards, K. (1985). Cooperative interaction in desegegated settings: A laboratory analogue. *Journal of Social Issues, 41,* 63–81.

Miller, N., & Davidson-Podgorny, G. (1987). Theoretical models of intergroup relations and the use of cooperative teams as an intervention for desegregated settings. In C. Hendrick (Ed.), *Group processes and intergroup relations* (pp. 41–67). Beverly Hills, CA: Sage.

Miller, N., & Harrington, H. J. (1990). A model of social category salience for intergroup relations: Empirical tests of relevant variables. In P. Drenth, J. Sergeant, & R. Takens (Eds.), *European perspectives in psychology* (Vol. 3, pp. 205–220). Chichester, UK: Wiley.

Miller, N., & Harrington, H. J. (1992). Social categorization and intergroup acceptance: Principles for the design and development of cooperative learning teams. In R. Hertz-Lazarowitz & N. Miller (Eds.), *Interaction in cooperative groups: The theoretical anatomy of group learning* (pp. 203–227). Cambridge, UK: Cambridge University Press.

Mummedey, A., & Schreiber, H.-J. (1983). Better or just different? Positive social identity by discrimination against or by differentiation from outgroups. *European Journal of Social Psychology, 13,* 389–397.

Newcomb, T. M. (1961). *The acquaintance process.* New York: Holt, Rinehart & Winston.

Noblit, G. W., & Collins, T. W. (1981). Gui bono? White students in a desegregated high school. *Urban Review, 13,* 205–216.

Oakes, P. J., Haslam, A., & Turner, J. C. (1994). *Stereotyping and social reality.* Oxford: Blackwell.

Park, B., Judd, C. M., & Ryan, C. S. (1991). Social categorization and the representation of variability information. In W. Stroebe & M. Hewstone (Eds.), *European review of social psychology* (Vol. 2, pp. 211–246). Chichester, UK: Wiley.

Perdue, C. W., Dovidio, J. F., Gurtman, M. B., & Tyler, R. B. (1990). "Us" and "Them": Social categorization and the process of intergroup bias. *Journal of Personality and Social Psychology, 59,* 475–486.

Pettigrew, T. F. (1967). Social evaluation theory: Convergences and applications. In D. Levine (Ed.), *Nebraska symposium on motivation* (Vol. 15, pp. 241–311). Lincoln: University of Nebraska Press.

Pettigrew, T. F. (1973). The case for the racial integration of the schools. In O. Duff (Ed.), *Report on the future of school desegregation in the United States* (pp. 52–93). Pittsburgh: University of Pittsburgh, Consultative Resource Center on School Desegregation and Conflict.

Pettigrew, T. F. (1981). Extending the stereotype concept. In D. L. Hamilton (Ed.), *Cognitive processes in stereotyping and intergroup behavior* (pp. 301–331). Hillsdale, NJ: Erlbaum.

Pettigrew, T. F. (1986). The intergroup contact hypothesis reconsidered. In M.

Hewstone & R. Brown (Eds.), *Contact and conflict in intergroup encounters* (pp. 169–195). New York: Blackwell.

Pettigrew, T. F., & Martin, J. (1987). Shaping the organizational context for black American inclusion. *Journal of Social Issues, 43,* 41–78.

Rehm, J., Lilli, W., & Van Eimeren, B. (1988). Reduced intergroup differentiation as a result of self-categorization in overlapping categories: A quasi-experiment. *European Journal of Social Psychology, 18,* 375–379.

Riordan, C. (1978). Equal status interracial contact: A review and revision of the concept. *International Journal of Intercultural Relations, 2,* 161–185.

Rist, R. C. (1979). *Desegregated schools: Appraisals of an American experiment.* New York: Academic Press.

Rogers, M., Miller, N., & Hennigan, K. (1981). Cooperative games as an intervention to promote cross-racial acceptance. *American Education Research Journal, 18,* 513–516.

Rokeach, M. (Ed.). (1960). *The open and closed mind.* New York: Basic Books.

Rose, T. L. (1981). Cognitive and dyadic processes in intergroup contact. In D. L. Hamilton (Ed.), *Cognitive processes in stereotyping and intergroup behavior* (pp. 259–302). Hillsdale, NJ: Erlbaum.

Rothbart, M. (1981). Memory processes and social beliefs. In D. L. Hamilton (Ed.), *Cognitive processes in stereotyping and intergroup behavior* (pp. 145–181). Hillsdale, NJ: Erlbaum.

Rothbart, M., & John, O. P. (1985). Social categorization and behavioral episodes: A cognitive analysis of the effects of intergroup contact. *Journal of Social Issues, 41,* 81–104.

Rothbart, M., & John, O. P. (1993). Intergroup relations and stereotype change: A social-cognitive analysis and some longitudinal findings. In P. M. Sniderman, P. E. Tetlock, & E. G. Carmines (Eds.), *Prejudice, politics and the American dilemma* (pp. 32–58). Stanford, CA: Stanford University Press.

Rothbart, M., & Lewis, S. (1988). Inferring category attributes from exemplar attributes: Geometric shapes and social categories. *Journal of Personality and Social Psychology, 55,* 861–872.

Rothbart, M., & Park, B. (1986). On the confirmability and disconfirmability of trait concepts. *Journal of Personality and Social Psychology, 50,* 131–141.

Sagar, H. A., & Schofield, J. W. (1984). Integrating the desegregated school: Problems and possibilities. In M. Maehr & D. Bartz (Eds.), *Advances in motivation and achievement: A research manual* (pp. 203–242). Greenwich, CT: JAI Press.

Saharso, S. (1989). Ethnic identity and the paradox of equality. In J. P. van Oudenhoven & T. M. Willemsen (Eds.), *Ethnic minorities: Social psychological perspectives* (pp. 97–114). Amsterdam: Swets & Zeitlinger.

Schofield, J. W. (1978). School desegregation and intergroup attitudes. In D. Bar-Tal & L. Saxe (Eds.), *Social psychology of education: Theory and research* (pp. 330–363). Washington, DC: Halsted Press.

Schofield, J. W. (1979). The impact of positively structured contact on intergroup behaviour: Does it last under adverse conditions? *Social Psychology Quarterly, 42,* 280–284.

Schofield, J. W. (1981). Uncharted territory: Desegregation and organizational innovation. *The Urban Review, 13,* 227–242.

Schofield, J. W. (1986). Causes and consequences of the colorblind perspective. In J. F. Dovidio & S. L. Gaertner (Eds.), *Prejudice, discrimination, and racism* (pp. 231–254). Orlando, FL: Academic Press.

Schofield, J. W. (1989). *Black and white in school: Trust, tension, or tolerance?* New York: Teachers College Press.

Schofield, J. W. (1991). School desegregation and intergroup relations: A review of the literature. In G. Grant (Ed.), *Review of research in education* (Vol. 17, pp. 335–409). Washington, DC: American Educational Research Association.

Schofield, J. W., & McGivern, E. (1979). Changing interracial bonds in a desegregated school. In R. G. Blumberg & W. J. Roye (Eds.), *Interracial bonds* (pp. 106–119). New York: General Hall.

Schofield, J. W., & Sagar, H. A. (1977). Peer interaction patterns in an integrated middle school. *Sociometry, 40,* 130–138.

Sharan, S. (Ed.). (1990). *Cooperative learning: Theory and research.* New York: Praeger.

Sherif, M. (1966). *Group conflict and cooperation.* London: Routledge & Kegan Paul.

Sherif, M., & Sherif, C. W. (1965). Research on intergroup relations. In O. Klineberg & R. Christie (Eds.), *Perspectives in social psychology.* New York: Holt, Rinehart & Winston.

Slavin, R. E. (1985). Cooperative learning: Applying contact theory in desegregated schools. *Journal of Social Issues, 41,* 45–62.

Smith, E. R. (1992). The role of exemplars in social judgment. In L. L. Martin & A. Tesser (Eds.), *The construction of social judgments* (pp. 107–132). Hillsdale, NJ: Erlbaum.

Srull, T. K. (1981). Person memory: Some tests of associative storage and retrieval models. *Journal of Experimental Psychology: Human Learning and Memory, 7,* 440–463.

St. John, N. H. (1975). *School desegregation: Outcomes for children.* New York: Wiley.

Stephan, W. G. (1978). School desegregation: An evaluation of predictions made in *Brown v. Board of Education. Psychological Bulletin, 85,* 217–238.

Stephan, W. G. (1985). Intergroup relations. In G. Lindzey & E. Aronson (Eds.), *Handbook of social psychology* (3rd ed., Vol. 2, pp. 599–658). New York: Random House.

Stephan, W. G. (1987). The contact hypothesis in intergroup relations. In C. Hendrick (Ed.), *Group processes and intergroup relations: Review of personality and social psychology* (Vol. 9, pp. 13–40). Newbury Park, CA: Sage.

Stephan, W. G., & Stephan, C. W. (1984). The role of ignorance in intergroup relations. In N. Miller, & M. B. Brewer (Eds.), *Group in contact: The psychology of desegregation* (pp. 229–255). New York: Academic Press.

Stephen, W. G., & Stephan, C. W. (1985). Intergroup anxiety. *Journal of Social Issues, 41*, 157–175.

Stephenson, G. M. (1981). Intergroup bargaining and negotiation. In J. C. Turner & H. Giles (Eds.), *Intergroup behavior* (pp. 168–198). Oxford: Blackwell.

Tajfel, H. (1959). Quantitative judgement in social perception. *British Journal of Psychology, 50*, 16–29.

Tajfel, H. (Ed.). (1978). *Differentiation between social groups.* London: Academic Press.

Tajfel, H. (1981). Social stereotypes and social groups. In J. C. Turner & H. Giles (Eds.), *Intergroup behaviour* (pp. 144–167). Oxford: Blackwell.

Tajfel, H. (1982). Social psychology of intergroup relations. *Annual Review of Psychology, 33*, 1–39.

Tajfel, H., & Turner, J. C. (1979). An integrative theory of intergroup conflict. In W. G. Austin & S. Worchel (Eds.), *The social psychology of intergroup relations* (pp. 33–47). Monterey, CA: Brooks/Cole.

Taylor, D. M., & Simard, L. (1979). Ethnic identity and intergroup relations. In D. J. Lee (Ed.), *Emerging ethnic boundaries.* Ottawa: University of Ottawa Press.

Taylor, S. E. (1981). A categorization approach to stereotyping. In D. L. Hamilton (Ed.), *Cognitive processes in stereotyping and intergroup behavior* (pp. 83–114). Hillsdale, NJ: Erlbaum.

Triandis, H. C. (1988). The future of pluralism revisited. In P. A. Katz & D. A. Taylor (Eds.), *Eliminating racism: Profiles in controversy* (pp. 31–50). New York: Plenum Press.

Turner, J. C. (1981). The experimental social psychology of intergroup behavior. In J. C. Turner & H. Giles (Eds.), *Intergroup behaviour* (pp. 1–32). Oxford: Blackwell.

Turner, J. C. (1987). *Rediscovering the social group: A self-categorization theory.* Cambridge, UK: Cambridge University Press.

Vanbeselaere, N. (1987). The effect of dichotomous and crossed social categorizations upon intergroup discrimination. *European Journal of Social Psychology, 17*, 143–156.

Vanbeselaere, N. (1991). The different effects of simple and crossed categorizations: A result of the category differentiation process or of differential category salience? In W. Stroebe & M. Hewstone (Eds.), *European review of social psychology* (Vol. 2, pp. 247–278). Chichester, UK: Wiley.

Van Knippenberg, A. (1984). Intergroup differences in group perceptions. In H. Tajfel (Ed.), *The social dimension: European developments in social psychology* (Vol. 2, pp. 560–578). Cambridge, UK: Cambridge University Press.

Van Oudenhoven, J. P., Groenewoud, J. T., & Hewstone, M. (1995). Cooperation, ethnic salience and generalization of interethnic attitudes. *European Journal of Social Psychology, 25*, 1–13.

Van Oudenhoven, J. P., & Willemsen, T. M. (Eds.). (1989). *Ethnic minorities: Social psychological perspectives.* Amsterdam: Swets & Zeitlinger.

Vivian, J., Brown, R., & Hewstone, M. (1995). Changing attitudes through intergroup contact: The effects of group membership salience. Manuscript under review.

Vivian, J., Hewstone, M., & Brown, R. J. (in press). Intergroup contact: Theoretical and empirical developments. In R. Ben-Ari & Y. Rich (Eds.), *Understanding and enhancing education for diverse students: An international perspective.* Ramat Gan, Israel: Bar-Ilan University Press.

Warring, D., Johnson, D. W., Maruyama, G., & Johnson, R. (1985). Impact of different types of cooperative learning on cross-ethnic and cross-sex relationships. *Journal of Educational Psychology, 77,* 53–59.

Weber, R., & Crocker, J. (1983). Cognitive processes in the revision of stereotypic beliefs. *Journal of Personality and Social Psychology, 45,* 961–977.

Weber-Kollmann, R. (1985). *Subtyping: The development and consequences of differentiated categories for stereotyped groups.* Unpublished doctoral dissertation, Northwestern University, Evanston, IL.

Wegner, D. M. (1989). *White bears and other unwanted thoughts: Suppression, obsession, and the psychology of mental control.* New York: Viking Press.

Werth, J. L., & Lord, C. G. (1992). Previous conceptions of the typical group member and the contact hypothesis. *Basic and Applied Social Psychology, 13,* 351–369.

White, R. M., & Zsambok, C. (1994). Biases in memory for and use of inconsistent beliefs in stereotyping. *British Journal of Social Psychology, 33,* 243–258.

Wilder, D. A. (1984). Intergroup contact: The typical member and the exception to the rule. *Journal of Experimental Social Psychology, 20,* 177–194.

Wilder, D. A. (1986a). Cognitive factors affecting the success of intergroup contact. In S. Worchel & W. G. Austin (Eds.), *Psychology of intergroup relations* (pp. 49–66). Chicago: Nelson-Hall.

Wilder, D. A. (1986b). Social categorization: Implications for creation and reduction of intergroup bias. In L. Berkowitz (Ed.), *Advances in experimental social psychology* (Vol. 19, 293–355). New York: Academic Press.

Wilder, D. A. (1993a). The role of anxiety in facilitating stereotypic judgment of outgroup behavior. In D. M. Mackie & D. L. Hamilton (Eds.), *Affect, cognition, and stereotyping: Interactive processes in group perception* (pp. 87–109). San Diego: Academic Press.

Wilder, D. A. (1993b). Freezing intergroup evaluations: Anxiety fosters resistance to counterstereotypic information. In M. A. Hogg & D. Abrams (Eds.), *Group motivation: Social psychological perspectives* (pp. 68–86). Hemel Hempstead, UK: Havester Wheatsheaf.

Wilder, D. A., & Shapiro, P. N. (1989). Role of competition-induced anxiety in limiting the beneficial impact of positive behavior by an out-group member. *Journal of Personality and Social Psychology, 56,* 60–69.

Wilder, D. A., & Thompson, J. G. (1980). Intergroup contact with independent manipulations of ingroup and outgroup interaction. *Journal of Personality and Social Psychology, 38,* 589–603.

Wilder, D. A., & Thompson, J. E. (1988). Assimilation and contrast effects in the judgement of groups. *Journal of Personality and Social Psychology, 54,* 62–73.

Williams, R. M. (1964). *Strangers next door: Ethnic relations in American communities.* Englewood Cliffs, NJ: Prentice-Hall.

Wilner, D. M., Walkley, R., & Cook, S. W. (1955). *Human relations in interracial housing: A study of the contact hypothesis.* Minneapolis: University of Minnesota Press.

11

Motivating Individuals to Change: What Is a Target to Do?

JENNIFER L. EBERHARDT
SUSAN T. FISKE

> The choice is between initiating some form of
> action on a limited scale or waiting until—
> miraculously—prejudice and discrimination
> disappear from our social scene.
> —TAJFEL (1981, p. 186)

The highest ranking female police officer in a large city in the southern United States wanted to know what advice social psychologists have for her. She described how her peers and supervisors had resisted her advancement at every turn. They consistently teased, tormented, and undervalued her. Once, her unit had even encouraged her to lead them into a life-threatening situation with "We're right behind you," only to abandon her completely without backup. "Can the stereotyping research tell me how to get a fair shake?" she asked. Abashed, the social psychologist admitted that the research had lots of implications, but these had not really been spelled out at the individual level. This chapter is therefore dedicated to seeing how well we can answer the question raised by this woman and by many other potential targets of stereotyping. This chapter focuses on processes that cut across many specific out-groups (elsewhere, Eberhardt & Fiske, 1994, stress some important differences between, for example, gender and race stereotypes). Given decades of research on stereotyping, do we know how one person can make a difference? How can a single individual take the resources personally available and motivate other individual people within a particular organization to change their treatment of at least that individual? In short, how is it that targets of stereotypes might promote one-on-one change?

Answering the police officer's question requires some background, so the bulk of this chapter is devoted to an overview of ideas about motivation and stereotyping. Both individual-level and group-level theories matter, but with an eye to each theory's implications for change, especially individual change. (Others, such as Fiske & Glick, 1995, and Hewstone, Chapter 10, this volume, examine group-level change.) Oddly, targets of stereotyping have not been studied as potential change agents. Nevertheless, social psychological theories do have implications for tactics available to targets. Thus, finally, we will get around to providing some advice to the police officer, admitting also the limits of what one individual alone can do.

MOTIVATION AND STEREOTYPING: SOME HISTORICAL PRECEDENTS AND CONTEMPORARY APPROACHES

Social psychology provides no generic or comprehensive theory of prejudice and stereotyping (Pettigrew, 1986). Instead, there are many theories, each focusing on a slightly different aspect of the problem. At best, researchers have attempted to develop integrative frameworks that capture the common theoretical and methodological conceptions of these different formulations across time (Ashmore & Del Boca, 1976, 1981; Brown, 1995; Duckitt, 1992a; Leyens, Yzerbyt, & Schadron, 1994). This section outlines a few influential theories that capture major trends in conceptions of stereotyping and prejudice over the last 40 years. The motivational aspects of each theory are salient for our purposes.

Each theory claims its own primary level of analysis. Some theories examine individual differences in prejudice and stereotyping. Others highlight the stereotyping and prejudice involved in intergroup contexts. But each has clear implications for individual stereotype change and prejudice reduction, some implying that change is practically impossible, and some prescribing change strategies. Changes in social climate dictate the popularity of theories that focus on individual differences as compared to intergroup relations (Duckitt, 1992a). Neither level of analysis defeats the other nor, fortunately, do they preclude each other.

Targets, hence, should develop sensitivity to both the individual person and the intergroup situation.

In examining the motivational side of theories at a variety of levels of analysis, one discovers a singular asymmetry that might disconcert our beleaguered police officer. Virtually all the theories describe racial and ethnic stereotypes. Analysis of gender stereotypes did not begin in earnest until the late 1970s, sparked by the women's movement and by the entrance of more women into social psychology, both of which coincided with the cognitive revolution in psychology. Hence, cognitive theories have been assumed to apply to the stereotyping of women, and have been abundantly tested therein, however with scant attention to motivational issues (but see Fiske & Stevens, 1993; Glick & Fiske, in press). Most prior theories of stereotyping have had little to say about gender. We will import gender where we can because traditionally it has been missed.

Individual Differences

Three influential theories focus on individual differences in prejudice and stereotyping: the theory of the authoritarian personality, developed in the early 1950s; the theory of modern racism, developed in the 1970s; and the dissociation model of prejudice, developed in the 1990s.

The Authoritarian Personality Theory (1950s)

Theory. The unprecedented and unthinkable tragedies of the Holocaust sparked a vigorous search to uncover a correlative personality type capable of such massive acts of brutality. Adorno, Frenkel-Brunswik, Levinson, and Sanford's (1950) theory of the authoritarian personality promised to expose the roots of prejudice and anti-Semitism. From an array of fixed-alternative questionnaires, in-depth interviews, and projective tests emerged the personality type prone to prejudice and afflicted with a dangerous psychological syndrome. Adorno and colleagues found symptoms characterizing the authoritarian: strict adherence to middle-class conventions, acts of aggression against those who do not live by conventional norms, blind submission to authority, and stereotypy (the tendency to think in rigid categories).

According to Adorno et al. (1950), the syndrome develops from interactions with parents who, because of severe status anxiety, adopt authoritarian childrearing strategies. The role of parent becomes one of domination; the role of child becomes one of obedience, conformity, submission, and unquestioned respect for parental authority. The children of these strict disciplinarians learn to repress the anger they harbor toward their parents, and these unconscious, unacceptable impulses are projected onto out-group members.

Unacceptable expressions of anger and fear become acceptable when directed toward safe out-group targets who seemingly deserve mistreatment. Thus, for the authoritarian, Jews become stereotyped as personally offensive, socially threatening, too seclusive, and too intrusive, and Blacks are best segregated into menial jobs. Authoritarians cannot handle ambivalence; they can only perceive others as bad people about whom they feel negatively or good people about whom they feel positively. As they denigrate out-groups, authoritarians glorify the parents who nurtured the hostility and prejudice that now consumes them.

Thus, the authoritarian personality develops from an unconscious, intrapsychic conflict. The need to express aggressive impulses and the reality of the costs involved in directing these impulses at the parental source create a tension that is resolved through displacing negative impulses onto out-group members and subsequently rationalizing this displacement.

Adorno et al.'s (1950) pioneering research on the authoritarian personality sparked the interests of many social scientists, who produced volumes of research findings on the topic (e.g., Harding, Proshansky, Kutner, & Chein, 1969; Katz, 1976). However, this enthusiasm was short-lived, as both methodological and conceptual problems soon became apparent (Brown, 1965; Hyman & Sheatsley, 1954), for example, low internal consistency across items and response set biases favoring acquiescence (Christie, 1991).

Yet methodological and conceptual problems were not solely responsible for the increasingly pessimistic attitudes regarding the theory's ability to explain prejudice. In general, theories influenced by psychodynamic principles became less fashionable in social psychology (Stroebe & Insko, 1989). Moreover, partly as a result of the 1960s civil rights movement in the United States (Duckitt, 1992a), the focus began to shift from a concern with the effects of individual differences on the propensity for stereotyping and prejudice, to sociocultural issues, such as the institutionalized segregation of Blacks and Whites in the southern United States.

Moreover, individual-level theories could not explain societal or regional differences in prejudice. People tended to score higher in prejudice in some regions than in others (Pettigrew, 1959). Furthermore, prejudice was not correlated strongly with authoritarianism in regions such as South Africa or the southern United States (Pettigrew, 1958). These limitations, coupled with unrelenting methodological and conceptual problems, contributed to the rapid decline in popularity of the authoritarian personality theory.

However, interest revived recently, due chiefly to a creative research program led by Altemeyer (1981, 1988). Altemeyer and colleagues eradicated many of the conceptual and methodological snags by restricting the symptoms of the authoritarian personality construct to the three that covary most highly (authoritarian submission to authority, authoritarian aggression, and conventionalism) and by developing a sound instrument to measure the syndrome (the Right Wing Authoritarian Scale).

Although the name of the scale implies a strong correlation between authoritarianism and conservatism, Altemeyer does not make this general claim (Altemeyer, 1988). Because conservatism is defined differently across regions (e.g., he compares Canadian and American samples), he does not use political party affiliation to predict authoritarianism. In contrast, inspired by the link between German Fascism and anti-Semitism, Adorno et al. (1950) expected authoritarianism and political conservatism to be highly correlated. The correlation between authoritarian personality and American conservatism (for the most part conceptualized as strong attachment to the status quo) indeed was in the predicted direction but relatively weak. Subsequent researchers have reported positive correlations as well (Altemeyer, 1981; Comrey & Newmeyer, 1965; Wilson, 1973). Yet, as Altemeyer (1988) notes, regional and societal differences may alter the strength of the relationship between conservatism and authoritarianism.

Applications to Gender. Work on the authoritarian personality has almost exclusively encompassed race and ethnicity. However, the authoritarian personality theoretically finds unacceptable other impulses besides aggression. Many of the original scale items relate to intolerance of sexuality, especially nontraditional sexuality. This has obvious implications for its relationship to homophobia, implications all but unexplored as far as we know (but see Bierly, 1985; Fiske, Canfield, & Von Hendy, 1994). It also has implications for ambivalence toward women, essentially contrasting the idealized mother with women who elicit strong sexual feelings. Frenkel-Brunswik described a pattern prevalent in high scorers on the ethnocentrism scale, "underlying disrespect-and-resentment toward the opposite sex, typically combined with pseudo-admiration" (Adorno et al., 1950, p. 391). A scale of authoritarian attitudes toward women followed this insight (Nadler & Morrow, 1959), but to our knowledge was not much used. However, its positively correlated scales assessing simultaneous chivalry and open subordination of women reappears in a more recent scale of ambivalent sexism, described later (Glick & Fiske, in press).

Implications for Change. If one accepts Adorno et al.'s (1950) theory of the authoritarian personality, one must also accept the potential for promoting stereotype change and reducing prejudice as minimal. Changing the prejudiced individual would require extensive psychotherapy. Yet, individuals who could most benefit from psychotherapeutic techniques would be least likely to seek them out. Authoritarians are not introspective. By definition, they cannot deal with the ambivalent feelings that introspection would render more salient. They view physical suffering as more real than psychological suffering. Authoritarians idealize the self and in-group; any problems are caused by out-group members or other external forces. The prejudices that authoritarians hold toward out-group members seem to them well justified; they are not problematic perceptions that require therapeutic assistance to alter. According to the theory, their cognitive flexibility is limited. Precisely because authoritarians cannot handle ambiguity in general, or the conflicting feelings about their parents in particular, they are engaged in unconscious, intrapsychic conflict in the first place. The rigidity, which allows them to resist altering negative stereotypes in the face of conflicting evidence, also makes it likely that they will resist psychotherapeutic intervention, much less intervention attempts by a coworker (and especially by a subordinate).

Modern Racism Theory (1970s)

Theory. Just as social scientists searching for the cause of prejudice at the individual level were disillusioned quickly, so were those who had begun searching at the sociocultural level. The civil rights movement dramatically altered sociostructural factors in the United States, yet racial prejudice remained. Changes initially thought to presage the disappearance of inequality resulted merely in more subtle expressions of racial bias (Crosby, Bromley, & Saxe, 1980; Dovidio & Gaertner, 1986; Pettigrew, 1979, 1985).

Not only had U.S. laws changed in the 1960s, racial attitudes appeared to be changing as well. Racial attitudes had begun to change in the 1940s, as the World War II horrors of Nazi Germany became known and as mounting evidence discredited biological theories of racial differences (Bobo, 1988; Schuman, Steeh, & Bobo, 1985; Sears, 1988). On the home front, Whites in public opinion polls began to show a decline in their acceptance of negative stereotypes about Blacks (Campbell, 1971; Greeley & Sheatsley, 1971). By the 1970s, White support for overt discrimination against Blacks in voting rights, public accommodation, employment, and housing had drastically declined (Kinder, 1986; Schuman et al., 1985). This shift in views, coupled with the legal changes brought about during the 1960s civil rights movement, led to a change in the social norms dictating the expression of racial stereotypes. Overt racism was disappearing from American society.

Yet anti-Black feeling and racial conflict continued (McConahay, 1986). Although White Americans were forced to comply with newly created laws, many did not (and some would argue, have yet to) fully internalize egalitarian standards. Gaertner and Dovidio (1986) describe this anti-Black feeling "not as hostility or hate. Instead, this negativity involves discomfort, uneasiness, disgust, and sometimes fear, which would tend to motivate avoidance rather than intentionally destructive behaviors" (p. 63). In fact, although support for negative racial stereotypes has been decreasing, support for post-civil-rights policies designed to bring about greater racial integration and to reduce inequality (e.g., busing, affirmative action) has not been increasing (Pettigrew, 1985).

In the 1970s, this new expression of racial bias was termed "symbolic racism" (Sears & Kinder, 1971; Sears & McConahay, 1973) and later described as "modern racism" by McConahay (McConahay & Hough, 1976). The Modern Racism Scale indirectly measures individual differences in racial attitudes. So, after close to two decades of neglect, the individual reappeared as a legitimate level of analysis.

Because this new form of racism is subtle and indirect, it is marked by attitudes that differ from traditional prejudice. By definition, modern racists believe Blacks are unfairly pushing themselves into places where they are not wanted and gaining undeserved attention and status. Modern racists do not acknowledge more subtle, post-civil-rights forms of prejudice and discrimination; they do not consider their own attitudes as racist; and they believe that discrimination is a thing of the past (McConahay, 1986). Whereas modern racists support laws against blatant discrimination, they simultaneously endorse such statements as "Over the past few years, the government and news media have shown more respect for Blacks than they deserve" or "Blacks are getting too demanding in their push for equal rights."

Modern racism is defined as "the expression in terms of abstract ideological symbols and symbolic behaviors of the feeling that blacks are violating cherished values and making illegitimate demands for changes in the racial status quo" (McConahay & Hough, 1976, p. 38). The abstract symbols used to express anti-Black feeling are those associated with conservatism and the Protestant ethic. From the perspective of the modern racist, to endorse such statements as "Over the past few years, Blacks have gotten more economically than they deserve," is to endorse "self-reliance" and "individualism" rather than to express anti-Black sentiment.

Modern racism is measured by a scale that accomplishes nonreactivity by disguising the link to racial prejudice. A nonracial explanation can be offered for one's responses to each item. For example, ambivalent people can explain their agreement with the item "Over the past few years, Blacks have gotten more economically than they deserve" in terms of the race-neutral principles of justice and fair play. The more often one's ambivalence is resolved in policy directions detrimental to Blacks, the higher one's score on the scale.

Although the Modern Racism Scale has been used widely by social psychologists as an individual difference measure, some researchers have disagreed with central aspects of the theory embodied by the scale (Bobo, 1983; Sniderman & Piazza, 1993; Sniderman, Piazza, Tetlock, & Kendrick, 1991; Sniderman & Tetlock, 1986; Sniderman, Tetlock, Carmines, & Peterson, 1993; Weigel & Howes, 1985). They argue, for instance, that modern racism theorists fail to recognize the continuing significance of overt racism, and that they detect covert racism in resistance to social policies that have as much to do with the role of government assistance as with negative affect directed at Blacks (Sniderman & Piazza, 1993; Sniderman et al., 1993).

Nevertheless, McConahay and other researchers have shown that modern racism predicts anti-Black feeling (McConahay & Hough, 1976), anti-Black voting behavior (McConahay & Hough, 1976; Sears & Kinder, 1971), social distance preferences (cf. Hardee & McConahay, 1981), and job applicant evaluations when race is an issue (McConahay, 1983). Thus, they argue that some form of racial sentiment is clearly being tapped (McConahay, Hardee, & Batts, 1981).

Although modern racism emerged in the midst of drastic changes in public racial sentiment, it shares some core characteristics with the "old-fashioned" racism depicted in the authoritarian personality type. Both modern racists and authoritarians are attached to the racial status quo, use their commitment to traditionally conservative values to rationalize their position, and react negatively to out-groups such as Blacks, whom they perceive to be violating conventional standards.

Moreover, as is the case for the authoritarian personality type, modern racists are thought to exhibit prejudice because of an unconscious, intrapsychic conflict. The conflict for the authoritarian arises from deep-seated ambivalent feelings toward the parents. The ambivalence experienced by modern racists arises from "a conflict between negative affect toward blacks and the person's values, cognitions, and/or need to maintain a positive/nonprejudiced self-image" (McConahay, 1986, p. 99). Anti-Black affect is not due to personal experience with Blacks or to direct competition, "threats to the good life" (Kinder & Sears, 1981). Negative affect is learned in early childhood socialization, is deeply embedded, and thus is difficult to change. Because the expression of anti-Black feelings is discouraged in the current social climate, modern racists do not necessarily acknowledge even to themselves the negative feelings they harbor toward Blacks. They express this negative affect in racially ambiguous situations only: when the norms for behaving in a nonprejudiced manner are not clearly defined, when they do not recognize that racial prejudice may be influencing their reactions, and when nonracial explanations for their reactions are readily available.

A primary distinction between the "old-fashioned" authoritarian and the modern racist is that authoritarians recognize and openly express their negative racial sentiment, whereas modern racists do not. Just as acknowledging ambivalent feelings toward the parents poses a ·psychological threat to authoritarians, acknowledging ambivalent feelings toward Blacks poses a threat to modern racists' nonprejudiced self-image. Whereas the repression of ambivalent feelings is fueled by family dynamics for the old-fashioned authoritarian, it is fueled by societal norms for modern racists.

Applications to Gender. Modern racism has been applied exclusively to Whites' reactions to Blacks. Recently, researchers have begun to discuss comparable forms of modern sexism, as sexist attitudes have moved from general social acceptance to more subtle, covert forms (Ashmore, Del Boca, & Bilder, 1994). Tougas, Brown, Beaton, and Joly (1995) and Swim, Aikin, Hall, and Hunter (1995) have simultaneously and independently developed modern sexism (or "neosexism") scales tapping perceptions that women are getting more than they deserve, are pushing themselves where they are not wanted, or are moving too fast— essentially items reworded from racism to sexism. Neosexism (Tougas, Brown, Beaton, & Joly, 1995) predicts opposition to affirmative action for women, just as modern racism predicts opposition to policies that benefit Blacks. Modern sexism (Swim et al., 1995) predicts preference for a male over a female senatorial candidate, just as modern racism predicts race-based voting preferences.

Although the parallels are a useful starting point, some would argue that people still are less fearful of and offended about being labeled "sexist" than they are about being labeled "racist" (Fiske & Stevens,

1993), so the parallels between modern sexism and racism are not complete. Moreover, the motivational basis for sexism and racism differs. As noted, the motivational basis for modern racism consists in the tension between anti-Black feelings and egalitarian norms. In modern sexism, egalitarian norms are less motivationally important than people's inherent and traditional ambivalence about women. For men, according to a theory of ambivalent sexism (Glick & Fiske, in press), three motives contribute: (1) paternalism, with its protective and dominative elements; (2) gender identity, with its complementary and competitive implications; and (3) heterosexual attraction, with its intimacy-seeking and hostility-potentiating sides. These three motives, each ambivalent in its own terms, result in correlated but affectively opposite dimensions of hostile and benevolent sexism. The separable dimensions of ambivalent sexism empirically predict stereotyping of women and theoretically predict both subtypes of women and corresponding subtypes of sexual harassment (Fiske & Glick, 1995).

Implications for Change. On the surface, the hopes for changing modern racists and sexists are just as dismal as the hopes for changing old-fashioned authoritarians. Modern bigots, for the most part, are unaware of the conflict they experience between negative affect and values. Furthermore, their anti-Black (or antifemale) affect theoretically is acquired early in childhood, is deep-seated, and is difficult to change.

Yet change indeed is possible for modern racists and sexists. Because the present social climate demands that they behave in a nonracist manner (and to some extent, a nonsexist manner), cognitive consistency pressures may push modern racists and sexists to bring lingering negative feelings into line with the egalitarian behaviors that they must exhibit. McConahay (1986) states that "there are grounds for limited optimism about the long-range future so long as the norm that 'nice people can't be racists and racists can't be nice people' establishes the climate for creative ambivalence" (p. 123). Research based on other theories (contact hypothesis and power relations) in a later section will further demonstrate the impact of changing norms.

The Dissociation Model (1990s)

Theory. The dissociation model developed by Devine and colleagues represents an even more contemporary individual-level approach to prejudice and stereotyping (Devine, 1989, 1995; Devine & Monteith, 1993). In the dissociation model, Devine (1989) draws a distinction between cultural stereotypes and personal beliefs. Devine argues that although most White Americans know about cultural stereotypes regarding Black Americans, some White Americans endorse these stereotypes (high prejudice), whereas others do not (low prejudice).

The dissociation model hinges on distinctions between the mental processing of social stereotypes as opposed to personal beliefs. Cultural stereotypes are automatically activated and processed, whereas personal beliefs are subject to controlled processing. The automaticity of cultural stereotypes arises from a long history of activation. Because stereotypes regarding Blacks exist in American society (and have for centuries), most White Americans as children gain knowledge of these stereotypes, as a part of being socialized into American culture. Devine (1989) argues that because White Americans gain knowledge of these stereotypes at such a young age, (1) they do not have the ability to evaluate critically the validity of the stereotypes as they learn them, (2) they begin to access these stereotypes across many situations, and (3) due to repeated activations, they begin to process the stereotypes automatically over time. The fact that cultural stereotypes are processed automatically means that they are spontaneously activated, are unintentional, and require no conscious effort.

White Americans may later form personal beliefs that are incongruent with cultural stereotypes; however, these beliefs are not accompanied by a long history of activations and are therefore accessed by the complex, inferential reasoning strategies of controlled processing. As White Americans grow older, they may begin endorsing notions of equality rather than endorsing the cultural stereotypes with which they have become most familiar. However, accessing personal beliefs in racial equality is intentional; it requires time, effort, cognitive capacity, and active attention.

Many Whites make conscious attempts to internalize nonprejudiced values and egalitarian norms. However, these efforts are not always immediately accompanied by overt behaviors consistent with these values (Devine & Monteith, 1993; Devine, Monteith, Zuwerink, & Elliot, 1991; Monteith, 1993; Monteith, Devine, & Zuwerink, 1993). This, in effect, establishes an intrapsychic conflict. However, the conflict that Devine and colleagues describe is between beliefs about how one should behave toward out-group members such as Blacks and beliefs about how one would actually behave toward these people. These should-would discrepancies generate negative affect for both high- and low-prejudiced individuals. For those whose egalitarian values are well internalized (i.e., they view these values as central to their self-concepts and are committed to responding consistently with them), discrepancies produce guilt and deliberate attempts to bring actual responses into line with ideal responses, and thus to reduce prejudice. For those whose egalitarian values come from external sources, discrepancies produce anger at out-groups.

The dissociation model resembles the modern racism idea: Both recognize that negative feelings and beliefs about out-group members are learned early in childhood, that people do not always act in ways consistent with their nonprejudiced standards, that people sometimes express prejudice unintentionally, and that people differ in their internalization of nonprejudiced values.

Yet the dissociation model departs from modern racism theory in some fundamental ways. First, according to the dissociation model, both high- and low-prejudiced people are well aware of the conflict they experience between their actual behaviors and their personal beliefs (Devine & Monteith, 1993; Devine et al., 1991). According to modern racism theory, only those high in prejudice experience a conflict; the conflict is between negative affect and values and is, for the most part, unconscious. Also, modern racism theory focuses more on highly prejudiced politically conservative subjects who attempt to resolve their internal conflict by appealing to abstract political and social issues. The dissociation model highlights the manner in which subjects low in prejudice resolve their conflict through self-regulatory processes that tend to decrease prejudice (for a more comprehensive review of self-regulation of prejudice, see Bodenhausen & Macrae, Chapter 7, this volume).

Applications to Gender. The dissociation model has been applied broadly to reactions to women (Klinger & Beall, 1992, as cited by Devine, 1995) and homosexuals (Devine et al., 1991; Monteith, 1993; Monteith et al., 1993), as well as to Blacks. The proposed theoretical mechanisms are assumed to be the same regardless of target group.

Implications for Change. The possibilities for changing prejudiced responses are great for individuals with well-internalized egalitarian values. Those values trigger a self-regulatory process that enables low-prejudice people to reduce prejudice. After making a conscious and deliberate choice to live by egalitarian principles, one may still behave in ways that are inconsistent with these values, because the activation of social stereotypes is so well-learned and automatic (Devine, 1989). However, acknowledging these discrepancies allows one to begin to reduce prejudice. Those with highly internalized nonprejudiced values will use the negative affect generated through acknowledging their discrepancies to reduce prejudiced responses (Devine & Monteith, 1993; Monteith, 1993). Specifically, negative affect inhibits social stereotypes that are cued automatically on categorizing the target and allows them to be replaced with belief-based responses. Through practice, low-prejudice people are able to strengthen the relationship between their belief-based response and the stimulus, while weakening the relationship between the social stereotype and the stimulus.

Summary

Three individual-level theories—authoritarian personality, modern racism, dissociation—differ significantly in their conceptualizations of stereotyping and prejudice. However, some important commonalities highlight (1) the primary focus of the theories (individual differences), (2) the motivation for stereotyping (intrapsychic conflict between personal desires/feelings/beliefs and appropriate or learned social outlets), and (3) the agent of stereotype change and prejudice reduction (the potential stereotypers themselves).

Moreover, in all of the theories, the prospects for targets motivating change and prejudice reduction are dismal. Because the motivational dynamics are intrapsychic, an acquaintance, from work, for example, is hardly in a position to intervene; only psychotherapy and close relationships might provide the long-term, secure setting in which change would occur for authoritarians, modern racists, and high-prejudice individuals. And then only if the stereotyper is motivated. Outside of committed relationships, change for those with well-internalized egalitarian norms appears promising. Change for those who have not fully internalized these norms appears rather unlikely.

Intergroup Dynamics

Whereas individual-level theories concentrate on the likelihood of particular perceptions or attitudes within individuals, group-level theories examine interactions among group members. We define "intergroup interactions" as do Tajfel and colleagues (Tajfel & Turner, 1979): interactions between members of different social groups, who perceive themselves and are perceived by others in terms of their group membership. For the purposes of this chapter, we often restrict our discussion of intergroup interactions to those between *individuals* of different groups (as opposed to interactions between whole groups or even several members of each group). Nevertheless, those individuals interact as mutually exclusive group members. In this, we have adopted the terms "stereotyper" and "target" as convenient shorthand, respectively, for a person who potentially stereotypes in this interaction and a person who is vulnerable to being stereotyped in this interaction. People may, of course, mutually stereotype, acting as stereotypers and targets simultaneously.

Initial group-level research, dating from the 1940s and persisting through the 1960s, focused on the contact hypothesis, which presumes that contact between members of different groups reduces prejudice and enhances opportunities for productive group relations, an assumption based, in part, on interpersonal attraction principles (Hewstone & Brown, 1986; Pettigrew, 1986). Contact affords people the opportunity to recognize that out-group members are similar to themselves, and that they share values and attitudes. According to the hypothesis in its more elaborated form, intergroup contact should reduce stereotyping and prejudice, at least under conditions in which the two groups actually do share values and positive initial attitudes, have equal status, and are located in stereotype-disconfirming roles. People are also more likely to change if the contact is intimate, frequent, socially or institutionally supported, and most important, if in-group and out-group members are cooperatively interdependent in the pursuit of common goals.

Looking beyond its original applications to race, the great unremarked irony in the contact literature is the failure of daily, prolonged, intimate, interdependent contact between the sexes to break down gender stereotyping and discrimination. Of course, men and women have ample contact, and of course gender stereotypes persist. Why? The ample contact between men and women often operates within prescribed roles, thus violating one of the basic requirements of successful intergroup contact. When women are brought into nontraditional roles, information about their (nonstereotypic) qualifications indeed can discourage stereotyping (Heilman, 1984; Heilman & Martell, 1986). Contact under the right circumstances can provide such disconfirmation of gender stereotypes.

Unlike many theories of stereotyping and prejudice, the contact hypothesis focuses primarily on attitude change. The central premise of the theory itself directly addresses implications for change. Contact should promote favorable intergroup attitudes. Research has qualified the initial, oversimple contact hypothesis to further a more sophisticated understanding of how and when contact works. Nevertheless, the contact hypothesis is less relevant in our current context, for it is not as such a motivational theory, and perhaps not even a theory (in its original forms; see Hewstone, Chapter 10, this volume, for an extensive treatment of the contact hypothesis). The remainder of this section therefore examines two more pertinent group-level theories of stereotyping and prejudice: social identity theory and a theory of interdependence and power relations.

Social Identity Theory (1970s)

In the 1970s, many researchers were disillusioned by the contact hypothesis that examined mid-range structural effects on prejudice and stereotyping. Some responded by re-examining individual differences (e.g., the theory of modern racism developed at this time). Others responded by remaining focused on intergroup relations, but by broadening this focus to include a greater understanding of the basic psychological processes individuals bring to these interactions, in the context of the larger society (Duckitt, 1992b). Social identity theory, developed by Tajfel, and colleagues (Tajfel, 1970, 1981, 1982; Tajfel & Turner, 1979, 1986; Turner, 1975), embodies this latter approach.

Theory. Tajfel defines "social identity" as "that part of individual self-concept that derives from knowledge of one's membership in a social group (or groups), together with the value and emotional significance attached to that membership" (1981, p. 255). According to social identity theory, stereotyping, prejudice, and discrimination result from both psychological processes and the structure of the relationship between groups. Group members are motivated to seek and maintain a positive social identity relative to other groups. Intergroup discrimination is most likely in situations that accentuate group distinctions and thus encourage social comparisons between groups.

Intergroup competition is no prerequisite to discrimination. Tajfel and Turner (1986) found that "the mere perception of belonging to two distinct groups . . . is sufficient to trigger intergroup discrimination favoring the in-group" (p. 13). Thus, intergroup biases arise from basic social categorization processes. The effect is quite robust (for a review, see Brewer, 1979). Simply assigning people to different groups in an experimental laboratory (a procedure known as the "minimal group paradigm") can lead to intergroup bias, even when these assignments are made randomly (Billig & Tajfel, 1973), arbitrarily (Turner, Sachdev, & Hogg, 1983), or on ostensibly trivial criteria (Tajfel, 1970; Tajfel, Flament, Billig, & Bundy, 1971).

Intergroup bias can take the form of evaluating in-group members more positively on a variety of trait dimensions (Doise & Sinclair, 1973; Kahn & Ryen, 1972), more positively evaluating the products created by in-group members (Rabbie & Wilkens, 1971), and allocating greater rewards to in-group members (Billig & Tajfel, 1973; Brewer & Silver, 1978; again, for a review see Brewer, 1979). Individuals distribute greater monetary rewards to members of the in-group, distribute fewer awards to out-group members, and work to maximize the difference between in-group and out-group profits (Tajfel et al., 1971). Moreover, individuals exhibit intergroup biases even at the expense of absolute monetary outcomes for the in-group or for the individual him or herself. Because intergroup boundaries are salient, individuals in this situation respond to others not as individuals but as members of a group. Interactions between individuals have become intergroup rather than interpersonal.

Intergroup bias may be prompted by group members' desires to maintain a positive social identity. Social identity is evaluated by comparing social perceptions about one's own group to social perceptions about relevant out-groups. Positive social identity is directly correlated with the number of favorable comparisons that can be made between groups on valued social dimensions.

If, on one hand, comparisons are favorable to the in-group, differences between groups may be highlighted or augmented so that social identity remains positive. Because people are motivated to make favorable comparisons, similarities between groups may lead to increased prejudice rather than a reduction in prejudice (as would be predicted by the contact hypothesis; Hewstone & Brown, 1986). As differences between groups are accentuated, differences within the out-group are downplayed, so that category membership more likely determines responses to out-group members (Tajfel, 1969; Wilder, 1978).

On the other hand, if group members have a negative social identity, they will be motivated to alter it. The strategies they employ will be determined by the structure of their relationship to the high status group. Specifically, perceptions of the legitimacy and stability of their relationship with the high status group will directly influence strategy choice. If the relationship is perceived as legitimate, low status members will attempt to exit their group by individually assimilating, a strategy that used to be called "passing." This process is an individual strategy and, as such, will not affect the status or perceptions of the group as a whole.

If the intergroup relationship is perceived as illegitimate, the low status group can implement group strategies that result in more widespread impact. Social creativity will be the strategy chosen for illegitimate relationships that low status members perceive as impossible to change. Social creativity involves attempting to achieve positive group distinctiveness through (1) changing the dimension on which social comparisons differentiate between the in-group and out-group, (2) assigning a positive value to a dimension previously thought of as negative (e.g., "Black is beautiful"), or (3) choosing for comparison another out-group that would result in a more positive group identity.

If the illegitimate relationship between the high status group and the low-status group is perceived as unstable, and therefore alterable, low status groups will directly challenge the status quo through social competition. Large-scale, organized social and political movements are examples of this strategy.

According to social identity theory, intergroup discrimination emerges from basic categorization processes. The motivation to seek and maintain a positive social identity interacts with the effect of social categorization on intergroup discrimination. Interestingly, as group members seek a positive social identity, the structure of the relationship between groups may influence the content of the social stereotypes that develop as a result. For example, Tajfel and Turner (1986) point out that whereas Black slaves in Brazil and the United States were stereotyped as "happy-go-lucky" and "child-like," when the racial status quo was threatened by the potential abolishment of slavery, social stereotypes about Blacks changed to reflect the fears that this new relationship brought with it for Whites. Blacks became stereotyped as "insolent" and "violent" (van den Berghe, 1967). Rather than attempting simply to dispel stereotypes and reduce prejudice through contact, social identity theory examines the functions that social stereotypes and group affiliations serve.

Applications to Gender. Social identity theory, sprung from Europe, has concentrated on ethnic and national identity (when not leaning on the minimal group paradigm). Only recently has it been applied to race relations in the United States. And there have been a few applications to gender, given the obvious importance of gender to social identity (Skevington & Baker, 1989). One application (Lorenzi-Cioldi, 1988, 1991) suggests that men and women are not symmetrical in their use of gender as a social identity; women, as a dominated group, rely more on their social identity contrasting men and women, whereas men, as a dominant group, rely on a more individual identity. Gender is an attribute women "have" more than do men, just as race is an attribute Blacks "have" more than do Whites (Eberhardt & Fiske, 1994).

Social-role analysis suggests that gender stereotypes reflect the division of men and women into prescribed social roles, the one more agentic or instrumental, the other more communal or social–emotional (Eagly, 1987). Gender stereotypes reflect to some extent measurable differences between the sexes, as people conform to the prescribed roles. Gender-role expectations fulfill themselves as prophecies by eliciting the predicted behavior, and gender-role performance enhances the gendered skills and abilities. Thus, gendered social identity, even if not based in a view of oneself as simply male or female, may be expressed in the paid or unpaid gender roles with which people explicitly identify. People's knowledge about gender roles, then, is a functional psychological process, just as are other uses of social identity.

Implications for Change. According to social identity theory, the underlying stereotyping process and the potential for prejudice cannot be altogether eliminated. Change, for any specific interaction, will be based on the degree of group boundary salience, which is greatly determined by broad sociostructural variables, such as perceived inequality, legitimacy, and stability of group relations. However, saliency also can be directly diminished in the more immediate social setting through re-categorization, which results from either crosscutting social categories or superordinate categories.

Social-group saliency for any one group can be decreased in the laboratory by crosscutting social categories to form subgroups (Deschamps & Doise, 1978). Relating to an ethnic or racial out-group member in terms of that person's profession or geographic origins would exemplify this. If an individual is placed in many subgroups simultaneously, loyalties to any one group will be diluted (especially if the groups have conflicting criteria for group membership), and the boundaries between "us" and "them" become less distinct.

Increasing the saliency of a more inclusive group category has also been shown to be an effective strategy for decreasing group boundary salience (Dovidio & Gaertner, 1993; Gaertner, Mann, Dovidio, Murrell, & Pomare, 1990). Relating to an out-group member as a colleague in the same field, for example, undercuts stereotyping. In creating a superordinate category, one group is created from many previously existing smaller groups, and every person is rendered an "in-group" member.

It is unclear whether either of these strategies for change (forming subgroups and superordinate groups) is practical. Both strategies have been implemented primarily in artificial groups in laboratory settings and may not replicate in real groups. Some characteristics may be too salient to alter easily. For example, crosscutting categories was much less effective in a study that examined Protestant–Catholic interactions in Northern Ireland (Commins & Lockwood, 1978). Moreover, some group identities may be too central to the self to relinquish.

Interdependence and Power Theory (1990s)

Theory. Social identity theory, along with the fieldwide explosion of social cognition approaches in the late 1970s and 1980s, paved the way for a new perspective on intergroup competition for control of resources. Earlier theories of realistic competition between groups (Levine & Campbell, 1972) took a sociological level of analysis to explain relations between waves of immigrants, focusing on blue-collar employment (Simpson & Yinger, 1985). At the individual, face-to-face level of analysis, the role of resource control had been ignored in theories of individual differences and even the face-to-face intergroup dynamics described by the contact hypothesis and social identity theory. As work progressed on the role of categorization in stereotyping (for a review, see Mackie et al., Chapter 2, this volume), it became evident that motivation to go beyond one's simple categories, that is, to stereotype or not, depends a lot on who holds the resources, that is, who depends on whom.

Social cognition approaches argued that normal processes of categorization can explain stereotyping (for examples, see Hamilton, 1981). Moreover, categorization seemed to be automatic and inevitable, projecting a dreary fatalism about the possibility of undermining stereotypes (Fiske, 1989; Jones et al., 1984). Since then, more sophisticated models of impression formation suggested that categorization is only a first, albeit relatively automatic, step. It is from this perspective that Devine's dissociation model comes, as previously described, and both Brewer (1988) and Fiske (Fiske & Pavelchak, 1986; Fiske & Neuberg, 1990) developed models of categorization and the motivation to go beyond categories to more individuated impressions. Fiske's continuum model, in particular, began to address the role of interdependence for valued resources.

According to the theory, initial categorization is the default option, and people only go beyond their categories when they have the capacity and the motivation. If people do go beyond initial categorization, they attend to the target's other, potentially individuating attributes. Attention thus is the key mediator between motivation and individuation. People cannot go beyond their stereotypes without paying attention to the other person. Attention is no guarantee of individuation; people can reconfirm their initial categories, subcategorize, or recategorize into other (negative) categories, all of which perpetuate stereotyping. But attention is a necessary condition for individuation.

One kind of motive that encourages attention and potential individuation is outcome dependency, that is, wanting resources controlled by another party. Sometimes outcome dependency is symmetrical, resulting in interdependence (mutual dependence or mutual control). In one-on-one settings, people attend to others with whom they are cooperatively (Erber & Fiske, 1984) and competitively (Ruscher & Fiske, 1990) interdependent. The motivation to be accurate is key here (Neuberg & Fiske, 1987), as interdependent people try to enhance their sense of prediction and control over their own outcomes. These principles apply equally to asymmetrical dependence, when one person controls the other's outcomes but not vice versa, again in one-on-one task settings (Stevens & Fiske, 1995).

Dependence on another encourages individuation only when people interact as individuals. When interacting as groups, competitors mutually stereotype (Ruscher, Fiske, Miki, & Van Manen, 1991), consistent with the results from the contact hypothesis and social identity theory. And when people asymmetrically depend on a homogeneous group, as opposed to a collection of individuals, they stereotype (Dépret & Fiske, 1994). People seem to believe that prediction and control can be enhanced by attending to a powerful individual who controls their outcomes, but they apparently feel that effort is useless with a powerful group, which is presumably less open to influence. This is consistent with the idea that individuating attention operates in the service of prediction and control.

People also do not attend and judge in an individuating fashion when prediction and control motivations defer to self-esteem maintenance. People apparently do not emphasize accuracy when they depend on another for an evaluation, either social–romantic (Fiske, Goodwin, Rosen, & Rosenthal, 1995) or task (Stevens & Fiske, 1995). In this instance, people's self-esteem is threatened, and they engage defensive rather than accuracy-oriented, control-enhancing motivational processes.

In purely task-oriented, individual interactions, however, people reliably attend to those who control their outcomes. Moreover, they attend to the most informative and potentially individuating cues, those inconsistent with their stereotype or prior expectancy. This suggests, then, that people are less likely to stereotype up a hierarchy; people are less likely to stereotype those powerful people who control outcomes.

This analysis also suggests the absence of accuracy motivations when people's outcomes are not controlled by others. According to a theory of stereotyping by the powerful (Fiske, 1993), the powerful are more likely to stereotype down the hierarchy. Because fewer of their outcomes are contingent on their subordinates and because people typically have more subordinates than superiors, the powerful do not attend down as much as the powerless attend up (Goodwin & Fiske, 1995; Goodwin, Fiske, & Yzerbyt, 1995). This phenomenon is mimicked by individual differences in power orientation (Goodwin & Fiske, 1995). This documented tendency of the powerful not to pay attention to their subordinates suggests that the powerful will be vulnerable to stereotyping their subordinates.

So how can one influence the powerful to individuate? If the powerful are not much influenced by outcomes controlled by their subordinates, they may be more influenced by outcomes controlled by their peers or their own superiors. The contingencies established for their career advancement (e.g., performing well for their own superiors) would follow a similar theoretical analysis as any other outcome-dependency situation; that is, the powerful person will attend to those who control relevant outcomes and resources. A chief executive officer who comes from an out-group may not be so easily stereotyped.

Besides their own dependency, the powerful may be influenced by perceived standards, either internal or external. If the powerful person's own superiors make outcomes and resources contingent on specific standards (e.g., the ability to nurture subordinates from underrepresented groups), the powerful person will attempt to meet the criteria. But the standards need not be provided by the powerful person's own superiors. For example, the tendency of the powerful not to attend to their subordinates can be reduced by their own previous public endorsement of consensual egalitarian norms (Goodwin & Fiske, 1995). Similarly, some people in positions of power respond in a more individuating fashion when the environment makes salient the individuating strategies used by others in a similar position (in effect, another manipulation of external standards), and others in power respond when the environment makes salient the powerful person's private self-concept as fair-minded (Fiske & Von Hendy, 1992). The common thread of these effects on the powerful is the standards made salient.

In a similar vein, accountability for the accuracy, or at least justifiability, of one's decision makes people more vigilant decision makers (Tetlock, 1992). Accountability for one's conduct is universal, and people seek approval and status provided by others, so they consider what others would say about their decisions and the process by which they arrived at those decisions. In effect, accountability—the potential requirement to subject one's decisions to outside scrutiny—makes people either (1) adopt opinions acceptable to others, for a known audience; (2) reason in a more integratively complex manner (explicitly balancing the pros and cons of evidence), for an unknown audience; or (3) generate reasons for chosen alternatives being right and for rejected alternatives being wrong, when people have irrevocably committed themselves to action. To translate these predictions to the language of standards, the decision maker may adopt acceptability (the standards of the audience), preemptive self-criticism (the standards of a rational and fair decision maker), or justifiability (the rationalizing standards of an actor who wants to appear to have chosen wisely). The outcomes controlled by accountability are other people's approval and respect.

Higgins has also described the effects on social cognitions of an audience's known standards (Higgins & Rholes, 1978), one's own standards internalized from significant others (Higgins, 1987), and judgment standards established by social comparison (Higgins & Stangor, 1988). There is no reason to suspect that the motivating effects of standards would be reduced for the powerful. The relevant outcomes again consist in part of social acceptance, but also the person's own emotional reactions to meeting or failing to meet internalized standards (cf. Devine's dissociation model).

Finally, according to social judgeability theory (Leyens, Yzerbyt, & Schadron, 1992), people have various rules for when they may or may not make a judgment at all. People try to meet rules for perceived adequacy of information (Yzerbyt, Schadron, Leyens, & Rocher, 1994; cf. Darley & Gross, 1983), as well as various social and cultural rules for when judgments are appropriate. Most relevant here, the powerful apparently feel more entitled to judge than do the less powerful (Caetano & Vala, 1993). To the extent that people monitor their judgments according to various specifiable internal and external standards, one can better predict when they will judge others stereotypically (Goodwin & Fiske, in press).

To summarize, people categorize (and probably stereotype) unless they are motivated to pay attention (and have the capacity to do so). Outcome control is one motivating factor, especially for task-oriented interactions between individuals. The powerful are therefore less motivated to attend to their subordinates than vice versa, so they are more vulnerable to stereotyping. The effects of power can be mitigated by a variety of standards, including perceived norms, social comparison, malleable self-concept, self-discrepancies, accountability, information adequacy, and social role.

Applications to Gender. Research on interdependence and power has included targets potentially stereotyped by individual stigma, ethnicity, social class, negative expectancy, and race. Conceptual discussions suggest the strong relevance of gender to power (Griscom, 1992; Unger, 1986; Yoder & Kahn, 1992). Preliminary empirical work supports the applicability to gender (Goodwin, Fiske, & Yzerbyt, 1994).

Implications for Change. People can change their own category-based responding through attention and motivation. However, because attention and motivation are greatly influenced by power relations, those stereotypes most in need of change are least likely to change.

Those who are relatively powerful are less motivated and have less capacity to attend than do the powerless. Power is empirically correlated with gender and race, so structural changes are implicated ultimately (Eberhardt & Fiske, 1994; Fiske & Glick, 1995).

Yet, structural changes are not sufficient without individual sensitivity to their dynamics, especially to the ways they can go wrong. Affirmative action for women and underrepresented minorities is a clear, real-world example of the kind of structural action necessary to change the concurrence of women or minorities with powerlessness. Changes in the power structure, however, may heighten group tensions and contribute to the stereotyping and prejudice they are attempting to eliminate. The theoretical does not perfectly predict the effects of practical solutions addressing the problem. The theory needs to specify the most effective processes by which change is to be accomplished.

The negative consequences of affirmative action can be prevented by the manner in which the policy is implemented. If unambiguous, concrete, and focused information is provided about the policies and the recipients' qualifications, reactions to affirmative action are more likely to be favorable (Major, Feinstein, & Crocker, 1994; Murrell, Dietz-Uhler, Dovidio, Gaertner, & Drout, 1994; Turner & Pratkanis, 1994). This information may also dispel stereotypes about recipients and calm the fears of the nontargeted who are members of more powerful groups. The positive effects of affirmative action can be bolstered by strong support from authority figures in the organization who highlight the common goals of the members in the organization (Murrell et al., 1994; Turner & Pratkanis, 1994). These organizational strategies have implications for individual strategies, which we address in the final section of this chapter.

Summary

Social identity theory and the interdependence–power theory share (1) their primary focus (i.e., interactions within a social context), (2) analysis of motivations for stereotyping (as driven by the social structure, given basic categorization processes and cognitive resource limitations), and (3) the identified change agent (i.e., the social environment that affects intergroup contact).

Prospects for change appear most encouraging when members of different groups are in situations that force them to work cooperatively, interdependently, and in pursuit of common goals. This was initially discovered from extensive research conducted on the contact hypothesis, yet the theory did not provide a convincing theoretical rationale for the effect.

Both social identity theory and the interdependence and power theories provide answers. According to social identity theory, positive attitude change will occur to the extent that situations are structured to eliminate the intergroup nature of the interaction by allowing individuals to perceive themselves as one single group. According to the interdependence and power theory, positive attitude change is possible because, as dependency on out-group members increases, the motivation to individuate out-group members increases as well.

Comparing Approaches

There is yet a broader framework to consider. A number of issues arise when comparing group-level theories to individual-level theories. First, distinctions between individual-level approaches and group-level approaches are becoming much more blurred. Individual-level theories have begun to consider the social context. Both modern racism theory and the dissociation model, for example, acknowledge the effects of cultural beliefs and norms on the individual. Group-level theories increasingly consider individual differences. Social identity theory accounts for individual differences in attitudes and behavior by considering how central an individual's social identity is to his or her self-concept. The power theory examines individual differences in the need for dominance among the powerful.

Quite possibly, the distinctions between individual- and group-level theories are so blurred because neither approach has yet to reign consistently superior to the other. Thus, the question turns to which theories are more appropriate and offer greatest explanatory power in which situations (Ashmore & Del Boca, 1976; Duckitt, 1992b; Pettigrew, 1958). Examining cultural norms that exist in a particular social setting may be informative in this regard. If there are strong cultural norms promoting prejudice (or condemning it), individual differences may have less impact (Pettigrew, 1958). If, however, cultural norms are weak, individual differences may have greater impact (Gaertner & Dovidio, 1986; McConahay, 1986). Individual differences are significant when social norms for behaving are ambiguous. This may be particularly likely when intergroup relations become unstable. Because instability is often marked by uncertainty, anxiety, and rapid transformation, old cultural norms cease adequately to dictate ongoing social interactions.

The norms for what is considered inappropriate behavior change over time (e.g., compare the antebellum American South to the post-civil rights era) and across situations (e.g., compare casual vs. intimate intergroup contact). Remaining cognizant of both the strength and nature of cultural norms may allow us to predict more accurately which strategies to implement to bring about stereotype change and prejudice reduction. If individual-level analyses have more explanatory power (i.e., cultural norms are weak), attempts should be made to change stereotypers directly. If group-level analyses have more explanatory power (i.e., there are strong social norms that condone prejudice), attempts should be made to change stereotypers indirectly by altering the structure of social interactions.

Finally, what becomes clear from our review of central theories is that the field has not extensively studied targets as agents of change. The agents of change in most social psychological theories of stereotyping and prejudice are the stereotypers themselves (in theories that focus on the individual) or the social environment (in theories that focus on the group). Intergroup theories have been much better at focusing on the attitudes of individual targets (Amir, 1976), yet there is limited research on the manner in which these attitudes and behaviors might encourage stereotypers to change.

TARGETS OF STEREOTYPES AS AGENTS OF CHANGE

Why Haven't Targets Been Studied?

Targets have received such limited attention in the social psychological literature on stereotyping and prejudice quite possibly because targets typically are not seen as causal agents who can impact their social environment in any meaningful way. In 1944, for example, Gunnar Myrdal located the American race problem in the attitudes of White Americans. His characterization of the "American Dilemma" as the disparity between White Americans' ideals and their practices generated an enormous amount of research on the factors that lead White Americans to employ category-based responding, as well as the factors that lead them to change their attitudes.

Research on targets' attitudes and behavior has also been limited because targets oftentimes do not control resources. If they do not control resources, the assumption is that they lack the ability to express their attitudes in ways that alter the social environment. Examining stereotypers seemed more crucial because they are not only viewed as causal agents, but also as agents who generally control the resources necessary to put their views into action.

Finally, many of the researchers have been members of groups not traditionally victimized by prejudice. Although the research may be altruistically motivated, it necessarily takes the perspective of powerful or majority group members as change agents, rather than targets as change agents.

In What Capacity Have Targets Been Studied?

The research that actually has focused on targets still does not examine how individual targets influence stereotypers. Instead, researchers have examined how stereotypers influence targets by (1) bringing about negative consequences for targets, (2) eliciting target behaviors that work to sustain the stereotyping process, or (3) giving rise to protective self-esteem mechanisms.

The negative consequences of being affiliated with a targeted group have been well documented (Jones, 1972, 1986; National Research Council, 1989; Simpson & Yinger, 1985). Doubtless, the nature and severity of these negative consequences may change with time and across specified targeted groups. Yet researchers have found that African Americans, for instance, are more likely to receive inferior health care (Cooper, Steinhauer, Schatzkin, & Miller, 1981; Woodlander et al., 1985), education (National Research Council, 1989), and housing (Massey & Denton, 1993) in comparison to dominant group members. Although the gap is narrowing in the United States, income levels of women and minorities tend to be lower (Crosby, 1994; Jones, 1986; Major, 1989) and occupational choices are more restricted than for dominant group members (Featherman & Houser, 1978; Kanter, 1977). Targets are less likely to hold political office (Pettigrew, 1985) and more likely to become victims of crime (National Research Council, 1989). Moreover, the probability of becoming both socially stigmatized and discriminated against is greater for targeted individuals than it is for dominant group members (Jones et al., 1984).

Researchers have shown that targeted individuals themselves may assist in perpetuating the stereotypes directed against them. Subordinate group members sometimes internalize dominant group members' negative perceptions of them (Tajfel, 1981). In fact, rather than exhibit ingroup favoritism, targeted individuals sometimes derogate their own low-status in-group (Simpson & Yinger, 1985; Tajfel & Turner, 1986). Moreover, targets may unintentionally behave in ways that confirm the beliefs of stereotypers (Snyder, 1981; Snyder & Swann, 1978; Word, Zanna, & Cooper, 1974). Stereotypers' expectations may guide their social interactions with the targeted in directions that lead to self-fulfilling prophecies (see Jussim & Fleming, Chapter 5, this volume).

However, targets do not always fulfill the negative expectations of stereotypers. Targets are particularly unlikely to fulfill expectations if they interpret stereotypers' negative responses as due solely to their subordinate group membership (Hilton & Darley, 1985). In these situations, individual targets will be motivated to protect their self-esteem by not complying with negative expectations.

Social identity theorists describe an alternative process of developing a positive social identity in terms of individual mobility. To the degree that a positive social identity cannot be attained through identification with one's own group, individuals may disidentify with their low-status group and attempt to exit. Individual targets may distance themselves from negative perceptions by assimilating into the high status group.

If the dominant group's negative perceptions are considered illegitimate, targets may distance themselves from those perceptions by attributing them to prejudice and discrimination. When targets receive negative feedback from dominant group members, rather than accepting this feedback as accurate and allowing it to affect self-perceptions, they can protect their self-esteem by forming negative external attributions about dominant group members (Crocker & Major, 1989; Crocker, Voelkl, Testa, & Major, 1991; Major & Crocker, 1993) and by disidentifying with the larger society that the dominant group represents (Steele, 1992).

Can Targets Influence Stereotypers?

Amir stated in 1969 what, in many respects, remains true in 1995: "The emphasis in American studies on attitudes and behavior of the white majority group has led to consideration of minority group members almost exclusively in their role as 'objects' and of the white majority group as 'subjects'" (p. 321). The picture that springs forth from the social psychological literature is one in which there is no room for individual targets to have an impact on their social environment. Instead, targets are depicted as passively responding to the fate they inherit, or almost futilely seeking to protect themselves from the social structure that oppresses them. The possibility that individual targets may significantly impact stereotypers has generated little theoretical discussion and has been neglected empirically (for notable exceptions see Frable, Blackstone, & Scherbaum, 1990; Ickes, 1984). The consequences of this neglect are considerable. By not permitting targets to function as subjects of study, we become blind to their capacity strategically to manipulate their social environment. As a result, we fail to consider seriously the complexities of target behavior and to apply this knowledge to our understanding of stereotyping and prejudice. We fail to bolster the strategies that individual targets employ by not giving them access to social psychological research findings that could significantly change how they are perceived and treated by stereotypers. Thus, we unintentionally aid in perpetuating the perception of targets as helpless, dependent, simplistic, and ineffective—the very perception we are working to eliminate.

Of the major social psychological theories reviewed, social identity theory most directly examines targets as agents of change, but again, primarily in terms of what Tajfel and Turner (1986) describe as "unified group action," in comparison to individual reactions to subordination. Unified group action attempts to bring about sweeping structural changes and would include such socially competitive strategies as the women's movement in the United States or the movement in South Africa to change the racial status quo. As we write, Black South Africans are voting for the first time in that country's history.

Yet, how will individuals of these subordinate groups continue to influence stereotypers in their day-to-day interactions? Is effective change possible on this level? More generally, given that targeted individuals must live in an imperfect social environment, how should they navigate through this and begin to make small-scale changes? How can targets protect themselves and simultaneously begin to affect those who control their outcomes? These are the questions for which we seek answers in the following section.

TACTICS FOR TARGETS

Although targets rarely have been the primary focus of social psychological study, much of the research conducted on stereotyping and prejudice has indirect implications for targets. Targets can use what researchers have already discovered about stereotypes and the stereotyping process to understand and predict the actions of those who use stereotypes as a source of control.

After many pages of review, we hope to begin to answer the female police officer and other trailblazers. We will address her and other members of underrepresented groups in organizations, but this advice extends beyond the workplace and ultimately deals with how targets might effectively change the nature of their relationship to stereotypers. The key for targets in each case is to motivate the other person to think harder about them, and preferably as people with shared interests.

Thinking Strategically: Applying Social Psychological Findings to Combat Prejudice and Discrimination in the Workplace

Gender and racial occupational inequalities are extensive (Braddock & McPartland, 1987; Kanter, 1977; Pettigrew & Martin, 1987). Not only are women and minorities more likely than White males to be tracked into low-skill, low pay, low prestige jobs, but also they often are further marginalized by being disconnected from the informal social networks and productive mentoring experiences that can be crucial to occupational advancement (Feagin & Sikes, 1994; Kanter, 1977). African Americans, in particular, perceive widespread discrimination in the workplace in the form of hiring, wages, task assignments, promotions, and performance evaluations (Feagin & Sikes, 1994; Pettigrew & Martin, 1987; Sigelman & Welch, 1991). The discrimination that targets face can be directly linked to gender and racial stereotypes. Targets report that they often are presumed incompetent by their superiors and coworkers. What little power they hold is resented. They are considered "poor risks," who "just won't fit in" regardless of performance (Feagin & Sikes, 1994).

Stereotyping theories provide practical advice to potential targets of stereotyping. Yet, theories do differ on the mechanisms and even the possibility of change. Each theory focuses on different aspects of the problem as well. Hence, from the target's perspective, it is best to be eclectic, dealing with many aspects of the potential problem simultaneously. Moreover, each theory suggests strategies that carry different types and levels of risk. We order the strategies, starting with those that probably pose the least risk to the individual target, and ending with those that seem to pose more risk to the individual. We do not address whether they benfit the whole group, as this is not our level of analysis here.

Eliciting Recategorization

People have a predilection for using categories. Given that people are likely to think about targets categorically (especially when they are minimally motivated), targets can decide whether they would rather be categorized according to one category rather than another. According to various cognitive theories emphasizing categorization, one can make different categories salient, and with them, the associated stereotypes, some of which may be relatively positive. For example, one might prefer to be respected and envied, even if not liked so much (e.g., a Harvard graduate, an overachiever), rather than liked but dismissed as incompetent (e.g., a nice, traditional woman).

Because women and ethnic minorities are underrepresented in numerous white-collar positions, often they have the burden of occupying "solo status" within organizations (see Pettigrew & Martin, 1987). Race and gender can be particularly salient in these situations. If this is the case, attempting to crosscut social categories might be most effective. For example, a single Puerto Rican male in a predominantly White organizational setting should recognize that many people may draw on negative stereotypes to categorize him. Yet, he can combat this by restructuring the content of the ethnic stereotype (e.g., emphasizing the positive aspects of his ethnic identity) and by rendering salient other categories simultaneously (e.g., his role as manager, his educational background). Highlighting numerous categories will cause others to rethink oversimplified negative stereotypes, at least as they pertain to that particular target.

Inviting Identification

Targets can also motivate others to categorize them as members of the in-group. People view in-group members as more varied, more positive, and more similar to themselves as a rule. People are more likely to individuate in-group members, to appreciate their unique attributes, under the umbrella of shared group membership.

Groups are defined, in large part, by shared goals. According to social identity theory and the contact hypothesis in particular, shared superordinate goals can dramatically redefine category boundaries. Groups are defined by shared goals, common fate, similarity, and proximity. If targets successfully capitalize on any of these, they invite other people to identify with them as a member of their in-group.

Making Use of Interdependence

Even if targets cannot be (or do not wish to be) in-group members, targets often are needed by in-group members. For example, people do not easily stereotype targets who are their bosses or teammates. Generally, people have little difficulty stereotyping those who are relatively powerless. People are more sensitive to avoid stereotyping those on whom they rely for outcomes that matter, because the negative consequences for stereotypers are more immediately and directly felt. According to both the contact hypothesis and interdependence theory, people learn more about people with whom they are cooperatively interdependent.

"We are in this together" is the message to get across. Targets can use this opportunity to highlight what they have to offer that might surprise people, that might contradict stereotypes about their group. Research has shown that people will especially attend to the target's inconsistencies with their stereotype and use them to make sense of the targeted individual. Of course, they can attend to the inconsistencies to discount them and reconfirm their stereotypes, or they can use the inconsistencies to dispute their stereotypes. But attending to inconsistencies is a necessary if not a sufficient condition for individuation.

If the relationship is not symmetrical, if the targeted individual is in authority over stereotypers or controls resources they desire, the targeted person will most certainly have their attention. What the target does with it matters greatly. This is an opportunity for targets to communicate who they are, in ways that both affirm and go beyond their stereotypic group membership. It is also important, however, for targets to highlight their shared identity, for if others perceive targets to be outgroup members with power over them, they will be prone to seeing conspiracies between powerful targets, allegedly to their detriment, and ultimately, realistically, to that of the targets, when they respond with undermining stereotypes and resentment.

If the relationship is asymmetrical in the other direction, the person in power has less incentive to attend to the target than vice versa. Some of the other strategies are likely to be more helpful here, simply because targets do not control many resources that matter to this person. It is, however, true that powerful people feel more dependent on their subordinates' performance than may sometimes be apparent. That is, the supervisor who delegates to targets depends on targets to get the tasks done competently. If targets can demonstrate more than sufficient competence, they make themselves indispensable, thereby also making use of interdependence. Regardless, then, of the asymmetry or symmetry of the outcome dependency, there are ways targets can make interdependence work for them.

Accentuating Accountability

If those in power are by definition not so outcome-dependent on targets, they still care about the good opinion of third parties. The third party's good opinion may carry approval and respect or even financial incentives, but all people have to justify their judgments and behavior on occasion. According to principles of interdependence and power, people attend to the third parties who control the coin of social acceptance.

If the third parties have a known opinion, then targets will be judged by the standards of those third parties, for better or worse. This also fits with the contact hypothesis idea that the goodwill of authorities facilitates constructive intergroup contact, whereas their ill will destroys it. If targets can make known the opinions of benevolent authorities, it may help.

If the third parties do not have a known opinion, but will be merely checking up on how the person in power judges and behaves toward targeted individuals, then the person in power will think more complexly about targets. This can be good if the person uses relevant information that also undercuts superficial first impressions and stereotypes. This can also be bad if there is extraneous, stereotypic, or damaging information. The person who is accountable to third parties with unknown opinions will use more information, even if that information is inappropriate. The person wants to have the appearance of making use of all potentially relevant information. And sometimes that can reinforce stereotypes. But all else equal, the accountable person is more likely to discover the truth of the ways that targets do and do not fit the stereotypic pigeonhole.

Accountability can be hazardous to a targeted individual's fate, if the decision maker has already made a (negative) judgment about the target and acted on it (or irrevocably committed to action on it). In that case, the person will generate reasons for the chosen response being right and for rejected alternatives being wrong, striving for approval and respect for what cannot be undone. Nevertheless, accountability, under the right circumstances, can make other people see targets for who they are.

Priming Shared Values

It is a short step from accountability to shared values. Shared values and prevalent norms represent the generalized other, the unidentified third parties who might approve or disapprove. Both the contact hypothesis and power theory would counsel targets to make salient egalitarian values. People subscribe to egalitarian values, even if they do not act on them consistently. Priming people's sense of fairness and responsibility demonstrably makes them act more in accord with those values.

This strategy was used effectively in the civil rights movement during the 1960s. Shared principles of fairness, justice, freedom, and equality were made quite salient, helping to bring about a massive change in the social norms dictating appropriate expressions of racial attitudes. Experimenters prime shared values by having subjects complete questionnaires endorsing responsibility, egalitarian values, and fair play. Doing this as an individual in an organization is hardly practical. But in conversation, at meetings, and in policy statements, targets can remind people of shared values, which brings out people's better sides.

Bringing Out the Best Self-Concept

The effectiveness of priming shared values depends in part on people's self-concept as nonracist, nonsexist, and egalitarian. Bringing out the best self-concept, like priming shared values, makes salient certain standards for behavior. If the standards are salient, people try to adhere to them. People's sense of themselves is flexible. A boss, a coworker, or a peer all can imagine themselves using category-based or individuating reponses, although individuation is easier for people to imagine.

Both power theory and modern racism theory predict that targets can motivate people by bringing out their best self-concept, which is unprejudiced. This is not hard to do: Targets can verbally appreciate people's fair-minded behavior and egalitarian views. People in positions of power may view targets as a risk. Although they may be tempted to "play it safe," targets can dare them to "take the risk" by reminding them that they are fair-minded people, that they are above relying on simplistic stereotypes, and that they are strong enough to stand up to those who might question this judgment. People like to be told they are good at treating people fairly, as unique individuals. Targets can help ensure that they are in fact treated fairly by reminding potential stereotypers that they possess this admirable quality. Praising people is relatively easy.

Pointing Out Should–Would Discrepancies

Being people's conscience is harder. The dissociation model suggests that when people notice the discrepancy between their ideal (should) and actual (would) behavior, they can be motivated to reduce the discrepancy. The problem is that this holds only for low-prejudiced people; in that case, they respond by feeling guilty. High-prejudice people respond by becoming angry at others. So this is not a technique to use with someone whom the target suspects of having a high degree of prejudice. Moreover, none of the studies have examined the impact that targets might have on alerting people to their should–would discrepancies; even seemingly low-prejudice people might be inclined to shoot the messenger. Those who think of themselves as egalitarian may feel quite betrayed and insulted by targets who directly address these discrepancies, especially if the target has relatively little power. This is a strategy to be used with caution.

Appealing to Stereotyper's Self-Interest

Another risky strategy points out the costs of stereotyping and discrimination for the stereotyper. In the abstract, targets could highlight the inefficiency of stereotyping, as underusing resources, and most people would agree. But most people also deny their stereotyping; they locate the cause of perceived deficiencies in the target, not in their own perceptions. A boss or coworkers are unlikely to feel spontaneously that they are being unfair to targets, so the indirect abstract strategy is not so likely to work.

A more aggressive strategy is threatening to litigate or pointing to the costs of litigation. Targets can use lawsuits successfully to fight for equitable wages and positions within an organization. However, lawsuits do little to curb subtle forms of racism and sexism, and may significantly hinder social relations in the workplace. Lawsuits polarize. They make people defensive, and defensive people do not become more fair-minded.

An intermediate strategy is appealing to self-interest by pointing out how something could look to other (allegedly wrong-headed) people: Treatment of a specific person or group of persons could be (supposedly mis)interpreted as discrimination. In effect, this strategy puts the target on the same side as the nontarget, trying to protect the nontarget's interests. Simultaneously, it allows targets to voice their own reservations about how things are going, without becoming the accuser.

In summary, theories and research about motivation and stereotyping suggest many avenues for the target who wishes to be treated fairly. Some of these tactics have been tested directly, and others are as-yet-untested implications. We hope the previous literature review makes it evident which is which.

Danger Signals to Monitor in the Other

Theory and research also issue some warnings. There are times to lie low and not atttempt to intervene. As implied between the lines in the preceding section, we also know some caveats about the deleterious effects of capacity and threat.

Time Pressure and Overload

Busy, stressed people are not the best candidates for psychic transformation. According to the impression formation models that underlie the theories of interdependence, power, and dissociation, people categorize in a relatively automatic fashion, using little capacity or intention. The associated stereotypes, prejudice, and discriminatory tendencies follow.

These can be averted only when people take the time to gather additional information and go beyond initial categorization. The implication for tactics employed by potential targets is obvious: Intervention attempts with someone who does not have the time or capacity to pay attention will not pay off. Tactics that require the other person to reflect, before gathering additional information about the target, will be particularly unsuccessful. Priming shared values, bringing out the best self-concept, and pointing out should–would discrepancies all compare judgments to a standard. This takes time and capacity. In contrast, interdependence and power, accountability, recategorization, and shared identity all are more primitive motivators that, from the research literature, seem not to require so much reflection. But subsequently, all these strategies rely on the person's ability to attend to additional information in order to individuate the target or targets. This cannot occur under time pressure.

Personal Threats to Self-Esteem

Theories of modern racism and authoritarian personality both would counsel targets to protect the other person's self-esteem, but for different reasons. Modern racism theory notes that people's own prejudice is aversive to them; they want to see themselves as unprejudiced, and they will deny or make excuses for actions that might appear prejudiced. Such psychic defenses resist frontal attack. Authoritarian personality theory suggests, in a compatible way, that prejudices serve long-term psychic functions, again implying resistance to change. Social judgeability theory, described in relation to interdependence and power, similarly argues that people make judgments that protect their own integrity.

One implication is that targets have to be careful in dealings with a person who has been under attack or experienced major failures; fragile self-esteem is probably not the best preparation for intervention attempts.

Threats to the Other's Group

Direct attacks on the other person's group should also be used with caution; people's judgments protect their group's integrity as well their own, according to social judgeability theory. According to social identity theory, people's group identification is a major source of self-esteem, so people will resist any overt or implied attacks on the group. Thus, competition between groups exacerbates stereotyping, as attested by the contact hypothesis, social identity theory, as well as interdependence and power theories. The person whose group is believed to be under attack will resist mightily if the targeted indivdual appears not to be on their side.

Individual Differences in Dominance and Rigidity

People who are consistently high in prejudice, dominance-oriented, or rigid in their thinking are unlikely candidates for change, according to authoritarian personality theory, the dissociation model, and the power theory. Such people do not pay careful attention to others. They tend to polarize their worlds into idealized and despised others, and thus react with anger to perceived discrepancies between their own actual and ideal behavior. Social psychological theories offer the least hope for changing these people. If at all possible, such people are best avoided if one is a potential target of their stereotyped beliefs.

CONCLUSION

Beyond the Single Intervention

Limited Generality from One Stereotyper to Another and from One Target to Another

Unlike group strategies that focus on institutional change, individual strategies have less widespread impact. Consequently, any of the strategies mentioned earlier must be employed over and over again by targeted individuals for each potential stereotyper. Stereotypers often are resistant to inconsistent information. Even if a target's intervention attempts are successful, they may not be long-lasting. Furthermore, the positive results of intervention attempts are not guaranteed to lead to improved treatment of other potential targets. Therefore, targets may need to prove themselves once again with different stereotypers and in different settings.

Strategies may differ in effectiveness, depending on the history of social relations among the particular groups involved, as well as the content of the stereotypes that arises from those relations. Many of the theories present "universal principles"; however, most have been tested narrowly: with particular groups, in particular situations, at particular points in time (Pettigrew, 1986). Not only may various ethnic and racial stereotypes differ in content and processing, but also gender and racial stereotypes may differ in fundamental ways (Eberhardt & Fiske, 1994; Fiske & Stevens, 1993). Researchers examining the role of motivation and prejudice in gender stereotyping have borrowed some principles from the social psychological literature on race, yet research on gender is still not as theoretically advanced.

Limited Access to Information

Potential targets may not always know precisely when they are, in fact, targets of stereotypes. Outside of the experimental laboratory, most social interactions are inherently ambiguous. The judgments nontargets make about potential targets often can be attributed to nonracial or gender-irrelevant factors. Low-prejudice people are particularly likely to make use of ostensibly race-neutral attributions to protect their egalitarian identities.

In the workplace, targets are likely to have only limited information on the wages and treatment of other people in similar positions within the organization. Without the relevant information, targets will be unable to recognize trends and accurately point to inconsistencies determined by discriminatory treatment of women and ethnic minorities. Wage inequalities between men and women are especially likely to go undetected by women (Crosby, 1984; Major, 1989).

Moreover, because targets tend to be locked out of informal social networks, they have less access to information that may be freely provided for nontargets and could significantly impact targets' understanding of the position they maintain within the organization, and the best strategies to renegotiate this.

Costs

The limitations of individual strategies can easily result in increased energy, time, vigilance, and frustration. Targets' self-protective techniques can become all-consuming. Additionally, many individual strategies require that targets protect stereotypers by not directly confronting stereotypers' prejudices and discriminatory behaviors. As a result, employing fairly indirect strategies to motivate change may lead to feelings of self-betrayal. Institutional change, indeed, may have much more adaptive impact. However, most individuals are not in the position to create change at the institutional level. Doubtless, the costs of relying on individual strategies for change are great, yet the costs of not relying on individual strategies, in addition to institutional strategies, may be greater. Individual strategies may not have an impact that extends to the target's entire group; however, they can have a significant impact for any one target across many life circumstances. This impact, from the individual target's perspective, may be a powerful beginning.

What Can Social Psychologists Learn by Focusing on Targets as Agents of Change?

Examining the behavior of targets is critical to any understanding of stereotyping, prejudice, and intergroup relations. Social psychologists should begin to examine not only the conditions under which targets might employ particular strategies, but look further to determine how consistent target responses are with what social psychological theories of motivation and stereotyping would predict. What strategies might be common to all groups that are targets of stereotypes? What strategies might be different, and what factors might predict these differences? The answers to these questions may not only provide us with a greater understanding of target behavior, but they may also point to as-yet unresearched factors that may influence stereotypers. Focusing on both stereotypers and targets of stereotypes will allow us to begin to understand the interactive processes involved in the creation, the maintenance, and the change of both stereotypes and the stereotyping process across time and cultures.

ACKNOWLEDGMENTS

The writing of this chapter was supported by National Institute of Mental Health Grant No. 41801 to Susan T. Fiske, and by funds from the University of Massachusetts at Amherst that supported Jennifer L. Eberhardt on a 1-year postdoctoral fellowship.

REFERENCES

Adorno, T. W., Frenkel-Brunswik, E., Levinson, D. J., & Sanford, R. N. (1950). *The authoritarian personality*. New York: Harper & Row.

Altemeyer, B. (1981). *Right-wing authoritarianism*. Winnipeg: University of Manitoba Press.

Altemeyer, B. (1988). *Enemies of freedom*. San Francisco: Jossey-Bass.

Amir, Y. (1969). Contact hypothesis in ethnic relations. *Psychological Bulletin*, *71*, 319–342.

Amir, Y. (1976). The role of intergroup contact in change of prejudice and ethnic relations. In P. Katz (Ed.), *Towards the elimination of racism* (pp. 245–308). New York: Pergamon Press.

Ashmore, R. D., & Del Boca, F. K. (1976). Psychological approaches to understanding intergroup conflict. In P. A. Katz (Ed.), *Towards the elimination of racism*. New York: Pergamon Press.

Ashmore, R. D., & Del Boca, F. K. (1981). Conceptual approaches to stereotypes and stereotyping. In D. L. Hamilton (Ed.), *Cognitive processes in stereotyping and intergroup behavior* (pp. 1–35). Hillsdale, NJ: Erlbaum.

Ashmore, R. D., Del Boca, F. K., & Bilder, S. M. (1994). *Construction and validation of the Gender Attitude Inventory (GAI), a structured inventory to assess multiple dimensions of gender attitudes.* Unpublished manuscript, Rutgers University, New Brunswick, NJ.

Bierly, M. M. (1985). Prejudice toward contemporary out-groups as a generalized attitude. *Journal of Applied Social Psychology, 15,* 189–199.

Billig, M., & Tajfel, H. (1973). Social categorization and similarity in intergroup behavior. *European Journal of Social Psychology, 3,* 27–52.

Bobo, L. (1983). Whites' opposition to busing: Symbolic racism or realistic group conflict? *Journal of Personality and Social Psychology, 45,* 1196–1210.

Bobo, L. (1988). Group conflict, prejudice, and the paradox of contemporary racial attitudes. In P. A. Katz & D. A. Taylor (Eds.), *Eliminating racism: Profiles in controversy* (pp. 85–114). New York: Plenum Press.

Braddock, J. H., Jr., & McPartland, J. M. (1987). How minorities continue to be excluded from equal employment opportunities: Research on labor market and institutional barriers. *Journal of Social Issues, 43,* 5–40.

Brewer, M. B. (1979). In-group bias in the minimal intergroup situation: A cognitive–motivational analysis. *Psychological Bulletin, 86,* 307–324.

Brewer, M. B. (1988). A dual process model of impression formation. In R. Wyer & T. Srull (Eds.), *Advances in social cognition* (Vol. 1, pp. 1–36). Hillsdale, NJ: Erlbaum.

Brewer, M. B., & Silver, M. (1978). In-group bias as a function of task characteristics. *European Journal of Social Psychology, 8,* 393–400.

Brown, R. (1965). *Social psychology.* New York: Free Press.

Brown, R. (1995). *Prejudice: Its social psychology.* Oxford: Blackwell.

Campbell, A. (1971). *White attitudes toward black people.* Ann Arbor, MI: Institute for Social Research.

Caetano, A., & Vala, J. (1993, September). *Status position and social judgeability.* Paper presented at European Association of Experimental Social Psychology, Lisboa, Portugal.

Christie, R. (1991). Authoritarianism and related constructs. In J. P. Robinson, P. R. Shaver, & L. S. Wrightsman (Eds.), *Measures of personality and social psychological attitudes* (Vol. 1, pp. 501–571). San Diego: Academic Press.

Commins, B., & Lockwood, J. (1978). The effects on intergroup relations of mixing Roman Catholics and Protestants: An experimental investigation. *European Journal of Social Psychology, 8,* 383–386.

Comrey, A. L., & Newmeyer, J. A. (1965). Measurement of radicalism–conservatism. *Journal of Social Psychology, 67,* 357–369.

Cooper, R., Steinhauer, M., Schatzkin, A., & Miller, W. (1981). Improved mortality among U.S. blacks, 1968–1978: The role of anti-racist struggle. *International Journal of Health Services, 11,* 511–522.

Crocker, J., & Major, B. (1989). Social stigma and self-esteem: The self-protective properties of stigma. *Psychological Review, 96,* 608–630.

Crocker, J., Voelkl, K., Testa, M., & Major, B. (1991). Social stigma: The affective consequences of attributional ambiguity. *Journal of Personality and Social Psychology, 60,* 218–228.

Crosby, F. J. (1984). The denial of personal discrimination. *American Behavioral Scientist, 27,* 380–386.

Crosby, F. J. (1994). Understanding affirmative action. *Basic and Applied Social Psychology, 15,* 13–41.

Crosby, F., Bromley, S., & Saxe, L. (1980). Recent unobtrusive studies of black and white discrimination and prejudice: A literature review. *Psychological Bulletin, 87,* 546–563.

Darley, J. M., & Gross, P. H. (1983). A hypothesis-confirming bias in labeling effects. *Journal of Personality and Social Psychology, 44,* 20–33.

Dépret, E. F., & Fiske, S. T. (1994). Social cognition and power: Some cognitive consequences of social structure as a source of control deprivation. In G. Weary, F. Gleicher, & K. Marsh (Eds.), *Control motivation and social cognition* (pp. 176–202). New York: Springer-Verlag.

Deschamps, J. -C., & Doise, W. (1978). Crossed category memberships in intergroup relations. In H. Tajfel (Ed.), *Differentiation in social groups: Studies in the social psychology of intergroup relations* (pp. 141–158). London: Academic Press.

Devine, P. G. (1989). Stereotypes and prejudice: Their automatic and controlled components. *Journal of Personality and Social Psychology, 56,* 5–18.

Devine, P. G. (1995). Prejudice and out-group perception. In A. Tesser (Ed.), *Constructing social psychology* (pp. 467–524). New York: McGraw-Hill.

Devine, P. G., & Monteith, M. J. (1993). The role of discrepancy-associated affect in prejudice reduction. In D. E. Mackie & D. L. Hamilton (Eds.), *Affect, cognition, and stereotyping: Interactive processes in group perception* (pp. 317–344). San Diego: Academic Press.

Devine, P. G., Monteith, M. J., Zuwerink, J. R., & Elliot, A. J. (1991). Prejudice with and without compunction. *Journal of Personality and Social Psychology, 60,* 817–830.

Doise, W., & Sinclair, A. (1973). The categorization process in intergroup relations. *European Journal of Social Psychology, 3,* 145–157.

Dovidio, J. F., & Gaertner, S. L. (1986). *Prejudice, discrimination, and racism.* San Diego: Academic Press.

Dovidio, J. F., & Gaertner, S. L. (1993). Stereotypes and evaluative intergroup bias. In D. E. Mackie & D. L. Hamilton (Eds.), *Affect, cognition, and stereotyping: Interactive processes in group perception* (pp. 167–193). San Diego: Academic Press.

Duckitt, J. (1992a). Psychology and prejudice: A historical analysis and integrative framework. *American Psychologist, 47,* 1182–1193.

Duckitt, J. (1992b). *The social psychology of prejudice.* New York: Praeger.

Eagly, A. H. (1987). *Sex differences in social behavior: A social-role interpretation.* Hillsdale, NJ: Erlbaum.

Eberhardt, J. L., & Fiske, S. T. (1994). Affirmative action in theory and practice:

Issues of power, ambiguity, and gender vs. race. *Basic and Applied Social Psychology, 15,* 201–220.

Erber, R., & Fiske, S. T. (1984). Outcome dependency and attention to inconsistent information. *Journal of Personality and Social Psychology, 47,* 709–726.

Feagin, J. R., & Sikes, M. P. (1994). *Living with racism: The Black middle-class experience.* Boston: Beacon Press.

Featherman, D. L., & Hauser, R. M. (1978). *Opportunity and change.* New York: Academic Press.

Fiske, S. T. (1989). Examining the role of intent: Toward understanding its role in stereotyping and prejudice. In J. S. Uleman & J. A. Bargh (Eds.), *Unintended thought* (pp. 253–283). New York: Guilford Press.

Fiske, S. T. (1993). Controlling other people: The impact of power on stereotyping. *American Psychologist, 48,* 621–628.

Fiske, S. T., Canfield, J., & Von Hendy, H. (1994, June). *Stereotyping and prejudice across out-groups: A search for individual differences.* Poster presented at the Convention of the American Psychological Society, Washington, DC.

Fiske, S. T., & Glick, P. (1995). Ambivalence and stereotypes cause sexual harassment: A theory with implications for organizational change. *Journal of Social Issues, 51,* 97–116.

Fiske, S. T., Goodwin, S. A., Rosen, L. D., & Rosenthal, A. M. (1995). *Romantic outcome dependency and the (in)accuracy of impression formation: A case of clouded judgment.* Unpublished manuscript, University of Massachusetts at Amherst.

Fiske, S. T., & Neuberg, S. L. (1990). A continuum model of impression formation: From category based to individuating processes as a function of information, motivation, and attention. In M. P. Zanna (Ed.), *Advances in experimental psychology* (Vol. 23, pp. 1–108). San Diego: Academic Press.

Fiske, S. T., & Pavelchak, M. A. (1986). Category-based versus piecemeal-based affective responses: Developments in schema-triggered affect. In R. M. Sorrentino & E. T. Higgins (Eds.), *Handbook of motivation and cognition: Foundations of social behavior* (Vol. 1, pp. 167–203). New York: Guilford Press.

Fiske, S. T., & Stevens, L. E. (1993). What's so special about sex? Gender stereotyping and discrimination. In S. Oskamp & M. Costanzo (Eds.), *Gender issues in contemporary society: Applied social psychology annual* (pp. 173–196). Newbury Park, CA: Sage.

Fiske, S. T., & Von Hendy, H. M. (1992). Personality feedback and situational norms can control stereotyping processes. *Journal of Personality and Social Psychology, 62,* 577–596.

Frable, D. E. S., Blackstone, T., & Scherbaum, C. (1990). Marginal and mindful: Deviants in social interaction. *Journal of Personality and Social Psychology, 59,* 140–149.

Gaertner, S. L., & Dovidio, J. F. (1986). The aversive form of racism. In J. F. Dovidio & S. L. Gaertner (Eds.), *Prejudice, discrimination, and racism* (pp. 61–89). San Diego: Academic Press.

Gaertner, S. L., Mann, J., Dovidio, J. F., Murrell, A., & Pomare, M. (1990). How does cooperation reduce intergroup bias? *Journal of Personality and Social Psychology, 59,* 692–704.

Glick, P., & Fiske, S. T. (in press). The Ambivalent Sexism Inventory: Differentiating hostile and benevolent sexism. *Journal of Personality and Social Psychology.*

Goodwin, S. A., & Fiske, S. T. (1995). *Power and motivated impression formation: How power holders stereotype by default and by design.* Unpublished manuscript, University of Massachusetts at Amherst.

Goodwin, S. A., & Fiske, S. T. (in press). Judge not, unless. . . . Standards for social judgment and ethical decisionmaking. In D. Messick & A. Tenbrunsel (Eds.), *Psychological aspects of business ethics.* Newbury Park, CA: Sage.

Goodwin, S. A., Fiske, S. T., & Yzerbyt, V. (1995, August). *Social judgment in power relations: A judgment monitoring perspective.* Poster presented at the annual meeting of the American Psychological Association, New York.

Greeley, A. M., & Sheatsley, P. B. (1971). Attitudes toward integration. *Scientific American, 223,* 13–19.

Griscom, J. L. (1992). Women and power: Definition, dualism, and difference. *Psychology of Women Quarterly, 16,* 389–414.

Hamilton, D. L. (1981). *Cognitive processes in stereotyping and intergroup behavior.* Hillsdale, NJ: Erlbaum.

Hardee, B. B., & McConahay, J. B. (1981). *Race, racial attitudes and the perception of interpersonal distance.* Unpublished manuscript, Randolph–Macon Woman's College, Lynchburg, VA.

Harding, J. B., Proshansky, H., Kutner, B., & Chein, I. (1969). Prejudice and ethnic relations. In G. Lindzey & E. Aronson (Eds.), *The handbook of social psychology* (2nd ed., Vol. 5, pp. 1–76). Reading, MA: Addison.

Heilman, M. E. (1984). Information as a deterent against sex discrimination: The effects of applicant sex and information type on preliminary employment decisions. *Organizational Behavior and Human Performance, 33,* 174–186.

Heilman, M. E., & Martell, R. F. (1986). Exposure to successful women: Antidote to sex discrimination in applicant screening decisions? *Organizational Behavior and Human Decision Processes, 37,* 376–390.

Hewstone, M., & Brown, R. (1986). Contact is not enough: An intergroup perspective on the "contact hypothesis." In M. Hewstone & R. Brown (Eds.), *Contact and conflict in intergroup encounters* (pp. 1–44). Oxford: Blackwell.

Higgins, E. T. (1987). Self-discrepancy: A theory relating self and affect. *Psychological Review, 94,* 319–340.

Higgins, E. T., & Rholes, W. S. (1978). "Saying is believing": Effects of message modification on memory and liking for the person described. *Journal of Experimental Social Psychology, 14,* 363–378.

Higgins, E. T., & Stangor, C. (1988). A "change-of-standard" perspective on the relations among context, judgment, and memory. *Journal of Personality and Social Psychology, 54,* 181–192.

Hilton, J. L., & Darley, J. M. (1985). Constructing other persons: A limit on the effect. *Journal of Experimental Social Psychology, 21*, 1–18.

Hyman, H. H., & Sheatsley, P. B. (1954). "The authoritarian personality": A methodological critique. In R. Christie & M. Jahoda (Eds.), *Studies in the scope and method of "The authoritarian personality"* (pp. 50–122). New York: Free Press.

Ickes, W. (1984). Compositions in black and white: Determinants of interaction in interracial dyads. *Journal of Personality and Social Psychology, 47*, 330–341.

Jones, E. E., Farina, A., Hastorf, A. H., Markus, H., Miller, D. T., & Scott, R. A. (1984). *Social stigma: The psychology of marked relationships.* New York: Freeman.

Jones, J. M. (1972). *Prejudice and racism.* Reading, MA: Addison-Wesley.

Jones, J. M. (1986). Racism: A cultural analysis of the problem. In J. F. Dovidio & S. L. Gaertner (Eds.), *Prejudice, discrimination, and racism* (pp. 279–314). San Diego: Academic Press.

Kahn, A. S., & Ryen, A. H. (1972). Factors influencing the bias towards one's group. *International Journal of Group Tensions, 2*, 33–50.

Kanter, R. M. (1977). *Men and women of the corporation.* New York: Basic Books.

Katz, P. (Ed.). (1976). *Towards the elimination of racism.* New York: Pergamon Press.

Kinder, D. R. (1986). The continuing American dilemma: White resistance to racial change 40 years after Myrdal. *Journal of Social Issues, 42*, 151–171.

Kinder, D. R., & Sears, D. O. (1981). Prejudice and politics: Symbolic racism versus racial threats to the good life. *Journal of Personality and Social Psychology, 40*, 414–431.

Klinger, M. R., & Beall, P. M. (1992, April). *Conscious and unconscious effects of stereotype activation.* Paper presented at the meeting of the Midwestern Psychological Association, Chicago.

Levine, R. A., & Campbell, D. T. (1972). *Ethnocentrism: Theories of conflict, ethnic attitudes, and group behavior.* New York: Wiley.

Leyens, J.-Ph., Yzerbyt, V., & Schadron, G. (1992). The social judgeability approach to stereotypes. *European Review of Social Psychology, 3*, 91–120.

Leyens, J.-Ph., Yzerbyt, V., & Schadron, G. (1994). *Stereotypes, social cognition, and social explanation.* London: Sage.

Lorenzi-Cioldi, F. (1988). *Individus dominants et groupes dominés: Images masculines et féminines.* Grenoble, France: Presses Universitaires de Grenoble.

Lorenzi-Cioldi, F. (1991). Self-stereotyping and self-enhancement in gender groups. *European Journal of Social Psychology, 21*, 403–417.

Major, B. (1989). Gender differences in comparisons and entitlement: Implications for comparable worth. *Journal of Social Issues, 45*, 99–115.

Major, B., & Crocker, J. (1993). Social stigma: The consequences of attributional ambiguity. In D. E. Mackie & D. L. Hamilton (Eds.), *Affect, cognition,* and stereotyping: Interactive processes in group perception (pp. 345–370). San Diego: Academic Press.

Major, B., Feinstein, J., & Crocker, J. (1994). Attributional ambiguity of affirmative action. *Basic and Applied Social Psychology, 15*, 113–141.

Massey, D. S., & Denton, N. A. (1993). *American apartheid: Segregation and the making of the underclass*. Cambridge, MA: Harvard University Press.

McConahay, J. B. (1983). Modern racism and modern discrimination: The effects of race, racial attitudes, and context on simulated hiring decisions. *Personality and Social Psychology Bulletin, 9*, 551–558.

McConahay, J. B. (1986). Modern racism, ambivalence, and the modern racism scale. In J. F. Dovidio & S. L. Gaertner (Eds.), *Prejudice, discrimination and racism* (pp. 91–125). San Diego: Academic Press.

McConahay, J. B., Hardee, B. B., & Batts, V. (1981). Has racism declined in America? It depends upon who is asking and what is asked. *Journal of Conflict Resolution, 25*, 563–579.

McConahay, J. B., & Hough, J. C., Jr. (1976). Symbolic racism. *Journal of Social Issues, 32*, 23–45.

Monteith, M. J. (1993). Self-regulation of prejudiced responses: Implications for progress in prejudice-reduction efforts. *Journal of Personality and Social Psychology, 65*, 469–485.

Monteith, M. J., Devine, P. G., & Zuwerink, J. R. (1993). Self-directed versus other-directed affect as a consequence of prejudice-related discrepancies. *Journal of Personality and Social Psychology, 64*, 198–210.

Murrell, A. J., Dietz-Uhler, B. L., Dovidio, J. F., Gaertner, S. L., & Drout, C. (1994). Aversive racism and resistance to affirmative action: Perceptions of justice are not necessarily color blind. *Basic and Applied Social Psychology, 15*, 71–86.

Myrdal, G. (1944). *An American dilemma*. New York: Harper & Row.

Nadler, E. B., & Morrow, W. R. (1959). Authoritarian attitudes toward women, and their correlates. *Journal of Social Psychology, 49*, 113–123.

National Research Council. (1989). *A common destiny: Blacks and American society*. Washington, DC: National Academy Press.

Neuberg, S. L., & Fiske, S. T. (1987). Motivational influences on impression formation: Outcome dependency, accuracy-driven attention, and individuating processes. *Journal of Personality and Social Psychology, 53*, 431–444.

Pettigrew, T. F. (1958). Personality and sociostructural factors in intergroup attitudes: A cross-national comparison. *Journal of Conflict Resolution, 2*, 29–42.

Pettigrew, T. F. (1959). Regional differences in an anti-Negro prejudice. *Journal of Abnormal and Social Psychology, 59*, 28–36.

Pettigrew, T. F. (1979). The ultimate attribution error: Extending Allport's cognitive analysis of prejudice. *Personality and Social Psychology Bulletin, 5*, 461–476.

Pettigrew, T. F. (1985). New black–white patterns: How best to conceptualize them? *Annual Review of Sociology, 11*, 329–349.

Pettigrew, T. F. (1986). The intergroup contact hypothesis reconsidered. In M. Hewstone & R. Brown (Eds.), *Contact and conflict in intergroup encounters* (pp. 169–195). Oxford: Blackwell.

Pettigrew, T. F., & Martin, J. (1987). Shaping the organizational context for Black American inclusion. *Journal of Social Issues, 43,* 41–78.

Rabbie, J. M., & Wilkens, C. (1971). Intergroup competition and its effect on intra- and intergroup relations. *European Journal of Social Psychology, 1,* 215–234.

Ruscher, J. B., & Fiske, S. T. (1990). Interpersonal competition can cause individuating impression formation. *Journal of Personality and Social Psychology, 58,* 832–842.

Ruscher, J. B., Fiske, S. T., Miki, H., & Van Manen, S. (1991). Individuating processes in conpetition: Interpersonal versus intergroup. *Personality and Social Psychology Bulletin, 17,* 595–605.

Schuman, H., Steeh, C., & Bobo, L. (1985). *Racial attitudes in America: Trends and interpretation.* Cambridge, MA: Harvard University Press.

Sears, D. O. (1988). Symbolic racism. In P. A. Katz & D. A. Taylor (Eds.), *Eliminating race: Profiles in controversy* (pp. 85–114). New York: Plenum Press.

Sears, D. O., & Kinder, D. R. (1971). Racial tensions and voting in Los Angeles. In W. Z. Hirsch (Ed.), *Los Angeles: Viability and prospects for metropolitan leadership* (pp. 51–88). New York: Praeger.

Sears, D. O., & McConahay, J. B. (1973). *The politics of violence: The new urban blacks and the Watts Riot.* Boston: Houghton Mifflin.

Sigelman, L., & Welch, S. (1991). *Black Americans' views of racial inequality: The dream deferred.* Cambridge, UK: Cambridge University Press.

Simpson, G. E., & Yinger, J. M. (1985). *Racial and cultural minorities: An analysis of prejudice and discrimination* (5th ed.). New York: Plenum, Press.

Skevington, S., & Baker, D. (Eds.). (1989). *The social identity of women.* Newbury Park, CA: Sage.

Sniderman, P. M., & Piazza, T. (1993). *The scar of race.* Cambridge, MA: Harvard University Press.

Sniderman, P. M., Piazza, T., Tetlock, P. E., & Kendrick, A. (1991). The new racism. *American Journal of Political Science, 35,* 423–447.

Sniderman, P. M., & Tetlock, P. E. (1986). Symbolic racism: Problems of motive attribution in political analysis. *Journal of Social Issues, 42,* 129–150.

Sniderman, P. M., Tetlock, P. E., Carmines, E. G., & Peterson, R. S. (1993). The politics of the American dilemma: Issue pluralism. In P. M. Sniderman, P. E. Tetlock, & E. G. Carmines (Eds.), *Prejudice, politics, and the American dilemma* (pp. 212–236). Stanford, CA: Stanford University Press.

Snyder, M. (1981). On the self-perpetuating nature of social stereotypes. In D. L. Hamilton (Ed.), *Cognitive processes in stereotyping and intergroup behavior* (pp. 183–212). Hillsdale, NJ: Erlbaum.

Snyder, M., & Swann, W. B. (1978). Behavioral confirmation in social interactions: From social perception to social reality. *Journal of Experimental Social Psychology, 14,* 148–162.

Steele, C. M. (1992). Race and the schooling of black Americans. *The Atlantic,* 269(4), 68–78.

Stevens, L., & Fiske, S. T. (1995). *Forming motivated impressions of a power-holder: Accuracy under task dependency and misperception under evaluation dependency.* Unpublished manuscript, University of Massachusetts at Amherst.

Stroebe, W., & Inkso, C. A. (1989). Stereotype, prejudice, and discrimination: Changing conceptions in theory and research. In D. Bar-Tal, C. F. Graumann, A. W. Kruglanski, & W. Stroebe (Eds.), *Stereotyping and prejudice: Changing conceptions* (pp. 3–34). New York: Springer-Verlag.

Swim, J. K., Aikin, K. J., Hall, W. S., & Hunter, B. A. (1995). Sexism and racism: Old-fashioned and modern prejudices. *Journal of Personality and Social Psychology, 68,* 199–214.

Tajfel, H. (1969). Cognitive aspects of prejudice. *Journal of Social Issues, 25,* 79–97.

Tajfel, H. (1970). Experiments in intergroup discrimination. *Scientific American, 223*(2), 96–102.

Tajfel, H. (1981). *Human groups and social categories: Studies in social psychology.* Cambridge, UK: Cambridge University Press.

Tajfel, H. (1982). *Social identity and intergroup relations.* Cambridge, UK: Cambridge University Press.

Tajfel, H., Flament, C., Billig, M. G., & Bundy, R. P. (1971). Social categorization and intergroup behavior. *European Journal of Social Psychology, 1,* 149–178.

Tajfel, H., & Turner, J. C. (1979). An integrative theory of intergroup conflict. In W. G. Austin & S. Worchel (Eds.), *The social psychology of intergroup relations* (pp. 33–47). Belmont, CA: Wadsworth.

Tajfel, H., & Turner, J. C. (1986). The social identity theory of intergroup behavior. In S. Worchel & W. G. Austin (Eds.), *Psychology of intergroup relations* (pp. 7–24). Chicago: Nelson-Hall.

Tetlock, P. E. (1992). The impact of accountability on judgment and choice: Toward a social contingency model. *Advances in Experimental Social Psychology, 25,* 331–376.

Tougas, F., Brown, R., Beaton, A. M., & Joly, S. (1995). Neo-sexism: Plus ça change, plus c'est pareil. *Personality and Social Psychology Bulletin, 21,* 842–849.

Turner, J. C. (1975). Social comparison and social identity: Some prospects for intergroup behaviour. *European Journal of Social Psychology, 5,* 5–34.

Turner, J. C., Sachdev, I., & Hogg, M. A. (1983). Social categorization, interpersonal attraction, and group formation. *British Journal of Social Psychology, 22,* 227–239.

Turner, M. E., & Pratkanis, A. R. (1994). Affirmative action as help: A review of recipient reactions to preferential selection and affirmative action. *Basic and Applied Social Psychology, 15,* 43–69.

Unger, R. K. (1986). Looking toward the future by looking at the past: Social activism and social history. *Journal of Social Issues, 42,* 215–227.

van den Bergh, P. L. (1967). *Race and racism.* New York: Wiley.

Weigel, R. H., & Howes, P. W. (1985). Conceptions of racial prejudice: Symbolic racism reconsidered. *Journal of Social Issues, 41,* 117–138.

Wilder, D. A. (1978). Reduction of intergroup discrimination through individuation of the out-group. *Journal of Personality and Social Psychology, 36,* 1361–1374.

Wilson, G. D. (1973). *The psychology of conservatism.* New York: Academic Press.

Woodlander, S., Himmelstein, D. U., Silber, R., Bader, M., Harnly, T., & Jones, A. A. (1985). Medical care and mortality: Racial differences in preventable deaths. *International Journal of Health Services, 15,* 1–22.

Word, C. O., Zanna, M. P., & Cooper, J. (1974). The nonverbal mediation of self-fulfilling prophecies in interracial interaction. *Journal of Experimental Social Psychology, 10,* 109–120.

Yoder, J. D., & Kahn, A. S. (1992). Toward a feminist understanding of women and power. *Psychology of Women Quarterly, 16,* 381–388.

Yzerbyt, V. Y., Schadron, G., Leyens, J.-Ph., & Rocher, S. (1994). Social judgeability: The impact of metainformational cues on the use of stereotypes. *Journal of Personality and Social Psychology, 66,* 48–55.

V

CONCLUSIONS

12

Modern Stereotype Research: Unfinished Business

DAVID J. SCHNEIDER

Stereotypes have been on the social psychology menu for generations. When social psychologists were deeply concerned about groups and race relations, stereotypes were seen as manifestations of a sour culture. When we tended to imagine that the problems of the world were due to ill-tempered people who were also a bit on the stupid side, we saw stereotypes as products of rotten and troubled minds. In today's cognitive world, stereotypes are just generalizations, for better or worse, the products of everyone's minds. We have removed much of the historical fat from stereotypes. They are no longer seen as necessarily sour or rotten; they are not even flavored by the spice of everyday interaction in a multicultural society. In contemporary social psychology, stereotypes have no flavor at all. The rest of this chapter explores the good and the bad in that.

TRADITIONAL AND NEW PERSPECTIVES

The Traditional View

"Stereotype," as a term, was first used by Walter Lippmann (1922) to refer to beliefs about groups. As is well known to most stereotype researchers, Lippmann argued that stereotypes are pictures in our heads (not unlike present day schemas) of people in other groups, created by culture, and used to give meaning to the behavior of others. Much later, Gordon Allport (1954) would defend a similar view.[1] However, neither Lippmann nor Allport thought that stereotypes were simply bloodless, cognitive generalizations. Both were struck by what they took to be an obvious fact, namely, that some people, indeed many people, have views about others that are flavored by such a strong emotional quality that they are strongly defended, even in the presence of disconfirming evidence.

However, Lippmann was not the essential figure in the early history of stereotype research. The pathbreaking research of Katz and Braly (1933, 1935) was far more important. Katz and Braly initiated a way of studying stereotypes empirically, one that had broad influence for many years. Generally, they assumed that although stereotypes were products of our cognitive systems, culture provided their content and impetus; therefore, "stereotypes" were defined as beliefs shared by a large number of people within a culture. Much of the subsequent research in this area for the next 20 or so years used exactly these same assumptions.

A bit later on, we demanded that beliefs be attached to people rather than cultures, and stereotypes were spiced with irrationality. *The Authoritarian Personality* (Adorno, Frenkel-Brunswik, Levinson, & Sanford, 1950) crystallized many of the common ideas concerning the negativity and illogicality of stereotypes. This tradition emphasized the assumption that prejudice and racism were both causes of and caused by stereotypes. Authoritarians were people who were driven by unconscious motives to see the world in simplified terms, and stereotypes were a device that fit these needs nicely. Stereotypes reinforce prejudical thinking, but prejudice itself results more directly from projection of unacceptable desires and thoughts to other groups; this prejudice would, in turn, reinforce stereotypes. Although the authors of this important book clearly recognized the possibility that we all hold culturally sanctioned stereotypes, their strong emphasis was on the use of stereotypes by highly prejudiced people, whose limited rationality was further clouded by deep-seated and largely unconscious ethnocentric needs.

So we have two basic and highly influential perspectives. The first considers stereotypes as shared products of our worst cultural tendencies, the second, as mostly the products of minds whose shallow rationality could not buffer deep insecurities. When all this is put together, we get what might be described as the traditional view of stereotypes. At a minimum stereotypes are beliefs about people in other groups, but they had to be negative to account for prejudice, and they had to be false to more or less degree because troubled minds do not process information correctly. They were resistant to empirical disconfirmation and were held rigidly as part of a general cognitive style, because they were driven more by emotion than by rationality. They had to be uniform in the sense of being shared widely within a given culture; culture provides the content and some of the rationale for these shared beliefs.

These views also fit the dominant liberal ideology that prejudice and stereotyping were due to faulty education and corrupt culture, things that could be changed through the arts and sciences of psychologists. At some level, social scientists wanted to see stereotypes as culprits of one kind or another, and they wanted them to be products of a racist society and of untutored minds. It was comfortable knowing that prejudice and stereotyping could be localized in the Archie Bunkers of the world.

The Social Cognition Perspective

Unfortunately this turned out to be an unhelpful perspective and to confound issues that might better be parsed apart. Brigham's (1971) influential review made it clear that there had been too much unprofitable contentious debate about what stereotypes are and not nearly enough research on how stereotypes function in our social lives. In the last 20 or so years of stereotype research, we have seen a return to asking some fundamental questions that might have been posed more effectively long ago had it not been for a value agenda that dictated to some extent the image of stereotypes as dark and ugly things, rotten and sour. What we have left is an unflavored but pristine notion. Within the now dominant social cognitive perspective, stereotypes are beliefs we have about people in groups. They may or may not be false, negative, held rigidly. They need not be shared with other people, and the assumption that stereotypes bear a close relationship with prejudice and discrimination is not to be made lightly.

I think this cleansing has been essential. We can see stereotypes as part of the human family of beliefs and understand that stereotypes are derived from the general cognitive processes we all share. We can and must make good use of the methodological and theoretical developments in cognitive psychology and social cognition. It is important that we be able to raise issues about stereotypes without looking over our shoulders constantly to assess whether they fulfill some larger social agenda.

But there are also costs. Having shed traditional notions of culture, negativity, rigidity, and the like, we now have to account for why so many of our stereotypes are, in fact, held widely in a given culture, clearly false at least at the level of being overgeneralizations, sometimes rigidly held and resistant to disconfirmation, and related to prejudice and discrimination. These are not trivial "add-ons," and they must not be ignored, as they tend to be these days.

Stereotypes (at least, as most people consider them) seem to be more than simple generalizations, and we need to determine what, if anything, we should add. But just to make life messy, stereotypes seem to be somehow less than generalizations as well. Sooner or later, we come to the uncomfortable realization that whereas all stereotypes are generalizations, not all generalizations seem to be stereotypes. Why do we call generalizations about women and professors stereotypes and not those about dogs, cars, and broccoli? Or, as I asked in a previous paper (Schneider, 1992), what is different about saying that red, ripe apples taste good and professors are politically liberal? Both are likely true as generalizations (obviously leaving aside troubling issues about definitions of terms), but the former somehow seems a benign generalization, whereas the latter seems more loaded. The former may be based mainly on personal experience, and the latter on hearsay, and so forth. Whether these differences are important is open to question, but we might at least begin with some healthy respect for the commonsense notion that some generalizations qualify as stereotypes, whereas others do not.

We can use terms however we wish. Definitions are not true or false; rather, they are more or less useful or functional. What is central from my point of view is that the definition we use should not entail any restrictions on our abilities to study stereotypes as fundamentally generalizations. But we must always keep in the back of our minds that we may, in so proceeding, ignore important issues at our intellectual and moral peril.

Present Business

This Book

The chapters in the present book do a nice job of laying out the essentials of the ways modern social psychologists think about stereotypes and stereotyping. Three features are striking about this collection. The first is that despite some overlap of coverage, these chapters manage to span a wide territory, and they do so without setting up rigid fences between areas. That, plus the lack of contentious arguing, is all to the good. However, there is a downside: a lack of integration at the boundaries, and a patchwork of underlying theoretical notions.

Second, there is little disagreement among authors about essential issues. There seems to be an underlying commitment to the notion that stereotypes are best studied as a set of beliefs about groups, and that modern cognitive psychology is the best way to understand the development and use of these beliefs. The social cognition perspective is the dominant paradigm.

Third, I am glad of attempts in many of the chapters in this volume to address traditional issues in this area. It is useful and challenging to see some of the traditional issues of accuracy, cultural effects, and the like, being taken on in these chapters, albeit gingerly.

In the rest of this chapter, I would like to focus more attention on important and traditional issues that seem to me missing or underrepresented in the modern study of stereotyping. I will generally argue that the missing features, such as negativity, rigidity, and inaccuracy, should not be thought of as defining features of stereotypes.[2] On the other hand, I think we cannot ignore the fact that both in the popular culture and in our own academic discipline, stereotypes are important precisely because they are more than garden variety generalizations. The issue before us, then, is how we can incorporate these traditional features without giving up the hard-won ground in the center, defined by social cognition. In asking whether we can have our cake and eat it too, I am relatively sure that we will neither have nor eat until we address these issues more carefully than we have done in recent years.

Social Cognition Biases

There are, of course, reasons why the social cognition approach has tended to ignore the traditional views. Social cognition has biases of its own (Schneider, 1991). Four such biases have deflected attention away from the traditional features. First, social cognition has been relatively oblivious to the content of our thoughts, beliefs, attitudes, and the like. Second, it has assumed that our cognitions are products of our experiences as filtered through our cognitive system, with the emphasis on the filtering. In this there has been little attention to the contexts, especially social, of cognition. Third, because so much emphasis has been placed on how our cognitive systems transform "raw" experiences, we have tended to assume that error is the hallmark of our beliefs. This has left us ill prepared to confront issues of accuracy and inaccuracy, because they have been swamped by what seem to be ubiquitous biases. Fourth, despite the fact that ultimately we study cognitions because of their effects on our behavior, modern social cognition tends to stop at the point at which external stimuli have been transformed into cognitions. We know relatively little about the cognition–behavior link.

CONTENT ISSUES

Traditional views of stereotypes were heavily content-laden. It was assumed that some groups were particularly prone to being stereotyped, and that traits were not randomly associated with such groups. Although it was never clear theoretically why some groups were stereotyped and others were not, in practice, social psychologists were primarily interested in racial stereotypes and stereotypes about various nationalities. Gender joined the party late (Eberhardt & Fiske, Chapter 11, this volume). Racial and national groups were targets because they were culturally salient and because they were convenient out-groups for ethnocentric thinking. There were also important content differences. Blacks were stereotypically lazy, and Germans stereotypically analytical and efficient. Blacks were not efficient, and Germans were not lazy. Furthermore, it was generally assumed that stereotypes were predominately negative.

Content issues are not easily addressed with the social cognition perspective, yet they are important (see Zebrowitz, Chapter 3, this volume). Social cognition assumes that cognitive processes are general and relatively oblivious to what is being cognized. Thus, categorization should work about the same whether one is categorizing furniture, animals, or people, and at a general enough level, memory systems should not care whether one is trying to recall information about organic compounds for a chemistry test, behaviors performed by a person, or names of elementary school teachers. In particular, there is no reason to believe that we process information about men and women differently than we process information about Hispanics, Germans, or lawyers. The assumption of processing homogeneity has been a productive one, but when applied indiscriminately, it leaves important content questions unexplored.

What Categories Do We Use for Stereotypes?

Obviously, if all stereotypes are basically the same (at the level of structure and implications for processing), then it makes very little difference except in terms of content which groups are stereotyped. In most of our research studies, subjects are presented with paper credentials of people, so that the investigator can achieve very careful control over which categories are accessed. For many purposes, this is not only useful but also mandatory. But when all is said and done, it is not at all obvious that the cognitive processes that affect the stereotyping of women will work the same way with age or ethnicity. However, this picks up when the process is well advanced and has not encouraged questions about how content affects process.

Prepotency of Categories

Issues of categorization and classification have been in the forefront of our study for the past quarter of a century. Nonetheless, there are crucial questions that need further answers. One concerns the prepotency of various categories. Given neutral contexts and random perceivers with random recent experiences, which categories are likely to be used (Zárate & Smith, 1990; Stangor, Lynch, Duan, & Glass, 1992)? Is a Black woman more likely to be seen as female or as Black?

Categories with strong visual cues for membership (Brewer, 1988) and those that have strong emotional significance (Zebrowitz, Chapter 3, this volume) may be especially prone to promoting active work on their behalf. Perhaps some categories such as race, gender, and age seem more "natural" as opposed to artifactual, and lead to more potent categorization (Rothbart & Taylor, 1992). Surely culture plays some role in reminding us often of the importance of some categories. For example, religious affiliation seems to be less salient in the category systems of Americans than it is for many European and Asian cultures.

Category Availability

Although some categories may have a leg up in the sense that we are biased to use them, much of the time the categories we use are affected by their availability and accessibility (Higgins, 1989). Is this person before me a woman, a Hispanic person, a mother, a lawyer, a wife, a political liberal, an AIDS activist, a patron of the arts? Obviously, part of the classification will be controlled by the situation. If I were to meet this woman at a hospice for people with AIDS, I might see her as an AIDS activist, a possibility that would not be salient when I meet her in her lawyer's office to make out a new will. No doubt, I will be more likely to see her as a mother at the local meeting of the parent–teacher organization, and as a woman when I see her surrounded by males at a business meeting. My own interests and values may play a role. If I am especially interested in issues affecting minority groups, I might readily see her as Hispanic. Recent experiences may activate some categories. Having just been talking politics with a some friends, I might now be especially interested in whether she is liberal or conservative. As Zebrowitz (Chapter 3, this volume) points out, many categories are associated with prominent visual (and by extension, other readily perceived) cues. Her form of dress might push me toward lawyer or mother categories. If she speaks with a pronounced Hispanic accent, I may find it easy to see her as Hispanic rather than as a mother.

Category use obviously is a necessary condition for the activation of stereotypes, but also as Brewer (Chapter 8, this volume) reminds us, the use of one category may diminish stereotypic thinking based on other categories. Thus, it may be a victory of sorts if we can learn to see this Hispanic woman as a lawyer rather than as a member of her gender or ethnic groups.

Subcategories

Another important question is one of subcategories. There has been a great deal of discussion (and relatively less research) on the uses of subcategories. Some of this work was stimulated by the work of Rosch (1978) and others on category hierarchies in which it was argued that subcategories, such as professional woman, may be more basic than the more general category of woman (Deaux, Winton, Crowley, & Lewis, 1985). Then, there have been suggestions that our stereotypes of more general categories often reflect subcategories (Devine & Baker, 1991; Eagly & Steffen, 1984; Feldman, 1972). In addition, some people have argued that many of us use subcategories as a way of getting rid of exceptions to our stereotypes (Weber & Crocker, 1983). There are also major issues about default categories. For example, as Eberhardt and Fiske (Chapter 11, this volume) point out, men are seen as generic people, whereas women are more strongly subtyped as a category; similarly for most White perceivers, people are White, and Black people are a distinct subcategory.

Compound Categories

This, in turn, raises an important issue of compound categories. I see before me a Hispanic, female lawyer. Traditionally, we have asked whether our first impulse is to think of her in terms of her gender, ethnic group, or occupation. But there is another possibility. We may have a distinct stereotype of a Hispanic female, a Hispanic lawyer, or even a female, Hispanic lawyer. These compound categories may or may not inherit features from their more general parents.

There are a couple of relevant possibilities. One is that compound categories create brand new stereotypes. So, a female lawyer is not much like a lawyer or a female, let alone a male lawyer or a female doctor. She is privileged to have her own category, with its own traits (Hastie, Schroeder, & Weber, 1990; Kunda, Miller, & Claire, 1990; Murphy, 1988). Alternatively, people may assume that a female lawyer is a kind of female, so that they start with the relevant female stereotype and tweak it here and there to adjust for the differences that result from the addition of occupation. Alternatively, a female lawyer may be thought to be a kind of lawyer, with adjustments made for gender. However, my hunch is that the lawyer who happens to be female is not the same person as the female who happens to be a lawyer. Because it seems likely that much of our useful categories are compound (with subcategories being a possible class of examples), we need more research on how people use such categories in everyday life.

Categories That Attract Stereotypes

In some ways, the most important category question is why we seem to have strong stereotypes for some categories and not for others. Why do we have explicit and strong stereotypes for gender and not for height? Why do we stereotype African Americans more than French Americans? There are some obvious answers. The first is that we have generalizations for all these groups, but we call only some stereotypes. In particular, generalizations that we do not like, or which seem to denigrate a group, are given a more pejorative label (i.e., stereotype) than more benign generalizations. That is possible, but it hardly seems sufficient. Another is that the kinds of prepotent categories, such as race, age, and gender, that seem to give rise easily to categorization are also ripe for stereotypes, in part because highly visible cues often remind us of what types of people are associated with various behaviors. A third possibility is that some group differences are, as a matter of empirical fact, more prominent than others. It might be argued that French Americans are really little different than German Americans but that African Americans have a distinct culture that encourages real behavioral and attitudinal differences from other groups. There are surely greater differences between some groups than others; it seems likely that men and women differ more than do tall and short people. On the other hand, we do not seem to make much stereotypic hay out of major and real differences between the young and the old, or between the rich and the poor. Thus, when confronting issues of group differences, one can always have the suspicion that real differences are greatly magnified by social and cultural forces. Generally, there may be no single reason why we stereotype some groups more than others, but we need more empirical attention to this issue.

Are All Stereotypes the Same?

Well, obviously not. We do not assume that women are like men or that either is exactly the same as professors, lawyers, or the mentally ill. Not only do we use different traits for different groups, but also traits themselves seem to take on different meanings for different groups; yet we have not focused on the differences between various kinds of stereotypes.

The social cognition approach to stereotypes is a processing account; the basic interest of most modern stereotype researchers is how stereotypes affect the ways we process information about people (Schneider, 1991). For the purposes of this account, it matters little whether one is studying stereotypes of women, African Americans, professors, schizophrenics, priests, gay men, winners of the lottery, computer hackers, cancer victims, mothers, or mass murderers. Obviously, the content of these stereotypes will differ considerably, but the cognitive effects will likely be the same. So, we would expect the person who holds a stereotype that men are logical to label ambiguous behaviors of males as logical and to recall more logical behaviors by men than is warranted, just as we would expect the person who believes that professors are lazy to code professor behaviors as lazy and to give priority in memory to lazy deeds.

Why does it matter whether people in a group are seen as nurturant or lazy? The most obvious reason is that social interactions are likely to be affected. Regardless of whether "lazy" and "nurturant" have the same effects on processing information about people, we are likely to behave differently to a nurturant than to a lazy person, or perhaps seek more interactions with the one than the other. Thus, stereotype content is important in the social worlds we all inhabit, and I would apologize for making such an obvious point except that it has all too often been ignored.

Traits and Language

Contemporary stereotype researchers have shown little or no interest in what traits and other features are assigned to stereotypes, even though there is a small but growing body of research on differences among traits (e.g., Funder & Dobroth, 1987; Gifford, 1975; Hampson, John, & Goldberg, 1987; Maass, Salvi, Arcuri, & Semin, 1989; Rothbart & Park, 1986; Schneider, 1971; Semin & Fiedler, 1991). Maas and Arcuri (Chapter 6, this volume) review this research, and point to some of the many ways language affects stereotyping.

Obviously traits differ in how positive or negative they are, but for our purposes they may differ in even more fundamental ways. Some traits seem to be highly dispositional in the senses that they define a person, seem central to personality, and the like, whereas other traits seem more peripheral to personality. Moreover, as Rothbart and Park (1986) have argued, some traits are easy to acquire and hard to lose. It seems intuitively obvious that this is important for stereotyping. For example, there is also some evidence that out-groups tend to be described in more dispositional terms, whereas in-groups tend to be described by terms that are less abstract. Perhaps dispositional and nondispositional traits also function differently in our total cognitive systems, perhaps even affecting what we remember and how we code behavior.

Are Stereotypes Negative?

For most people, an essential feature of stereotypes is that they are negative, and that is one reason they seem so offensive. Still, it is easy enough to think of positive stereotypes. For example, generalizations that Asian Americans are smart and hardworking, that Hispanics are family oriented, that Blacks are good athletes, and that women are kind and caring, are positive ascriptions, and yet most of us would see these as stereotypes. One of my Asian American students reports that she is upset about what she calls the stereotype that Asian American students are hardworking and good at math and science.[3] So I argue by example that at least some stereotypes are positive, and therefore by implication, negativity cannot be part of the defining essence of stereotypes, although it may still be part of prototypic stereotypes.

One question is whether negativity is an important, if secondary, feature of stereotypes, whether, in other words, generalizations about people are empirically more negative than positive. There is no simple empirical answer to this question, because no one has done a census of stereotypes, and even if one had, there might still be debate about which generalizations qualify as stereotypes. A more important and basic question is whether negative stereotypes are different in kind from positive ones. Or put more broadly, is there any reason to believe that negative generalizations are arrived at differently, involve different cognitive processes, than positive generalizations? I do not believe that we have good answers to that set of questions.

It may also be that while we have approximately equal numbers of positive and negative generalizations about groups of people, we tend to label those that are negative as stereotypes, whereas the positive ones get recorded as simple generalizations. I think that is not quite right, because, as my Asian American student suggests, some people sometimes object to positive generalizations as being stereotypes. A better amplification would be that stereotypes are generalizations that elicit controversy (see Brigham, 1971, for a similar definition). Most of us are perfectly willing to wear the positive generalizations we get with pride, but we bristle when people assign us negative traits. However, even positive generalizations can feel wrong or can seem to provide an unwelcome message. Black students might object to the positive generalization that Blacks are superior athletes on the grounds that it fits only a minorty of them and that it seems to suggest that Blacks make good athletes but are less gifted at academic pursuits. It is understandable that such double-edged positive generalizations would be greeted with open hostility, however valid or invalid they might be.

CULTURAL AND SOCIAL CONTEXTS

Social cognition is often not especially social in its orientation (Schneider, 1991). To be sure, we often study how people think about social events and people, but actual research often employs stimuli so devoid of social and cultural significance that they are hardly distinguishable from physical stimuli. There are other constrains of our typical laboratory procedures that limit generalizability to the social world (see Brewer, Chapter 8, this volume). However, while it is always possible to find good empirical studies that do examine the cognition of culturally rich stimuli in socially rich environments, it has proved harder to study the effects of social and cultural contexts on cognition (Levine, Resnick, & Higgins, 1993). It remains, of course, an open question as to whether social stimuli require a special cognitive psychology and whether cultural contexts generally make a major difference in the ways we think.

Are Stereotypes Individual or Collective?

Much of the traditional research work on stereotypes assumed that stereotypes are beliefs that have some cultural legitimacy or are at least subscribed to by a large number of people. Still, there has been relatively little discussion of the theoretical costs and benefits of making this assumption. The issue is, of course, not whether some beliefs about other groups are held widely—clearly many are—but rather whether this should be a defining feature of stereotypes.

The modern social cognition tradition assumes that stereotypes are products of individual cognitive processes. In some cases, this has been assumed explicitly (Ashmore & Del Boca, 1981; Hamilton & Trolier, 1986), but the Trolier assumption has been implicit, ubiquitous, and underdebated. Most recent studies of stereotyping begin with the assumption that people have stereotypes (with little concern about origins), and then investigate how they are used as aids in processing information about people in relevant groups. This program of study does not require any assumptions about the collective representation of stereotypes, and indeed social cognitive psychologists would find this a limiting assumption.

I want to avoid any implication that the individual and collective approaches are mutually antagonistic. Unfortunately, the cognitive perspective has simply ignored the culture in which stereotypes are embedded, whereas those who believe that stereotypes must be understood as collective representations have tended to exhibit a level of hostility to the dominance of the cognitive perspective that might lead the unwary to assume that the two perspectives are mutually incompatible. They are not, and we need both.

There are problems with the traditional view that stereotypes reflect culture. In the first place, this idea was never adequately tested; it was merely assumed. Furthermore, there were few proposals about viable mechanisms for the cultural tuition that must take place; metaphors to the contrary, cultures are not merely absorbed. In some ways, an even more basic problem was that most stereotypes are not uniformly held. In the early Katz and Braly studies (as well as most studies that have followed), there are very few traits that even a majority of subjects are willing to ascribe to members of particular groups, so the evidence for collective representations is weak. Or perhaps the evidence is strong that collective representations weakly exist.

Stangor and Schaller (Chapter 1, this volume) have a number of sensible suggestions for how we might think about the importance of culture; they show that mechanisms familiar to most social psychologists can be used in this account. Social forces affect the words we use to describe things, and they push us to enact roles that support culturally derived stereotypes. At times, they encourage us to hold certain stereotypes (or at least to express our agreement with them) through well understood social influence processes. Maass and Arcuri (Chapter 6, this volume) also discuss the important issue of group labels and language as cultural products. As we are all aware in these days of political correctness, various groups have been fighting for rights to identify themselves in neutral ways.

Social psychologists are not skilled at integrating cultural and individual level analyses; we have few successful models. Much of what passes for cultural analysis these days is barely disguised political rhetoric, and the role of culture in our everyday lives is a highly contro-versial issue in the modern academy. However, we can make a few points that would be generally agreeable to a broad spectrum of social scientists.

Direct Effects on Content

In the first place, it is hard to escape the notion that cultures provide much of the content of stereotypes; they tell us what to think. They do so in a direct way when we are clearly taught what to believe about certain groups. Families, religious institutions, the mass media, and schools all contribute to messages about what stereotypes are currently in or out of favor. Despite the fact that we know relatively little about how effective these messages actually are and the exact mechanisms for their transmission and learning, there is no doubt that some stereotypes do acquire cultural legitimacy and even consensus. We also receive power-ful cultural messages about what stereotypes can be expressed publicly and under what conditions.

Indirect Effects on Content

That is the easy part, and unfortunately we often stop there. However, each of us is cognitively more than a passive receptacle for cultural wis-dom. Through effects on their behavior, cultures also indirectly affect our experiences with members of various groups. Eagly (1987) has re-minded us that stereotypes of women and men surely result in some part from the kinds of roles that men and women are encouraged to enact in our society. This point is obviously more general. When we look around us, there is ample evidence that members of different groups do not sort themselves randomly into roles, jobs, neighborhoods, classrooms, or any other cognitive or physical locations. That this is due in part, per-haps in large part, to culture is beyond dispute, and this is one (indirect) way that culture influences individual experiences. Any reasonably ob-servant child or adult is going to find out that incompetent plumbers and electricians are overwhelming male (and where I live, White); that unscrupulous lawyers are usually White; that caring nurses are usually women, although these days officious doctors are often female; and those gods of adolescents everywhere, take-charge football quarterbacks and their coaches, are male. That these traits largely are attached to roles and not to people, and that categories of people are differentially attached to the roles, is all too often forgotten (Schaller & O'Brien, 1992).

Direct Effects on Processing

So cultural forces suggest (but do not dictate) the content of stereo-types—what we think about various groups—by directly promoting some stereotypes and indirectly by encouraging and discouraging behaviors by certain groups of people. But cultural analysis requires more. We need not get into the more extreme forms of postmodern cultural analysis to understand that cultures limit our cognitive options, and they often do so actively by handing us a culturally approved cognitive tool kit. We are told not only what to think but also how to think about it. For example, students in secondary schools are usually taught a limited version of classic economics and history that all but guarantees that they will come to see people (disproportionately minorities) who do not have jobs in the economic mainstream as lazy or otherwise largely responsible for their plight. Many religions support traditional family roles, and recent flag-waving around the theme of family values suggests that thinking in traditional ways about traditional gender roles is alive and well in a large portion of our society.

Indirect Effects on Processing

I am also struck by how much of our "cultural conditioning" in these matters is constructed around what is not said. Culturally approved cognitive tool kits exclude as well as include and do not encourage a larger dialogue about why the things that are cannot be different. High school students who are constantly reminded about the importance of individual initiative and responsibility in their high school social studies classes will not be encouraged to ponder or be given the analytic tools to deal with the larger social, political, and economic forces that differentially affect the opportunities of people in our society. Individual initiative and responsibility are important, but so are the more abstract and larger scale factors. Those of us who have been trying to teach bright and nominally sophisticated college students about the complexities of race and gender in our society soon realize how limited their modes of thinking often are about such matters.

Culture affects the "how" as well as the "what" of thinking, directly and indirectly, so even those who favor the study of stereotyping over stereotypes must take account of cultural matters. We need not assume that all stereotypes are collectively held or culturally given (let alone define them in that way) to know that our social worlds aid and abet stereotypes. As social psychologists, we ought to care more about this than we seem to do.

How Do We Acquire Stereotypes?

This is seemingly a derivative issue. After all, if stereotypes are products of cultures, then we must acquire them in about the same ways that we acquire most any other culturally ingrained idea. If they are products of individual experiences, then they are created in the usual way by our individual cognitive systems as blends of raw experiences and previous knowledge. Unfortunately, we have few good ideas about how any of this actually works. If cultural ideas were easy to transmit, people who watch television would be even more greedy and hostile than they are, teaching school would be an easy profession, and parents would not have to worry about their lessons being undercut by the company their children keep. By the same token, it is too easy to assume that the reason one person has a negative stereotype about a group and another does not is that the former has had more negative experiences in his interactions with individual members of the group, or that one person's schema leads to a different interpretation of the same behavior than does another person's. It cannot be that simple. Culturally prescribed labels lurk around and about such pristine cognitive activity. The mere possibilities that terms such as "lazy" are more accessible labels in the work environment than are "happy" or "kind," or that "lazy" is a trait strongly seeking behavioral confirmation for members of minority groups, suggests that we also need to think about social and cultural forces.

One reason why we know so little in this area has been the division of labor that exists between social and developmental psychologists. Those who have studied stereotypes most intensively have been inclined to leave the problem of acquisition to those who have not. However, a more important reason is that we have parsed the situation as if there are individual experiences or cultural effects, when, as we have just suggested, the two reinforce one another in many ways. It is not just that our ubiquitous tendencies to categorize people into groups combined with our tendencies to assign traits to groups, creates conditions for culture to fill in the blanks with traits.

Consider the vexed issue of how children acquire gender stereotypes; this also happens to be the domain for which we have the best empirical data. As the chapter by Mackie, Hamilton, Susskind, and Rosselli (Chapter 2, this volume) makes clear, before children can develop stereotypes about men and women, they must be able to categorize people by gender, a skill that children have very early. Then they must acquire the features that they assign to different genders. That they should learn early on to categorize by gender should not come as a great surprise. Small children are reminded often of their gender, and most languages have various ways of distinguishing gender (in English this is conveyed mostly through the use of personal pronouns). Styles of dress and other appearance cues make this an easy discrimination for children to make. Even in the most gender-neutral families, males and females do different things (although not necessarily the culturally traditional things), and as the child comes in contact with the larger culture, she or he will discover that men and women are not alike, at least in terms of the behaviors they perform.

The reason, then, that it is impossible to separate cultural and individual experiences is because they shape one another. There are many ways in which people differ perceptually, but gender is surely one of the most obvious. Our culture makes much of this difference, which further reinforces the child's categorizations on this basis. The fact that children easily pick up a language of gender differences reinforces parents and others for reminding the child of gender. There is much temptation to blame the larger culture, especially the mass media, for whatever mischief exists in this area, but there is remarkably little direct and compelling evidence that television creates gender stereotypes or even plays a major role in reinforcing them. Like childrearing practices and roles within the home, television both reflects and reinforces prevailing cultural tendencies. Before the days of television and the consumption of mass media, children managed to learn their gender and racial stereotypes just fine, and they probably did so by doing what they do now—observing the world around them. That is not to say that efforts to rid the mass media of stereotypes are misguided—we all should do what we can to change supports for the worst forms of stereotyping—but neither are they likely to make a major difference.

The fact that there has been so much attention devoted to the development of gender stereotypes should not blind us to the possibility that stereotypes for racial categories, occupations, and religions are acquired in different ways. It is quite possible, for example, that some of our stereotypes are based almost solely on our personal experiences without benefit of the larger culture. I developed my stereotypes of Rice students, for example, quite quickly and without benefit of any discussion with my colleagues about students.[4] On the other hand, stereotypes of politicians seem to be quite strong, despite the fact the most people have probably never talked to a politician for more than a few minutes. In this case, the mass media play a major role in the ways we think about such people. By extension, there is not even any reason to believe that each individual develops her or his stereotypes in the same ways. A child who grows up in a home where parents work hard to reduce gender stereotypes may have fewer or different gender stereotypes than the child who grows up in a more traditional home, just as the person who works in Washington may have different stereotypes of politicians than one who lives in Iowa, or just as the person who watches Rush Limbaugh might have different stereotypes of feminists than one who watches news on PBS.

ADEQUACY ISSUES

One of the traditional assumptions of stereotype researchers has been that as generalizations, stereotypes were somehow inadequate. At a minimum, psychologists assumed that stereotypes were inaccurate, and because they were developed using flawed cognitive processes that were badly infected by emotions and culture, they were assumed to be rigidly held and relatively invulnerable to disconfirmation through experiences. The more modern social cognition perspective, of course, treats stereotypes as basically the same as any other generalization. As such, they may be true or false, rigid or labile.

Are Stereotypes False?

At the empirical level, it is manifestly obvious that at least some stereotypes are false (just as it should be obvious that others are not). In addition, most of us have moral and political commitments that discourage thinking about differences among people, especially when many of those comparisons seem to support the kinds of continuing discrimination we abhor.

The fact of the matter is, however, that we know little about whether stereotypes are true or false, because there have been few attempts to study their accuracy, and those studies that have been done have mostly been poorly conducted or have multiple interpretations (Judd & Park, 1993). The chapter by Ryan, Park, and Judd (Chapter 4, this volume) follows that earlier paper in making a strong case for the study of the accuracy of stereotypes and in discussing many of the measurement and methodological problems in this area. The emphasis of this work on isolating different attributes of accuracy is an important one, because discussions (especially heated ones) about the truth of stereotypes frequently confound various types of inaccuracy. Sometimes our stereotypes are inaccurate when we assume that a given group has too much or too little of a trait, and sometimes we do underestimate the variability of the group with regard to the trait. Valence inaccuracy in which we overestimate the prevalence of negative traits and underestimate that of positive (as well as the reverse) is also common but perhaps somewhat more derivative and indirect. Ryan and colleagues focus on inaccuracies of group stereotypes, but there is another kind of error that is also important, and that is the ascription of group traits to individuals to whom they do not belong.

The Ryan et al. chapter clarifies a number of important issues, but it is, I think, too facile about criterion issues (Schneider, Hastorf, & Ellsworth, 1979). Many traits are inherently vague. How could we ever decide whether a person (let alone a group) is lazy?[5] Imagine that a person, Sara, asserts that professors are lazy, and since you suspect that Sara is a person of limited experiences and is guided by her prejudices, you wish to investigate the accuracy of this claim empirically. How would you begin? I suspect that before you were very far along you would begin to have the sense of trying to shape water; Sara's cognitive molds do not keep her thoughts in place, and her mind begins to spring leaks everywhere. Sara can offer a never-ending list of examples of lazy behaviors that she has observed performed by professors.[6] When you point out that nonprofessors (say secretaries) also perform many of these same behaviors, she asserts that they don't perform them as often. When you point out what you take to be nonlazy behaviors by professors, she tells you that they are atypical or really lazy behaviors in disguise. You try to pin her down. What counts as a lazy behavior? Well, sitting around when others are typing and answering the phones. But you point out that lots of lawyers, say, spend little time typing while their secretaries do type, and she replies that the nontyping is really different when a lawyer does it; she is thinking and being creative. And Sara has you there: One of the guideposts of social psychology is that behaviors mean different things depending on goals, intentions, situational contexts, and the like. The point is this: Sara may have limited experiences and biased ways of thinking, but her cognitive bag of tricks may also be as resourceful as yours or mine, and we need not assume that she is necessarily inaccurate because we do not agree with her. Indeed, for this trait I would hard pressed to know how to determine whether professors are or are not lazy. Her definition of laziness is no better than mine and is less likely to be self-serving.

Ryan, Park, and Judd get around such criterion issues to some extent by using attitude measures. Not only are attitudes less subject to criterion problems, but they constitute important parts of many stereotypes. We can find out a great deal about the whys and wherefores of stereotype accuracy by studying accuracy of attitude ascription, but the fact remains that measurement of the accuracy of trait attributions (which are central to most stereotypes) has additional, and major, problems that are avoided in their discussion.

There seems no good reason for assuming that stereotypes are generally false. Traditionally, it was implicitly assumed that because most stereotypes arose from cultural tuition rather than individual experiences, they were tainted. However, it is not clear that those stereotypic beliefs we get from our culture are any more or less accurate that those we generate from our own experiences. My stereotype that astronauts are intelligent and analytical is based solely on what I have read and heard, and yet I suspect that this generalization is true. My own experiences suggest that Asian Americans are hardworking, but I occasionally remind myself that my exposure to this group has been somewhat parochial.[7]

It is important that we know more about the conditions that foster inaccuracy. The salient fact is this: Most people assume that their stereotypes are accurate. An appropriate response by social scientists would be to take that bit of data seriously. The fact that social scientists have been embarrassed by the political incorrectness of the accuracy issue has cut us off from important data about the ways stereotypes function in our social lives.

Are Stereotypes Rigidly Held?

One traditional feature that nearly everyone agreed on was that stereotypes are more rigidly held than other generalizations. The tradition of the authoritarian personality research simply amplified that common assumption and provided an elaborate conceptual rationale for it. Stereotypes were products of corrupt minds, and we hold rigid and negative stereotypes of people from other groups as a way of protecting ourselves from confronting our inadequacies. There is, of course, no shortage of Archie Bunkers at any given time. The question is whether there is an Archie in all of us waiting to come out.

Earlier theorists were not always clear what they meant by the putative rigidity of stereotypes. Because they took the racists and authoritarians of the world as holding prototypic stereotypes, at least two features of stereotypes were confounded. The first was the notion that stereotypes do not allow for exceptions—they apply to everyone, or nearly everyone, in the relevant group. The second was that stereotypes are held with such conviction and passion that they are invulnerable to disconfirmation. These notions will be confounded for theorists who believe that stereotypes owe more to needs and desires than to experience, but they are easily and appropriately separated within the cognitive tradition.

Simple observation—dangereous as a technique, but useful for all that—suggests that stereotypes, at least for most of us, are not rigid in either of the above senses. Most of us, when we confront our own stereotypes, realize that they do allow for many exceptions. Indeed, a conversation with an otherwise racist person will reveal that even he or she does not believe that *all* Blacks or Jews are anything. Furthermore, most of us assume (and can offer appropriate examples) that we do change our stereotypes when they do not fit the available data. I am certainly aware that my negative stereotypes of some groups have changed, and changed radically, as I have become better acquainted with individuals from those groups. How else could matters be? If behavioral data do not count for something, we would all be forever captive to the first generalizations we learned as small children. I do not mean to paint an overly rosy picture, because we all know far too many examples of people who do have at least some stereotypes that are rigid and uncompromising, and that are impervious to experiential disconfirmation. But we sell ourselves short when we emphasize lack of change as though change were nearly impossible.

Rigidity as Resistance to Change

Consider, first, the issue of whether some stereotypes are invulnerable to experiential change. Some seem to be, but unless we want to define stereotypes narrowly in terms of this feature, we also need to recognize that many are not. Therefore, the central question is what makes some stereotypes easier to change than others. There are at least four reasonable answers, I think.

The first is that the unyielding stereotypes are accurate at least in terms of mean tendencies. I doubt that spending even thousands of (boring) hours watching female bodybuilders would change my stereotype that men are stronger than women. As these things are generally measured, differential strength is a fact, although one that is not an important part of my own gender stereotypes. Generally our most important stereotypic ascriptions are probably not as well anchored in reality as this example would imply, but the fact remains that some of our stereotypes are difficult to change precisely because they are true.

Second, we have cultural considerations. I sometimes wonder about gender relations and stereotypes of a century ago,[8] and I try to imagine what one might have done to change the general stereotypes of women that were widely held by both men and women at that time. I suspect that whatever factual information and arguments one might have presented would have paled in the face of overwhelming cultural support to the contrary. As we consistently rediscover in theory and in our personal lives, culturally based realities are hard to change. That is another reason why we should be devoting more attention to the cultural flavoring of stereotypes.

Third, some of our stereotypes probably do fit the Archie Bunker, authoritarian personality mold. We do (or at least, I do) catch ourselves putting down other people from time to time as a way of asserting our own superiority and that of our reference groups. There is no doubt that our prejudices, however derived, can sometimes drive our stereotypes and make them resistant to change. Sometimes emotional experiences can create stereotypes that are locked into a rigid pattern. For example, we can all sympathize with the rape victim who finds all men frightening, or the boy who gets beat up by a minority gang and has trouble ridding himself of negative images of members of that race. The problem with the traditional view is that these sorts of emotionally laden stereotypes tended to be taken as prototypic when they are probably less typical than our garden variety generalizations.

Fourth, stereotypes are beliefs, and like other beliefs they are embedded in a rich cognitive structure. Obviously a feminist will think differently about gender differences than someone who supports traditional family values from a conservative Christian or Muslim perspective. Articulate Black writers from varying perspectives (e.g., Gates, 1992; Steele, 1990; West, 1993) see differences between Whites and Blacks differently than do conservative White politicians. And to be fair, we also need to point out that a refusal to recognize group differences or the desire to "excuse them away" may be as deeply embedded in moral and political values as the desire to view them in their most naked and detrimental light. In any event, the main point is simple enough. When beliefs about groups are deeply attached to other central and important beliefs, they will be the devil to change. In that way stereotypes are no different from our other beliefs. That is just as true for those of us who imagine ourselves to be fair, open, and rational as for those whose stereotypes lie closer to their overt prejudices.

Do Stereotypes Admit Exceptions?

Obviously they do, but some do so more than others, and we need to know why. Part of the answer may be social. Perhaps my stereotypes about Asian Americans and women, in these times of political correctness, are not rigidly held because they have been challenged more often than my stereotypes about rodeo riders or lovers of hot Thai food.

It is also possible (in what we might call the "Archie Bunker hypothesis") that the stereotypes held by some people are different than those held by others. Professor Jones says that all students are lazy, that none of them work as hard as he did when he was a student—and he was lazy enough—that the very rare exceptions only prove the rule. Professor Smith declares that whereas students are on average a bit on the lazy side, many work hard. Do Smith and Jones have the same stereo-type? One is tempted to say that they do, but that Jones simply has the stronger (and more rigid) stereotype. It is likely that Jones will rate students in general as more lazy than will Smith, and surely he will see students as more homogeneous than she will. Is this all there is to it? Is rigidity then reduced to matters of mean ratings and variances? If so, we have a major victory, because we know a lot about such business these days (e.g., Kraus, Ryan, Judd, Hastie, & Park, 1993; Linville & Fischer, 1993). Means and variances of ratings are important, but the key issue seems to me whether Jones and Smith think differently about students. There may be a giveaway in Jones's comment that students do not now work as hard as they did when he was a student. We hear a note of anger, perhaps envy, in his voice as he says this. His waters of resentment may run deeper than we might, at first, think. Should we ignore this extra baggage that Jones seems to bring with him?

What does this say about conditions of granting exceptions? Professor Smith says that students are basically lazy, but when questioned, she is perfectly happy to allow that many are not. Indeed, when pressed, she reports that about 60% of students in her experience have been lazy. Now we have the right to wonder: How does she make use of this extraordinary statistic? She meets her annual group of freshman advisees, and say, for the sake of computational ease, that she has ten of them. Does she privately say to herself that six of these kids are lazy as hell, and the other four will be okay? Does she assume that each student is 60% lazy, pending her getting the behavioral data sorted out? Or does she just play the odds and assume that they are all lazy until she finds out otherwise? And just to complicate matters even more, it is possible that what Smith really means is that 60% of the behaviors she observes are lazy ones. She does not really have the time or cognitive resources to recall which behaviors went with which students, but she is able to keep track of how many student behaviors seem to be lazy. Maybe she has a clear conception that student laziness is near 100% early in the semester but drops to near 20% just before major exams, averaging out to 60% over the semester. It is not easy to know how Smith handles this seemingly clear 60% estimate. These issues are partially about how people store behavioral information, but they are also about how they use the information to make judgments.

Dealing with Individuals

Whatever other disagreements social psychologists have on conceptual and moral issues connected with stereotypes, I suspect all of us would agree that there is all manner of psychological, moral, social, and political mischief when we apply our stereotypes to individuals (Fiske & Neuberg, 1990; Brewer, 1988). It is all too easy to transform judgments about group characteristics into judgments about individual proclivities. Whereas one may feel angry at having one's own group negatively stereotyped, that anger will be magnified when the trait is applied to ones self especially inaccurately.[9] Many people seem to assume that because Black males commit more violent crimes proportionately than do White males, Blacks in general are violence prone, and individual blacks are also more violence prone.[10] Perceived homogeneity of groups may encourage applications of stereotypes to group members. Obviously, with the rare exception of stereotypes that are universally true, there will always be exceptions to our most treasured generalizations about others, but that only creates a necessary condition for our realization that a given stereotype may not fit this member of the group. If one accepts the notions of McCauley and Stitt (1978) that stereotypes are simply ways in which groups are perceived to differ, stereotypic traits may not even fit most members of a group.

Eberhardt and Fiske (Chapter 11, this volume), Brewer (Chapter 8, this volume), and Bodenhausen and Macrae (Chapter 7, this volume) all deal with the important issue of how our stereotypes, true or false, ought to inform our judgments about individuals in stereotyped groups. Perhaps the most common suggestion has been that we try to individuate people and cease letting our stereotypes do our thinking for us. That is certainly a useful and important strategy, one that we should always urge upon those who have the power to make decisions about people. We would all be appalled by the college admissions director who refused to admit Black students because of her stereotypes that they perform poorly academically, and we would be equally upset if a talented White youngster were denied a tryout for the football team on the basis of his race.[11]

Generalizations Are Valid Cues for Decisions

Matters are not quite that simple, however, because often group judgments are perfectly acceptable and even rational. When she puts her course syllabus together, Professor Smith may be justified in building in many exams, because by so doing she will, at least for this course, lower the rate of lazy behaviors. It may be immaterial to her that some students are dispositionally lazy and others are hardworking, because she wants to raise the general mean.[12] We do not object in principle to selective colleges using narrow (e.g., SAT scores) and sometimes vague (e.g., well-roundedness) criteria to admit students, knowing full well that many students who could do well are not going to be admitted. Most of us would not criticize a person who avoided a known, dangerous minority neighborhood at midnight, even though the majority of people in that neighborhood are likely to be law-abiding and nonthreatening. I would generally not ridicule a person who refused to fly on an airline that leads the industry in accidents per mile flown, even though the probability of an accident occurring on a given flight is vanishingly small. Sometimes it is prudent, rational, and culturally (if not politically) correct to use generalizations as guides to thought and behavior, even though they have major and known exceptions. Other times we use generalizations at our moral, political, and bodily peril.

Individualized Information May Be Invalid

We may also make decisions based on group information because we think that individualized information is invalid or unfair. For example, those of us involved in admissions to our graduate programs have all had the experience of rejecting someone on the basis of, say, low GRE scores, only to be greeted with the claim: "If you'll only admit me, I'm sure I can prove to you that I can be a great graduate student."[13] Such claims are probably undiagnostic. It might also be argued that regardless of its diagnostic value, using such information for one student may be unfair to those who did not have opportunities to make a case for their individualized attributes.

Diagnosticity of Information

It is important to place all this in the context of what kinds of information are most diagnostic. It is, to be sure, often hard to compare the relative validities of group membership and information based on more individualistic cues. One can applaud the hard work and determination that a student from a deprived background brings to the graduate program admissions table, but still feel that her low GRE scores and inadequate research experience count more strongly as predictive aids.

Logical Status of Individualized Information

There is a further problem, and one that cuts deeper. Sometimes we suggest that individualized information has a stronger moral, if not predictive, force because it is somehow different than generalizations about group membership. But at one level this must be wrong on logical grounds. Persons who use gender as a predictive, aid in admitting graduate students may be on dubious moral ground, and may be using information that has little predictive validity. But it does not follow that when they use information about grades, GRE scores, and letters of recommendations, they have suddenly climbed to the moral or statistical high ground. After all, when they decide to use a careful reading of letters of recommendations instead of gender, as a basis for admitting students, they have really just switched stereotypes (or generalizations, if you prefer). The generalization that people with strong letters of recommendation do well in graduate school may be more morally and statistically sound than the one that males do better than females, but it still a stereotype and is subject to the same diagnostic tests. If, as I suspect, such letters are, in fact, more diagnostic than gender, so be it. But the superiority of letters lies in that statistical fact, and not in some diffuse and romantic notion that letters are more individualized. If it has any validity at all, then so called individualized information is really another generalization in a thick (and sometimes thin) disguise. Obviously some generalizations are more accurate than others in that they provide more valid predictions of individual behavior, and some are less politically and morally incorrect than others. I am certainly well aware that generalizations about men and women elicit more controversy than those about people who score high or low on GRE tests. All I want to say here is that using individuated information while appealing on moral grounds operates psychologically according to the same rules as the use of stereotypes.[14]

BEHAVIORAL EFFECTS OF STEREOTYPES

Social psychology, like most scientific endeavors, is gripped by fads and passions. One manifestation is that we often fail to finish projects. The original justification for person perception and social cognition more generally was the assumption that people are more affected by their perceptions of the social world than by its reality. Almost all of us make that phenomenological assumption, and for good reason—it is as true as anything is in these days of deep mistrust of ultimate truths. We study the relationship between objective stimuli and our thoughts because thoughts affect behavior. It is highly unlikely that we would have the interest in stereotypes we presently have were it not for this assumption. Yet, unfortunately, we have far better answers for questions about how external stimuli affect our thoughts than for how our thoughts affect our behaviors, especially in the area of stereotyping and prejudice.

How Are Stereotypes Related to
Prejudice and Discrimination?

The original reason for studying stereotypes was that they would help explain prejudice and discrimination. Yet as many people have commented (Brigham, 1971; Stangor, Sullivan, & Ford, 1991), there has been far too little attention devoted to the interrelations among these variables, and what studies we do have point to weak and inconsistent relationships.

Stereotypes, prejudice, and discrimination are surely related in complex ways, and there is no reason to believe that they are related the same way for everyone across all situations. Dovidio, Brigham, Johnson, and Gaertner (Chapter 9, this volume) and Eberhardt and Fiske (Chapter 11, this volume) have exceptionally lucid and thought provoking discussions of the issues involved, and I have no essential criticisms of their insightful analyses. However, I would make three general comments.

The first is that "prejudice" and "discrimination," like "stereotype," are not especially clear terms, and they pack in a lot of political baggage. In particular, prejudice has suffered from many of the limiting assumptions that have plagued stereotypes. There seems, for example, no a priori reason to assume that prejudice is a negative attitude, anymore than we have to define stereotypes as inevitably negative. Whether the positive and negative attitudes we have toward others differ in fundamental ways ought to be more a matter for empirical observation than for assumption. The same might be said for discrimination. Favoring certain groups may be as common as rejecting others. There are suggestions here and there (e.g., Brewer, 1979; Martell, 1991) that at least some, and perhaps most, of the differential feelings about and treatment of different groups may be driven more by favoritism of one group than by rejection of another. This may, of course, be a distinction without difference for those members of groups that do not get their share of jobs, places in college classes, or the like. I should doubt that it makes little difference to a Black woman who has been denied a promotion for which she feels qualified when her boss tells her (if he were so stupid in this day and age), "It's not that I dislike you, but I just like White workers better." Nevertheless it is important to understand the differences between positive and negative prejudices and stereotypes, both at the theoretical level and at a practical level that includes questions about how to change patterns of discrimination.

Second, it is quite possible that at least part of the reason we typically find such low correlations among these variables is that they are not defined or measured in congruent ways. As the most obvious example, educated as we all have been by the seminal work of Fishbein and Ajzen (1974), we might not expect general stereotypes of a group to predict prejudice against a single member of that group or a single act of discrimination. Also, given that measures of prejudice, discrimination, and stereotypes have been developed to fit different practical as well as theoretical agendas, there is no special reason to believe that a randomly selected measure of stereotypes might correlate with a randomly selected measure of prejudice. To believe that they should is to have a great deal of unwarranted faith in the ability of our tests to tap into stable and general underlying cognitive and affective states.

People who develop stereotype measures have not, in general, done so with an eye toward their abilities to predict prejudice or behavior. It would make good sense, for example, to use different measures of stereotypes for predicting their effects on memory and on discrimination. Similarly, we might want to use different measures of discrimination if we wanted to study the effects of stereotypes on hiring and on differential evaluation of work performance. It follows, or so I claim, that if we want to examine the relationships between stereotypes and prejudice, we should develop measures that are honed for exactly that task. A general pattern of research on this important issue (as opposed to the single study, hit-and-miss strategy that has been the norm) might begin by examining the whole issue about the interrelationships among beliefs, affect, and behavior, unconstrained by previous attempts to work around data created by measurement instruments that were not ideally suited to the purpose. In other words, I am going beyond the narrow suggestion that we create new and specialized measuring devices to the broader suggestion that we reconceptualize all three areas within a single paradigm. There is good work to be done in this area, and chapters in the present book point in useful directions.

My third point would be that not only is this work worth doing, but it is also essential that it be done. When all is said and done, the study of stereotypes, although interesting in its own right, is important primarily for the light it sheds on behavior. Do we ever really care (except as a matter if idle curiosity) about what others think and believe, apart from the effects it might have on their behavior? We care about the beliefs of others primarily (and I think solely) because we expect that such beliefs will lead to behaviors that have consequences for our social lives.

There is a further pragmatic reason for studying how our stereotypes affect our behavior. As Chapter 5 by Jussim and Fleming in the present volume makes clear, our behaviors within the context of a particular cultural set of understandings, create behaviors in others that will sometimes further reinforce the thoughts that guided our behaviors. Jussim's (1991) research program has suggested that such self-fulfilling prophecies are neither as strong nor as straightforward as previous discussions had assumed, but the fact remains that to the extent that stereotypes guide our verbal and nonverbal behavior, the social milieu that we create will never be a neutral one with regard to those thoughts. Obviously, for a full appreciation of that important fact, we will have to look more carefully than we have heretofore done at the social and cultural milieu of our cognitive activity.

Control of Stereotypes

Most of us would like to control our stereotypes; we want to be fair. There is some debate about whether this is possible (Devine, 1989; Fiske, 1989; Gilbert & Hixon, 1991). I do not propose to enter into that debate, but there would be general agreement that controlling stereotypic thought is a nontrivial cognitive achievement. One problem is that people are probably most likely to engage in stereotypic thinking when they are busy, distracted, or hurried—the very conditions that make control of stereotypes most difficult (Bodenhausen & Macrae, Chapter 7, this volume). But there are at least two other problems that require our attention: suppression of stereotypes and mental calibration.

Suppression

One problem outlined by Bodenhausen and Macrae is that trying to suppress our stereotypes may lead to untoward effects of the sort examined by Wegner (1994) and his colleagues. For example, Macrae, Bodenhausen, Milne, and Jetten (1994) have shown that trying to suppress stereotypic thought may actually make it stronger, an example of the rebound effect of suppression (Wegner, Schneider, Carter, & White, 1987). There are now abundant data and speculations that mental control is far from an easy achievement, and that it often has ironical and paradoxical effects (Wegner & Pennebaker, 1993).

Mental Calibration

It is frequently unclear how we should compensate for our stereotypes. I frequently tell people that we all have stereotypes, and that an initial step in getting beyond them is to bring them to front stage where their performance can be brutally critiqued. So far so good, but now what?

Suppose I am aware that I think women make worse graduate students in psychology.[15] And suppose for whatever blend of moral, legal, and political reasons, I want to be fair and not act on that stereotype. I weigh and think and stew, and finally decide that a particular female candidate would be my second choice behind a particular male. Suppose I may have been biased on gender grounds, and I want to correct for that. Exactly how do I set about making that correction? My life would be quite simple if my final decision were that he has eight application goody points, she has seven, and I know that my bias has lowered her evaluation by exactly two points. So I give her the two missing points she deserves and admit her, feeling all the more righteous for this correction. Unfortunately, I can only say that I have never confronted a decision, at least an important one, that resolved itself quite this way, but if one comes along, I stand ready with my corrective tools. Mental calibration is difficult under the best of circumstances and well nigh impossible in the complex world most of us inhabit (Wilson & Brekke, 1994). Our desires to do the right thing do not make it easy.

CONCLUSIONS

The ancient world of stereotyping had become sterile by the time of Brigham's (1971) review. People continued to argue about the nature of stereotypes and what counted as essential qualities, even after the nature of psychology and our national dialogue about discrimination had passed them by. The renaissance of stereotype research, begun in the middle 1970s and fueled by the effects of the cognitive revolution on social psychology, was a true breath of fresh air. My strong sense is that we have learned far more about stereotypes in the past 20 years than we learned in the previous 40. Blessed are those of us who have modern theories and powerful methods.

In this chapter I have tried to be respectful of those gains while still trying to make a case for what I fear we have lost in the transition. My position has been that rather than assume that stereotypes have this or that quality, assumptions that have generally not led to self-correcting research, we should begin with the most basic assumption that stereotypes are simply generalizations and then see where we might go. That strategy does, however, require that we be alive to the traditional issues.

I have tried to make the case, often by example, that stereotypes are not in any essential way negative, wrong, rigid, collectively held, and so forth. However, having cleansed our stables of various unproductive controversies, we ought to feel even more responsible to investigate as empirical claims what was once assumed. The assumptions we used to make are still made generally by the public at large, and they are not (and were never) stupid or silly. Moreover, we must face the fact that the stereotypes we most care about are ones that are negative, wrong, and culturally conditioned.

Many of the chapters in the present book are sensitive to issues such as these. As we broaden our ways of thinking about stereotypes, we have also identified new issues and concerns, not all of which fit comfortably within the traditional social cognitive perspective. I have tried to discuss some of these as well, in the hope that such discussion will stimulate an even broader look.

NOTES

1. That is no accident. Lippmann had been immensely influenced by William James while an undergraduate at Harvard. Gordon Allport came to Harvard too late to have met James, but he did his graduate work in a milieu that was still Jamesian through and through.

2. In this, I harken back to the important review by Brigham (1971), which made similar arguments.

3. Because this young woman is both, I was somewhat perplexed at why she reacted negatively to these positive generalizations, and why she felt they were stereotypes. I was promptly told that the real problem with stereotypes was that they constrained people's opportunities, and that she wanted the freedom to goof off and study pop singing (at which she is also outstanding) casually, without people looking at her as if she had broken some taboo.

4. Faculty do, of course, discuss such stereotypes, but I was amazed to discover how many of what I took to be my own stereotypes were widely shared by other faculty.

5. I would be the first to agree that some traits are more vague than others, and that it may be possible to get something like an "objective" definition for highly visible and observable traits. However, many of our stereotypes are saturated with traits such as lazy, rational, and nurturant that seem to me to fall on the vague side of the dimension.

6. More properly, she might observe an absence of many hardworking behaviors, because I suspect that laziness is often defined by behavioral sins of omission rather than of commission. Let's just keep matters simple for the sake of the example.

7. I recently had a lengthy conversation with a law enforcement professional who worked extensively with Asian American gangs that are now prevalent in Houston. His stereotype of Asians and Asian Americans certainly did not include "hardworking" as a central attribute.

8. The scholarly literature on late Victorian period gender conceptions is voluminous, but I can recommend the Thomas and Charlotte Pitt mysteries of

Anne Perry as interesting descriptions of gender stereotypes and behavioral relations of the times.

9. I once collected data on stereotypes of college professors by students at a state university. One trait that was rated as strongly characteristic by a minority of students (and on average by the students generally) was "lazy." I found that mildly amusing until I read a comment by one student, who said something to the effect that I was a particularly good exemplar of the lazy professor and since I was never around my office to help him with his problems, he hoped that my golf game was improving. I'm not sure whether I was more insulted at having been called "lazy" or at playing golf, which I have not done since I was a lazy lad.

10. Sometimes I am taken with the notion that many people assume that because Blacks are, say, four times more likely to commit violent crimes (about the figure for murder), individual Blacks are four times more likely to be violent. This kind of fallacy is hard to pin down.

11. The seminal papers of Brewer (1988) and Fiske and Neuberg (1990) on the issues surrounding individualized versus stereotypic information really are attempts to suggest that there may be information other than group memberships that is important to consider. Brewer's notions of personalization suggest that we think of a person not as an exemplar of a single category but as a member of several categories, with perhaps differing implications for various forms of behavior. Whereas in the subsequent discussion I am critical of what I take to be a relatively mindless appeal to individualized information, I would certainly agree that we should all be reminded that all of us have attributes, and important ones at that, which transcend particular categories. Black males are more than Black and male, just as liberal college professors are more than liberals who teach university courses

12. On the other hand, she might also want to reflect on the effects of this global policy on those 40% of the students who might have been inclined to work hard in any case and now feel they do not get sufficient credit for their dispositional claims to academic sainthood.

13. Obviously, sometimes students can offer additional diagnostic information that supports their claims, but depressingly often, they cannot.

14. There are matters of fact, and then there are matters of value. I have no quarrel with the notion that we should try to use generalizations other than those based on race, gender, sexual preference, and the like, especially when we have strong reason to believe that such group generalizations have low predictive power. And I do not even object to using information that has lower predictive power than group membership, so long as one recognizes that in so doing one is making a moral choice rather than a statistical one. The criteria of success for our various predictions are usually loose and vague (What does success in graduate school really mean anyway?), and there are many things besides local and ill-defined success criteria that are important in our complex world. That does not, however, justify confusing predictive power and moral concerns, as we often do these days. More than ever, we need clear thinking about such issues.

15. Just for the record my experience has generally been the reverse.

REFERENCES

Adorno, T. W., Frenkel-Brunswik, E., Levinson, D. J., & Sanford, R. N. (1950). *The authoritarian personality.* New York: Harper & Row.

Allport, G. W. (1954). *The nature of prejudice.* Garden City, NY: Doubleday/ Anchor.

Ashmore, R. D., & Del Boca, F. K. (1981). Conceptual approaches to stereotypes and stereotyping. In D. L. Hamilton (Ed.), *Cognitive processes in stereotyping and intergroup behavior* (pp. 1–35). Hillsdale, NJ: Erlbaum.

Brewer, M. B. (1979). In-group bias in the minimal intergroup situation: A cognitive-motivational analysis. *Psychological Bulletin, 86,* 307–324.

Brewer, M. B. (1988). A dual process model of impression formation. In T. K. Srull & R. S. Wyer, Jr. (Eds.), *Advances in social cognition* (Vol. 1, pp. 1–36). Hillsdale, NJ: Erlbaum.

Brigham, J. C. (1971). Ethnic stereotypes. *Psychological Bulletin, 76,* 15–33.

Deaux, K., Winton, W., Crowley, M., & Lewis, L. L. (1985). Level of categorization and content of gender stereotypes. *Social Cognition, 3,* 145–167.

Devine, P. G. (1989). Stereotypes and prejudice: Their automatic and controlled components. *Journal of Personality and Social Psychology, 56,* 5–18.

Devine, P. G., & Baker, M. (1991). Measurement of racial stereotype subtyping. *Personality and Social Psychology Bulletin, 17,* 44–50.

Eagly, A. H. (1987). *Sex differences in social behavior: A social-role interpretation.* Hillsdale, NJ: Erlbaum.

Eagly, A. H., & Steffen, J. J. (1984). Gender stereotypes stem from the distribution of men and women into social roles. *Journal of Personality and Social Psychology, 46,* 735–754.

Feldman, J. M. (1972). Stimulus characteristics and subject prejudice as determinants of stereotype attribution. *Journal of Personality and Social Psychology, 21,* 333–340.

Fishbein, M., & Ajzen, I. (1974). Attitudes toward objects as predictors of single and multiple behavioral criteria. *Psychological Review, 81,* 59–74.

Fiske, S. T. (1989). Examining the role of intent: Toward understanding its role in stereotyping and prejudice. In J. S. Uleman & J. A. Bargh (Eds.), *Unintended thought* (pp. 253–286). NY: Guilford Press.

Fiske, S. T., & Neuberg, S. L. (1990). A continuum of impression formation, from category-based to individuating processes: Influences of information and motivation on attention and interpretation. In M. Zanna (Ed.), *Advances in experimental social psychology* (Vol. 23, pp. 1–74). Orlando, FL: Academic Press.

Funder, D. C., & Dobroth, K. M. (1987). Differences between traits: Properties associated with intrajudge agreement. *Journal of Personality and Social Psychology, 52,* 409–418.

Gates, H. L. (1992). *Loose canons: Notes on the culture wars.* New York: Oxford University Press.

Gifford, R. K. (1975). Information properties of descriptive words. *Journal of Personality and Social Psychology, 31,* 727–734.

Gilbert, D. T., & Hixon, J. G. (1991). The trouble of thinking: Activation and application of stereotypic beliefs. *Journal of Personality and Social Psychology, 60*, 509–517.

Hamilton, D. L., & Trolier, T. K. (1986). Stereotypes and stereotyping: An overview of the cognitive approach. In J. F. Dovidio & S.L. Gaertner (Eds.), *Prejudice, discrimination, and racism* (pp. 127–163). Orlando, FL: Academic Press.

Hampson, S. E., John, O. P., & Goldberg, L. R. (1986). Category breadth and hierarchical structure in personality: Studies of asymmetries in judgments of trait implications. *Journal of Personality and Social Psychology, 51*, 37–54.

Hastie, R., Schroeder, C., & Weber, R. (1990). Creating complex social conjunction categories from simple categories. *Bulletin of the Psychonomic Society, 28*, 242–247.

Higgins, E. T. (1989). Knowledge accessibility and activation: Subjectivity and suffering from unconscious sources. In J. S. Uleman & J. A. Bargh (Eds.), *Unintended thought* (pp. 75–123). New York: Guilford Press.

Judd, C. M., & Park, B.(1993). Definition and assessment of accuracy in social stereotypes. *Psychological Review, 100*, 109–128.

Jussim, L. (1991). Social perception and social reality: A reflection–construction model. *Psychological Review, 98*, 54–73.

Katz, D., & Braly, K. (1933). Racial stereotypes in one hundred college students. *Journal of Abnormal and Social Psychology, 28*, 280–290.

Katz, D., & Braly, K. (1935). Racial prejudice and racial stereotypes. *Journal of Abnormal and Social Psychology, 30*, 175–193.

Kraus, S., Ryan, C. S., Judd, C. M., Hastie, R., & Park, B. (1993). Use of mental frequency distributions to represent variability among members of social categories. *Social Cognition, 11*, 22–43.

Kunda, Z., Miller, D. T., & Claire, T. (1990). Combining social concepts: The role of causal reasoning. *Cognitive Science, 14*, 551–557.

Levine, J. M., Resnick, L. B., & Higgins, E. T. (1993). Social foundations of cognition. *Annual Review of Psychology, 44*, 585–612.

Linville, P. W., & Fischer, G. W. (1993). Exemplar and abstraction models of perceived group variability and stereotypicality. *Social Cognition, 11*, 92–125.

Lippmann, W. (1922). *Public opinion.* New York: Harcourt Brace.

Maas, A., Salvi, D., Arcuri, L., & Semin, G.R. (1989). Language use in intergroup contexts: The linguistic intergroup bias. *Journal of Personality and Social Psychology, 57*, 981–993.

Macrae, C. N., Bodenhausen, G. V., Milne, A. B., & Jetten, J. (1994). Out of mind but back in sight: Stereotypes on the rebound. *Journal of Personality and Social Psychology, 67*, 808–817.

McCauley, C., & Stitt, C. L. (1978). An individual and quantitative measure of stereotypes. *Journal of Personality and Social Psychology, 36*, 929–140.

Martell, R. F. (1991). Sex bias at work: The effect of attentional and memory demands on performance ratings of men and women. *Journal of Applied Social Psychology, 21*, 1939–1960.

Murphy, G. L. (1988). Comprehending complex categories. *Cognitive Science, 12*, 529–562.

Rosch, E. (1978). Principles of categorization. In E. Rosch & B. B. Lloyd (Eds.), *Cognition and categorization* (pp. 27–48). Hillsdale, NJ: Erlbaum.

Rothbart, M., & Park, B. (1986). On the confirmability and disconfirmability of trait concepts. *Journal of Personality and Social Psychology, 50*, 131–142.

Rothbart, M., & Taylor, M. (1992). Category labels and social reality: Do we view social categories as natural kinds? In G. R. Semin & K. Fiedler (Eds.), *Language, interaction, and social cognition* (pp. 11–36). London: Sage.

Schaller, M., & O'Brien, M. (1992). "Intuitive analysis of covariance" and group stereotype formation. *Personality and Social Psychology Bulletin, 18*, 776–785.

Schneider, D. J. (1971, August). *Non-linguistic aspects of trait implications.* Paper presented at a symposium, "Recent Approaches to the Study of Implicit Personality Theories" at the American Psychological Association Convention, Washington, DC.

Schneider, D. J. (1991). Social cognition. *Annual Review of Psychology, 42*, 527–561.

Schneider, D.J. (1992). Red apples, liberal college professors, and farmers who love Bach. *Psychological Inquiry, 2*, 190–193.

Schneider, D. J., Hastorf, A. H., & Ellsworth, P. E. (1979). *Person perception.* (2nd ed.). Reading, MA: Addison-Wesley.

Semin, G.R., & Fiedler, K. (1991). The linguistic category model, its bases, applications, and range. In W. Stroebe & M. Hewstone (Eds.), *European review of social psychology* (Vol. 2, pp. 1–30). London: Wiley.

Steele, S. (1990). *The content of our character.* New York: Harper.

Stangor, C., Lynch, L., Duan, C., & Glass, B. (1992). Categorization of individuals on the basis of multiple social features. *Journal of Personalility and Social Psychology, 62*, 207–218.

Stangor, C., Sullivan, L. A ., & Ford, T. E. (1991). Affective and cognitive determinants of prejudice. *Social Cognition, 9*, 359–380.

Weber, R., & Crocker, J. (1983). Cognitive processes in the revision of stereotypic beliefs. *Journal of Personality and Social Psychology, 45*, 961–977.

Wegner, D. M. (1994). Ironic processes of mental control. *Psychological Review, 101*, 34–52.

Wegner, D. M., & Pennebaker, J. W. (Eds.). (1993). *Handbook of mental control.* Englewood Cliffs, NJ: Prentice-Hall.

Wegner, D. M. , Schneider, D. J., Carter, S., III, & White, L. (1987). Paradoxical effects of thought suppression. *Journal of Personality and Social Psychology, 53*, 5–13.

West, C. (1993). *Race matters.* Boston: Beacon Press.

Wilson, T. D., & Brekke, N. (1994). Mental contamination and mental correction: Unwanted influences on judgments and evaluations. *Psychological Bulletin, 116*, 117–142.

Zárate, M. A., & Smith, E. R. (1990). Person categorization and stereotyping. *Social Cognition, 8*, 161–185.

Index

Accentuation theory, 21
Accountability, 245–246, 389–390,
    399–400
Accuracy of stereotypes, 268, 388
    assessment research and theory,
        121–124
    correlates of, 138–140
    current conceptualizations, 436–438
    in-group/out-group differences,
        144–148
    intensity of group identification as fac-
        tor in, 149
    physical appearance-related, 87–89,
        106–107
    self-fulfilling prophecies and, 177–178
    subsequent group-relevant judgments,
        151–152
    types of inaccuracy, 131–134, 148. See
        also Assessment of stereotype accu-
        racy
Affective processes
    behavioral manifestations of prejudice,
        286–287
    emotion-appearance overgeneralization
        effects, 98–100
    evaluative role of stereotypes, 282–283
    in racial stereotyping and prejudice,
        292–293, 297–302, 308–311
    in stereotype change, 341
    in stereotype formation, 51–55, 67,
        281–282
Affirmative action, 176, 185, 391
Affordances, 81
Anger, 372
Animal characteristics, 104–106
Anti-Semitism, 371
Anxiety, 337

Appearance cues, 87–88
Arbitrary groups, 56
Assessment
    attitude–behavior relationship,
        290–292, 446
    authoritarian personality, 373
    discrimination, 446
    of group prototype mental representa-
        tions, 8
    of prejudice, 278–279, 287–288, 446
    racial attitudes, 375, 376
    of racial attitudes and prejudice,
        292–302
    stereotype–discrimination relationship,
        304–306
    of stereotypes, 281, 284, 310–311
    theoretical basis, 25–26
Assessment of stereotype accuracy
    cognitive representations of social cate-
        gories, 140–143
    full-accuracy design for, 134–140
    future research directions, 139–140,
        148–153
    measures of perceived group variability,
        128–130
    methodological issues, 128–130, 437
    problems in, 123–128
    role of perceived group variability, 143
    social stereotypes, 144–148
    types of inaccuracy, 131–134
Attention, 7, 387
Attention-deficit-hyperactivity disorder,
    173–174
Attitude
    assessment of, 287–288
    behavior and, 289–292
    forms of racism, 288–289

Attitude *(continued)*
  prototypes, 270
  racial, discrimination and, 285–292
  of stereotype targets, 394
  vs. stereotype, 283
Attitudes Toward Women Scale, 237–238
Attribution error, 57
Authoritarian personality, 55, 122, 302,
    371, 374, 403, 420
Aversive racism, 288, 289

Babyface appearance, 88, 89–98
Benign generalizations, 422, 429–430,
    442–443

Categorization, 140–143, 256
  assessment of, 269
  compound categories, 426–427
  conceptual challenges, 424–427
  cross-cutting, 266–267, 344–348, 386
  diagnostic, 173
  group prototypes model, 8–9
  individuating information and, 257–261
  interdependence model, 387
  linguistic activities in, 11, 196–197
  outcome dependency in, 267–268
  pathway to active stereotyping,
    255–256
  physical appearance as basis for, 79, 80,
    85
  social cognition models, 387
  social context, 66
  social policies and, 269–270
  in social settings, 261–262, 425–426
  stereotype change interventions,
    343–344
  stereotype-disconfirming information in,
    338
  stereotype flexibility, 15–16
  in stereotype formation, 44–47, 254
  subcategorization, 426
Children
  acquisition of gender stereotypes,
    434–435
  babyface stereotype, 89–98
  biased attributions, 58
  categorization, 46–47
  conditioning of stereotypes in, 53
  correspondence bias in, 49
  cultural mechanisms of stereotype trans-
    mission, 60–63
  development of authoritarian person-
    ality, 371–372
  hyperactive, self-fulfilling prophecies
    about, 173–174
  illusory correlation bias in, 51

language-mediated stereotype transmis-
    sion, 194, 195–196
  mere exposure effects, 54
  self-fulfilling prophecies among, 176
Civil rights movement, 372, 374–375,
    400
Cognitive processes
  abstractions, 141
  activation of social category representa-
    tion, 198–199, 203–204, 230–231,
    308–309
  attitude–behavior processes, 289–292
  authoritarian personality theory,
    371–374
  automatic, 229–230
  category-based judgment, 269–270
  cognitive load, 260–261
  cognitive miser, 228–229
  collective stereotypes, 10–14, 16–18,
    281
  commonalities of individual and collec-
    tive models of stereotyping, 19–25
  construction of meaning, 227–228
  contact hypothesis, 338–341
  control of stereotypes, 235–242,
    447–448
  cross-cutting categorization, 344
  definition of stereotype, 42–43
  discrimination and, 302–306
  dissociation model of prejudice,
    378–381
  epistemic functions of stereotypes,
    20–22
  esteem-related functions of stereotypes,
    23–25
  evaluative role of stereotypes, 282–283
  future research, 25–27
  individuated mental representations,
    241–242
  linguistic intergroup bias, 213–216
  mechanism of stereotype formation,
    44–51
  organizing function of language,
    196–199
  in racial stereotyping and prejudice,
    292–302
  representations of social categories,
    140–143
  research and conceptual trends,
    122–123, 279–280
  self-awareness of prejudice, 232–233
  self-regulation of mental processes,
    233–235
  stereotypes as individual beliefs, 5–10,
    14–16, 430–433
  traditional conceptualizations of stereo-

typing, 419–421. *See also* Information processing; Social cognitive approach
Common in-group identity, 349–352
Compound categories, 426–427
Conformity processes, 63–64
Consensualness, 17, 25, 26–27
Conservatism, 373, 376
Contact hypothesis
cognitive analysis of, 338–341
evaluation of, 328, 341–343
gender stereotypes and, 382
intergroup processes, 332–337
negative consequences, 327–328
personalization processes and, 329–332, 394
theoretical basis, 327
Cooperative learning, 331
Correspondence bias, 48–49, 56–57, 58–59, 64–66
Criminal stereotypes, 97–98
Cross-cutting categorization, 266–267, 344–348, 386
Culture
conceptual challenges in stereotype research, 430–433
current conceptualizations of stereotyping, 421–422
dissociation model of stereotyping and prejudice, 378–381
esteem-related functions of stereotypes, 23–25
functional determinants of stereotypes, 19–25
implications for stereotype research, 25–27
individual vs. collective stereotypes, 4–5, 14–18, 280–281, 430–433
language-mediated stereotype transmission, 194
mechanisms of stereotype formation, 60–66
social consequences of self-fulfilling prophecies, 162, 163, 166
in stereotype acquisition, 434–436
stereotype change and, 439
stereotype consensus, 17, 25, 26–27
stereotype content and, 80
stereotypes as collective belief systems in, 10–14
theoretical basis for stereotype models, 18
traditional conceptualizations of stereotyping, 420–421

Decategorization, 326

in bias reduction, 349
personalization effects, 331–332, 342
Desegregation, 181–182, 185, 328
Diagnostic categories, 173
Discrimination
definition, 279
in modern racism, 375
prejudice and, 283, 284–292, 307–311, 445–447
stereotyping and, 283–284, 302–311, 445–447
stereotyping as consequence of, 277, 310
Dispersion inaccuracy, 280
Dispositional inferences, 48–49, 209
Dissociation model, 378–381, 387, 401

Ecological theory, 81–82, 89, 107–108
Education, 18
desegregation effects, 328
self-fulfilling prophecy in school settings, 163–164, 168–170, 181–185
Egalitarian values, 232–233
aversive racism and, 288
conscious effort to internalize, 379–380
priming, as change strategy, 400
Elderly people, 90, 92, 100, 218
Emotion overgeneralization effects, 98–100
Ethnicity/race
child consciousness of, 61
dissociation model of prejudice, 378–381
ethnophaulisms, 199, 200
forms of racism, 288–289
historical and social significance, 277–278
mass media content analysis, 61–62
modern and symbolic racism, 288–289, 374–378
physical stereotypes, 95–98
self-fulfilling nature of stereotypes, 165–166
stereotype formation in children, 47
Ethnocentrism, 136
Exceptions, 440–441
Exemplars, 6, 9–10, 103–104, 140–141
Expectancies
biased language use, 213–216
group prototype model, 8–9
as part of stereotype concept, 43
social norms, 13–14
target noncompliance with, 395
Expectancy disconfirmation effect, 55
Experimenter effects, 163
Exposure effects, 53–55

Face recognition, 83–84
Facial expressions
  emotion-related, 98–100
  fitness-related, 100–101
Familiarity, 50–51, 54, 86
  as factor in perceived group variability,
    140–143
  stereotype accuracy and, 139
Fear, 372

Gender stereotypes
  authoritarian personality theory and,
    373–374
  babyface generalizations, 93–94
  conceptualizations of modern racism
    and, 377–378
  development in children, 46–47,
    434–435
  dissociation model applied to, 380
  emotion–appearance generalizations,
    99–100
  interdependence and power models, 390
  intergroup contact effects, 382
  physical appearance and, 85
  research trends, 371
  self-fulfilling nature of, 166–169
  sexist language, 201–204, 244–245
  social identity theory, 385–386
  social norms in development of, 13
  social role as basis for, 65
  sociomotivational justification, 58–59
Generalizations
  accepted use of, 442–443
  current conceptualizations of stereotyp-
    ing, 422
  vs. stereotyping, 427
Group boundaries, 43, 398
  common in-group identity, 349–352
  personalization strategy, 332

Heuristic, stereotyping as, 9

Illusory correlation, 50–51, 86
Impression formation, 255–261, 268,
  402–403
In-group/out-group differentiation, 44,
  45–46
  degree of confirmability/disconfirmabili-
    ty, 204–208
  language of, 198
  mere exposure effects, 54–55
  perception of individuals and, 264–267
  as personalization, 329–332
  in social identity theory, 56–58
  stereotype accuracy, 144–148
  types of trait attributes used in,

216–217
In-group-protective motives, 214–215
Individual differences
  capacity to change, 404
  conformity tendencies and prejudice, 63
  group dynamics vs. in stereotype
    change, 392–393
  models of prejudice and stereotyping,
    371–381
Individuated mental representations,
  241–242, 259
  determinants of, 269–271
  group stereotypes and, 441–442
  impression formation, 255–261
  in-group/out-group differentiation and,
    264–267
  interdependence model of categoriza-
    tion, 387–389
  as personalization, 329–332
  social contexts, 261–267
  social relationship effects, 267–269
Induced mindfulness, 246
Information processing
  accepted use of generalizations,
    442–443
  biased, 231, 233–234
  categorization mechanisms, 44–45, 46
  cognitive representations of social cate-
    gories, 140–143
  conceptualization of stereotype forma-
    tion, 280, 428
  ecological theory, 81–83
  epistemic functions of stereotypes,
    20–21
  group prototypes model, 8–9
  illusory correlation bias, 50–51
  individuating information, 255–261
  induced mindfulness, 246
  pathways to active stereotyping,
    255–256
  schematic models, 7–8, 197, 280
  social cognitive model of stereotypes,
    5–6, 16, 66
  social contexts, 261–267
  stereotype-disconfirming information in,
    338–341
  stereotype inaccuracies and, 149–150
  stereotype suppression, 233–242
  stereotyping as heuristic, 9. *See also*
    Cognitive models of stereotyping
Interdependence effects, 267–269
Interdependence model of intergroup bias,
  386–391, 398–399
Intergroup bias, 46, 279, 383–384
  linguistic, 209–217
Intergroup competition, 60, 215–216,

267, 383, 386–387
Intergroup conflict, 64, 65–66, 349–352
Intergroup contact, 332–337
  affective response, 53
  models of prejudice and stereotyping, 381–392
  as personalization, 329–332
  in stereotype change, 18
  in stereotype development, 17. *See also* Contact hypothesis
Intrapersonal processes
  esteem-related functions of stereotypes, 23–25
  functional determinants of stereotypes, 19–25
  implications for stereotype research, 25–27
  social cognitive models of stereotyping, 5–10, 42–43
  vs. collective processes in stereotyping, 4–5, 14–18, 280–281, 430–433
Intrapsychic conflict
  adoption of egalitarian values, 379–380
  in concept of modern racism, 376–377
  model of prejudice, 122
  stereotype change and, 381
  in stereotype formation, 55–56

Justification
  for action and inaction, 22
  attribution errors, 57
  for negative events, 21–22
  for status quo, 58–60

Kernel of truth, 27, 81, 108, 153

Labeling, 11–12
  automatic activation of social category representation, 198–199, 203–204, 230–231
  cognitive organizing function of, 197–198
  developmental capacity, 46
  in facilitation of dispositional infer- ences, 209
Language
  animal comparisons, 105
  breadth of trait descriptors, 208–209
  in category-based processing, 260–261
  in cultural model of stereotype develop- ment and change, 11–12
  disconfirmation of favorable vs. unfa- vorable traits, 205–208
  ethnic/racial slurs, 200
  function of stereotypes in simplifying communication, 22

identity-expressive function, 217–219
intergroup bias model, 209–217
organizing function, 196–199
psychological process of stereotyping, 216–217, 220
research trends, 193–194
response-language confounds, 124–125, 135
sexist, 201–204, 244–245
stereotype consensus and, 17
in stereotype maintenance, 204, 206–207, 209
in stereotype transmission, 193, 194–196

Mass media, 12–13, 61–62, 195, 211–212
Memory
  exemplars, 9–10
  face recognition, 83–84
  ironic effects of stereotype suppression, 236–237
  physiologic processes, 83–84
  proactive inhibition, 202
  schematic processing, 7–8
  social cognitive model of stereotypes, 6
  stereotype-confirming bias in, 231
Minimal group paradigm, 383
Mistaken identity effects, 102–104
MODE model, 289–290
Modern racism, 288–289, 374–378, 401, 403
Modern Racism Scale, 297, 304, 375, 376
Modern sexism, 377–378
Motivated stereotyping, 55–60, 150
  accuracy as goal of, 268
  individuation processes, 387–388
  linguistic intergroup bias, 214–216
  in modern racism/sexism theory, 378
  in self-fulfilling cognitions, 174–175

Nonverbal cues, 62–63, 286
  in appearance-trait correlations, 87–88
  automatic activation of social category representation, 230–231
  in category-based processing, 260–261

Out-group homogeneity, 140–143, 144, 266. *See also* Perceived group vari- ability
Outcome dependency effects, 267–268

Perceived group variability
  accuracy of, 124, 131–134, 144–148
  cognitive representation of social cate- gories, 140–143
  individual attributions and, 441–442

Perceived group variability *(continued)*
  measures of, 128–130
  as outcome measure of stereotype
    change, 326
  research trends, 140
  stereotype process, 143–144
Personalization, 326
  contact hypothesis, 329–332, 342
  in integrative intervention for stereotype
    change, 352, 354
Physical appearance, character inferred
    from
  accuracy in judgments, 87–89, 106–107
  animal analogies, 104–106
  attractiveness as quality in, 88–89,
    101–102, 171–173
  babyface overgeneralizations, 89–98
  current popular beliefs, 84–85
  emotion overgeneralizations, 98–100
  functional associations, 106
  height and weight stereotypes, 94–95
  historical concepts, 84
  illusory correlation effect, 86
  metaphorical associations, 106
  mistaken identity effects, 102–104
  national stereotypes, 95–98
  overgeneralizations in, 89, 106–107,
    108
  perceptual attunement, 82–84, 87–88
  prominence of features, 85–86
  research trends, 79–80
  sickness similarities, 100–102
  stability as factor in, 86
  stereotype development and, 79, 85,
    88–89, 263
Physiologic processes
  fitness-related appearance, 100–101
  memory, 83–84
  neural basis for emotion recognition, 99
Political contexts
  authoritarian personality type and, 373
  use of stereotypes in, 22
Power model of intergroup bias, 386–391
Prejudice
  acknowledgment of, 245
  affective-cognitive relationships in,
    292–293
  assessment of, 278–279, 287–288
  authoritarian personality theory,
    371–374
  aversive racism, 288
  conformity and, 63–64
  discrimination and, 283, 284–292,
    307–311, 445–447
  dissociation model, 378–381
  functional role of stereotypes in, 21–22

  nature of, 278
  racial stereotypes, 292–302
  research trends, 122–123, 370–371
  in response to perceived threats, 24
  school tracking and, 181–182
  self-awareness of, 232–233
  self-esteem and, 23, 24
  social identity theory, 383–386
  stereotype accuracy and, 139
  stereotype development and, 67–68,
    276–277, 283–285, 307–311,
    445–447
  stereotype rigidity and, 440
  target awareness, 405
Proactive inhibition, 202
Prosopagnosia, 83–84
Prototypes, 6, 8–9, 27, 340

Rebound phenomenon, 238–241, 447
Recategorization, 349–352, 386, 397–398
Representativeness, 109
Response-language confounds, 124–125,
    135

Salience
  common in-group identity, 351–352
  contact variables and, 335–336
  in-group/out-group differentiation,
    265–266
  of physical features, 85–86
  of social categorization, linguistic diver-
    gence effects, 219
  social-group, 386
Scapegoating, 122, 150
Schemas/schematic processing, 6–8, 197,
    280
Self-categorization theory, 343
Self-concept
  awareness of prejudice, 232–233
  change strategy targeted at, 401
  identity-expressive function of language,
    217–219
  individuating processes and, 388
  linguistic intergroup bias effects,
    214–216
  non-prejudiced, as obstacle to assess-
    ment, 288
  self-esteem, 23–25, 56–58, 403
  self-stereotypes, 15
  stereotype accuracy/inaccuracy and,
    149, 152
  of stereotype target, 175. *See also* in-
    group/out-group differentiation;
    Social identity theory
Self-fulfilling prophecies, 107, 161, 176,
    178, 447

about hyperactive children, 173–174
conditions necessary for occurrence of,
164
discrimination and, 185–186
in educational settings, 163–164,
168–170, 181–185
ethnicity stereotypes as, 165–166
gender stereotypes as, 166–169
group-level processes, 180–181
historical experience, 161–162, 185
in maintenance of social stereotypes,
177–178, 186–187
perceiver characteristics in, 174–175
physical attractiveness as basis for,
171–173
research trends, 162, 163–164
in school tracking practices, 181–182
social class stereotypes as, 169–171
social significance, 162, 163, 166, 176,
178–181, 187
target behaviors/characteristics,
175–176, 394–395
Simplification, 123
categorization for, 44
conservation of cognitive resources in
stereotypes, 229
function of stereotypes in, 21, 22
Social class, 64–65
linguistic convergence effects in interactions between, 218–219
self-fulfilling stereotypes, 169–171
Social cognitive approach, 5–10, 421–
422
categorization in, 387
conceptual problems of, 423
definition of stereotype in, 42–43
semantic labeling processes, 203–204
social component of, 430–433
stereotype acquisition in, 434–436
stereotype content issues, 424
Social identity theory, 45, 56–58, 139,
214–215, 324, 343, 344–345,
383–386, 391–392, 395, 396
Social judgeability, 258, 390
Social learning, 61–63
Social norms, 13–14, 63–64
assessment of racial attitudes and,
293–296
attitude assessment and, 287
civil rights movement, 374–375
cognitive change, 244
egalitarian values, 232–233
shared values between stereotyper and
target, 400
Speech accomodation theory, 217
Stereotype change

authoritarian personality theory and,
374
behavior change and, 444–448
categorization-based, 343–344, 352,
354
choosing intervention for, 404–405
common in-group identity for, 349–352
conceptual approaches to, 324
cross-cutting social categorization in,
344–348, 386
as cultural process, 10, 11, 18
danger signals in process of, 402–404
determinants of, 67
disconfirmation of favorable vs. unfavorable traits, 205–208
dissociation model, 380–381
future research, 325
generalizability of interventions,
324–325
granting exceptions, 440–441
individual differences in capacity for,
404
individual-level vs. group-level interventions, 392–393, 405
integrative approach, 352–357
interdependence and power theory,
386–392
intergroup contact and, 18, 332–337,
382, 391–392
intrapsychic origins of stereotype and,
381
mechanisms, 325
modern racism/sexism conceptualization
and, 378
outcome measures, 325–326
personalized contact in, 328–332, 354
social cognitive model, 6, 14–15
social identity theory and, 386,
391–392
stereotype-disconfirming information in,
338–341
stereotype rigidity, 438–441
target-oriented intervention, 370,
393–406
theoretical basis, 325, 356–357
workplace interventions, 397–402
Stereotype content
categorization and, 424–427
culturally-determined, 432
current theories, 80–81
ecological theory, 81–82
positive stereotypes, 429–430
research trends, 79–80, 276, 424
social learning, 61–63
as subject of language research,
193–194

Stereotype development
  affective mechanisms, 51–55, 67,
    281–282
  attitude development and, 283
  cognitive mechanisms, 44–51
  as collective process, 10, 11, 13, 25,
    430–433
  as consequence of discrimination, 277,
    310
  cultural mechanisms, 60–66, 433
  determinants of, 42, 66–68, 254–255,
    270–271, 434–436
  evaluative role, 282–283
  exemplar approach, 9–10
  experiential factors, 16
  functional determinants of, 19–25, 67
  group prototypes model, 8–9
  group schemas in, 7–8
  intergroup contact in, 17
  as intrapersonal process, 6, 14–15, 25
  language role in, 216–217, 220
  physical appearance and, 85, 88–89,
    107–108
  prejudice and, 67–68, 283–285,
    307–311, 370–371
  research needs, 67, 276, 419–421
  role of perceived group variability,
    143–144
  self-fulfilling prophecies in, 177–178
  sociomotivational mechanisms, 55–60
  subtyping, 141–143, 150, 262–263,
    339–340
  trait characteristics and likelihood of,
    428–429. See also Stereotyping
Stereotype disconfirmation, 15, 150
  cognitive evasions in presence of,
    231–232
  cognitive processes in, 338–341
  degree of confirmability/disconfirmabili-
    ty, 204–208
  development of self-fulfilling prophecies
    and, 177–178
  language as protection against, 204
Stereotype flexibility, 15–16
Stereotype maintenance
  intractability, 323–324
  language role in, 204, 209
  self-fulfilling prophecies in, 177–178,
    186–187
Stereotyping
  assessment, 280–281, 284
  cognitive load in, 260–261
  cognitive pathways, 255–256
  current conceptual challenges, 422–423
  discrimination and, 283–284, 302–306,
    307–311
  in-group/out-group differentiation,

  264–267
  individuating information and,
    257–261, 270–271
  in intergroup contexts, 262–264
  prejudice and, 276–277, 292–302,
    307–311
  research and conceptual trends,
    279–280, 448–449
  social relationship effects, 267–269
  stereotypes and, 254–255
Subgrouping, 355, 386
Subtypes/subtyping, 141–143, 150,
    262–264, 339–340, 355, 426
Superordinate categories, 349–352
Suppression of stereotypes
  accountability, 245–246
  in concept of modern racism, 377
  conscious effort to adopt egalitarian val-
    ues, 379–380
  determinants of success, 242–247
  forms of racism, 288–289
  ironic outcomes, 235–242
  processes of mental self-regulation,
    233–235
  rebound effect, 238–239, 447
  response suppression, 244
  settings for, 232–233
  social change, 244
  vs. recognition of prejudice, 245
Symbolic racism, 288, 375
Symbolic Racism Scale, 297

Targets of stereotypes, 21–22, 59–60
  awareness of prejudice, 405
  in change research, 370, 393–395, 406
  influence on stereotypers, 395–396
  monitoring of stereotypers by, 402–404
  noncompliance with stereotype, 395
  self-fulfilling prophecies in, 175–176
  tactics for change, 396–402
Threats, 24, 139, 403–404
Trait attributions, 46, 48–49, 64–65
  breadth of trait descriptors, 208–209
  degree of confirmability/disconfirmabili-
    ty, 204–208
  out-group stereotypes, 216–217
  research challenges, 428–429
Typicality
  contact effects, 334–336, 337
  perceived, 339–340, 342

Valence inaccuracy, 126, 132, 136, 149,
    150, 151, 205–208, 436–437
Vocal cues, 62, 87–88

Workplace, 64–65, 103–104, 176, 183,
    397–402, 432